# INTERLEUKIN-5

## FROM MOLECULE TO DRUG TARGET FOR ASTHMA

# LUNG BIOLOGY IN HEALTH AND DISEASE

*Executive Editor*

**Claude Lenfant**
*Director, National Heart, Lung and Blood Institute*
*National Institutes of Health*
*Bethesda, Maryland*

1. Immunologic and Infectious Reactions in the Lung, *edited by Charles H. Kirkpatrick and Herbert Y. Reynolds*
2. The Biochemical Basis of Pulmonary Function, *edited by Ronald G. Crystal*
3. Bioengineering Aspects of the Lung, *edited by John B. West*
4. Metabolic Functions of the Lung, *edited by Y. S. Bakhle and John R. Vane*
5. Respiratory Defense Mechanisms (in two parts), *edited by Joseph D. Brain, Donald F. Proctor, and Lynne M. Reid*
6. Development of the Lung, *edited by W. Alan Hodson*
7. Lung Water and Solute Exchange, *edited by Norman C. Staub*
8. Extrapulmonary Manifestations of Respiratory Disease, *edited by Eugene Debs Robin*
9. Chronic Obstructive Pulmonary Disease, *edited by Thomas L. Petty*
10. Pathogenesis and Therapy of Lung Cancer, *edited by Curtis C. Harris*
11. Genetic Determinants of Pulmonary Disease, *edited by Stephen D. Litwin*
12. The Lung in the Transition Between Health and Disease, *edited by Peter T. Macklem and Solbert Permutt*
13. Evolution of Respiratory Processes: A Comparative Approach, *edited by Stephen C. Wood and Claude Lenfant*
14. Pulmonary Vascular Diseases, *edited by Kenneth M. Moser*
15. Physiology and Pharmacology of the Airways, *edited by Jay A. Nadel*
16. Diagnostic Techniques in Pulmonary Disease (in two parts), *edited by Marvin A. Sackner*
17. Regulation of Breathing (in two parts), *edited by Thomas F. Hornbein*
18. Occupational Lung Diseases: Research Approaches and Methods, *edited by Hans Weill and Margaret Turner-Warwick*
19. Immunopharmacology of the Lung, *edited by Harold H. Newball*
20. Sarcoidosis and Other Granulomatous Diseases of the Lung, *edited by Barry L. Fanburg*

21. Sleep and Breathing, *edited by Nicholas A. Saunders and Colin E. Sullivan*
22. *Pneumocystis carinii* Pneumonia: Pathogenesis, Diagnosis, and Treatment, *edited by Lowell S. Young*
23. Pulmonary Nuclear Medicine: Techniques in Diagnosis of Lung Disease, *edited by Harold L. Atkins*
24. Acute Respiratory Failure, *edited by Warren M. Zapol and Konrad J. Falke*
25. Gas Mixing and Distribution in the Lung, *edited by Ludwig A. Engel and Manuel Paiva*
26. High-Frequency Ventilation in Intensive Care and During Surgery, *edited by Graziano Carlon and William S. Howland*
27. Pulmonary Development: Transition from Intrauterine to Extrauterine Life, *edited by George H. Nelson*
28. Chronic Obstructive Pulmonary Disease: Second Edition, Revised and Expanded, *edited by Thomas L. Petty*
29. The Thorax (in two parts), *edited by Charis Roussos and Peter T. Macklem*
30. The Pleura in Health and Disease, *edited by Jacques Chrétien, Jean Bignon, and Albert Hirsch*
31. Drug Therapy for Asthma: Research and Clinical Practice, *edited by John W. Jenne and Shirley Murphy*
32. Pulmonary Endothelium in Health and Disease, *edited by Una S. Ryan*
33. The Airways: Neural Control in Health and Disease, *edited by Michael A. Kaliner and Peter J. Barnes*
34. Pathophysiology and Treatment of Inhalation Injuries, *edited by Jacob Loke*
35. Respiratory Function of the Upper Airway, *edited by Oommen P. Mathew and Giuseppe Sant'Ambrogio*
36. Chronic Obstructive Pulmonary Disease: A Behavioral Perspective, *edited by A. John McSweeny and Igor Grant*
37. Biology of Lung Cancer: Diagnosis and Treatment, *edited by Steven T. Rosen, James L. Mulshine, Frank Cuttitta, and Paul G. Abrams*
38. Pulmonary Vascular Physiology and Pathophysiology, *edited by E. Kenneth Weir and John T. Reeves*
39. Comparative Pulmonary Physiology: Current Concepts, *edited by Stephen C. Wood*
40. Respiratory Physiology: An Analytical Approach, *edited by H. K. Chang and Manuel Paiva*
41. Lung Cell Biology, *edited by Donald Massaro*
42. Heart–Lung Interactions in Health and Disease, *edited by Steven M. Scharf and Sharon S. Cassidy*
43. Clinical Epidemiology of Chronic Obstructive Pulmonary Disease, *edited by Michael J. Hensley and Nicholas A. Saunders*
44. Surgical Pathology of Lung Neoplasms, *edited by Alberto M. Marchevsky*
45. The Lung in Rheumatic Diseases, *edited by Grant W. Cannon and Guy A. Zimmerman*

46. Diagnostic Imaging of the Lung, *edited by Charles E. Putman*
47. Models of Lung Disease: Microscopy and Structural Methods, *edited by Joan Gil*
48. Electron Microscopy of the Lung, *edited by Dean E. Schraufnagel*
49. Asthma: Its Pathology and Treatment, *edited by Michael A. Kaliner, Peter J. Barnes, and Carl G. A. Persson*
50. Acute Respiratory Failure: Second Edition, *edited by Warren M. Zapol and Francois Lemaire*
51. Lung Disease in the Tropics, *edited by Om P. Sharma*
52. Exercise: Pulmonary Physiology and Pathophysiology, *edited by Brian J. Whipp and Karlman Wasserman*
53. Developmental Neurobiology of Breathing, *edited by Gabriel G. Haddad and Jay P. Farber*
54. Mediators of Pulmonary Inflammation, *edited by Michael A. Bray and Wayne H. Anderson*
55. The Airway Epithelium, *edited by Stephen G. Farmer and Douglas Hay*
56. Physiological Adaptations in Vertebrates: Respiration, Circulation, and Metabolism, *edited by Stephen C. Wood, Roy E. Weber, Alan R. Hargens, and Ronald W. Millard*
57. The Bronchial Circulation, *edited by John Butler*
58. Lung Cancer Differentiation: Implications for Diagnosis and Treatment, *edited by Samuel D. Bernal and Paul J. Hesketh*
59. Pulmonary Complications of Systemic Disease, *edited by John F. Murray*
60. Lung Vascular Injury: Molecular and Cellular Response, *edited by Arnold Johnson and Thomas J. Ferro*
61. Cytokines of the Lung, *edited by Jason Kelley*
62. The Mast Cell in Health and Disease, *edited by Michael A. Kaliner and Dean D. Metcalfe*
63. Pulmonary Disease in the Elderly Patient, *edited by Donald A. Mahler*
64. Cystic Fibrosis, *edited by Pamela B. Davis*
65. Signal Transduction in Lung Cells, *edited by Jerome S. Brody, David M. Center, and Vsevolod A. Tkachuk*
66. Tuberculosis: A Comprehensive International Approach, *edited by Lee B. Reichman and Earl S. Hershfield*
67. Pharmacology of the Respiratory Tract: Experimental and Clinical Research, *edited by K. Fan Chung and Peter J. Barnes*
68. Prevention of Respiratory Diseases, *edited by Albert Hirsch, Marcel Goldberg, Jean-Pierre Martin, and Roland Masse*
69. *Pneumocystis carinii* Pneumonia: Second Edition, Revised and Expanded, *edited by Peter D. Walzer*
70. Fluid and Solute Transport in the Airspaces of the Lungs, *edited by Richard M. Effros and H. K. Chang*
71. Sleep and Breathing: Second Edition, Revised and Expanded, *edited by Nicholas A. Saunders and Colin E. Sullivan*
72. Airway Secretion: Physiological Bases for the Control of Mucous Hypersecretion, *edited by Tamotsu Takishima and Sanae Shimura*

73. Sarcoidosis and Other Granulomatous Disorders, *edited by D. Geraint James*
74. Epidemiology of Lung Cancer, *edited by Jonathan M. Samet*
75. Pulmonary Embolism, *edited by Mario Morpurgo*
76. Sports and Exercise Medicine, *edited by Stephen C. Wood and Robert C. Roach*
77. Endotoxin and the Lungs, *edited by Kenneth L. Brigham*
78. The Mesothelial Cell and Mesothelioma, *edited by Marie-Claude Jaurand and Jean Bignon*
79. Regulation of Breathing: Second Edition, Revised and Expanded, *edited by Jerome A. Dempsey and Allan I. Pack*
80. Pulmonary Fibrosis, *edited by Sem Hin Phan and Roger S. Thrall*
81. Long-Term Oxygen Therapy: Scientific Basis and Clinical Application, *edited by Walter J. O'Donohue, Jr.*
82. Ventral Brainstem Mechanisms and Control of Respiration and Blood Pressure, *edited by C. Ovid Trouth, Richard M. Millis, Heidrun F. Kiwull-Schöne, and Marianne E. Schläfke*
83. A History of Breathing Physiology, *edited by Donald F. Proctor*
84. Surfactant Therapy for Lung Disease, *edited by Bengt Robertson and H. William Taeusch*
85. The Thorax: Second Edition, Revised and Expanded (in three parts), *edited by Charis Roussos*
86. Severe Asthma: Pathogenesis and Clinical Management, *edited by Stanley J. Szefler and Donald Y. M. Leung*
87. *Mycobacterium avium*–Complex Infection: Progress in Research and Treatment, *edited by Joyce A. Korvick and Constance A. Benson*
88. Alpha 1–Antitrypsin Deficiency: Biology • Pathogenesis • Clinical Manifestations • Therapy, *edited by Ronald G. Crystal*
89. Adhesion Molecules and the Lung, *edited by Peter A. Ward and Joseph C. Fantone*
90. Respiratory Sensation, *edited by Lewis Adams and Abraham Guz*
91. Pulmonary Rehabilitation, *edited by Alfred P. Fishman*
92. Acute Respiratory Failure in Chronic Obstructive Pulmonary Disease, *edited by Jean-Philippe Derenne, William A. Whitelaw, and Thomas Similowski*
93. Environmental Impact on the Airways: From Injury to Repair, *edited by Jacques Chrétien and Daniel Dusser*
94. Inhalation Aerosols: Physical and Biological Basis for Therapy, *edited by Anthony J. Hickey*
95. Tissue Oxygen Deprivation: From Molecular to Integrated Function, *edited by Gabriel G. Haddad and George Lister*
96. The Genetics of Asthma, *edited by Stephen B. Liggett and Deborah A. Meyers*
97. Inhaled Glucocorticoids in Asthma: Mechanisms and Clinical Actions, *edited by Robert P. Schleimer, William W. Busse, and Paul M. O'Byrne*
98. Nitric Oxide and the Lung, *edited by Warren M. Zapol and Kenneth D. Bloch*

99. Primary Pulmonary Hypertension, *edited by Lewis J. Rubin and Stuart Rich*
100. Lung Growth and Development, *edited by John A. McDonald*
101. Parasitic Lung Diseases, *edited by Adel A. F. Mahmoud*
102. Lung Macrophages and Dendritic Cells in Health and Disease, *edited by Mary F. Lipscomb and Stephen W. Russell*
103. Pulmonary and Cardiac Imaging, *edited by Caroline Chiles and Charles E. Putman*
104. Gene Therapy for Diseases of the Lung, *edited by Kenneth L. Brigham*
105. Oxygen, Gene Expression, and Cellular Function, *edited by Linda Biadasz Clerch and Donald J. Massaro*
106. $Beta_2$-Agonists in Asthma Treatment, *edited by Romain Pauwels and Paul M. O'Byrne*
107. Inhalation Delivery of Therapeutic Peptides and Proteins, *edited by Akwete Lex Adjei and Pramod K. Gupta*
108. Asthma in the Elderly, *edited by Robert A. Barbee and John W. Bloom*
109. Treatment of the Hospitalized Cystic Fibrosis Patient, *edited by David M. Orenstein and Robert C. Stern*
110. Asthma and Immunological Diseases in Pregnancy and Early Infancy, *edited by Michael Schatz, Robert S. Zeiger, and Henry N. Claman*
111. Dyspnea, *edited by Donald A. Mahler*
112. Proinflammatory and Antiinflammatory Peptides, *edited by Sami I. Said*
113. Self-Management of Asthma, *edited by Harry Kotses and Andrew Harver*
114. Eicosanoids, Aspirin, and Asthma, *edited by Andrew Szczeklik, Ryszard J. Gryglewski, and John R. Vane*
115. Fatal Asthma, *edited by Albert L. Sheffer*
116. Pulmonary Edema, *edited by Michael A. Matthay and David H. Ingbar*
117. Inflammatory Mechanisms in Asthma, *edited by Stephen T. Holgate and William W. Busse*
118. Physiological Basis of Ventilatory Support, *edited by John J. Marini and Arthur S. Slutsky*
119. Human Immunodeficiency Virus and the Lung, *edited by Mark J. Rosen and James M. Beck*
120. Five-Lipoxygenase Products in Asthma, *edited by Jeffrey M. Drazen, Sven-Erik Dahlén, and Tak H. Lee*
121. Complexity in Structure and Function of the Lung, *edited by Michael P. Hlastala and H. Thomas Robertson*
122. Biology of Lung Cancer, *edited by Madeleine A. Kane and Paul A. Bunn, Jr.*
123. Rhinitis: Mechanisms and Management, *edited by Robert M. Naclerio, Stephen R. Durham, and Niels Mygind*
124. Lung Tumors: Fundamental Biology and Clinical Management, *edited by Christian Brambilla and Elisabeth Brambilla*
125. Interleukin-5: From Molecule to Drug Target for Asthma, *edited by Colin J. Sanderson*

## ADDITIONAL VOLUMES IN PREPARATION

The Lung at Depth, *edited by Claes Lundgren and John N. Miller*

Daignostic Pulmonary Pathology, *edited by Philip T. Cagle*

Immunotherapy of Asthma, *edited by Jean Bousquet and Hans Yssel*

Air Pollutants and the Respiratory Tract, *edited by David L. Swift and Michael Foster*

Viral Infections of the Respiratory Tract, *edited by Raphael Dolin and Peter F. Wright*

Pediatric Asthma, *edited by Shirley J. Murphy and H. William Kelly*

LAM and Other Diseases Characterized by Smooth Muscle Proliferation, *edited by Joel Moss*

GERD and Airway Disease, *edited by Mark R. Stein*

Neurobiology of Sleep and Circadian Rhythms, *edited by Fred Turek and Phyllis Zee*

Multimodality Treatment of Lung Cancer, *edited by Arthur T. Skarin*

Cytokines in Pulmonary Infectious Disease, *edited by Steven Nelson and Thomas Martin*

Asthma's Impact on Society: The Social and Economic Burden, *edited by Kevin B. Weiss, A. Sonia Buist, and Sean D. Sullivan*

Anticholinergics in Clinical Allergy Practice, *edited by Sheldon L. Spector*

Control of Breathing in Health and Disease, *edited by Murray D. Altose and Yoshikazu Kawakami*

Chronic Lung Disease of Early Infancy, *edited by Richard D. Bland and Jacqueline J. Coalson*

Exercise-Induced Asthma, *edited by E. R. McFadden, Jr.*

*The opinions expressed in these volumes do not necessarily represent the views of the National Institutes of Health.*

# INTERLEUKIN-5

## FROM MOLECULE TO DRUG TARGET FOR ASTHMA


*Edited by*

Colin J. Sanderson

*TVW Telethon Institute for Child Health Research*
*West Perth, Western Australia*



MARCEL DEKKER, INC. NEW YORK • BASEL

**Library of Congress Cataloging-in-Publication Data**

Interleukin-5: from molecule to drug target for asthma / edited by
Colin J. Sanderson.
p. cm. -- (Lung biology in health and disease ; 125)
Includes bibliographical references and indexes.
ISBN 0-8247-0190-9 (alk. paper)
1. Interleukin-5—Physiological effect—Congresses.
2. Interleukin-5—Pathophysiology—Congresses. 3. Asthma—Molecular aspects—Congresses. 4. Asthma—Chemotherapy—Congresses.
I. Sanderson, Colin J. II. Title: Interleukin five.
III. Series.
[DNLM: 1. Interleukin-5—physiology. 2. Receptors, Interleukin—-physiology. 3. Interleukin-5—antagonists & inhibitors.
4. Asthma—immunology. QW 568 I5722 1999 / W1 LU62 v. 125 1999]
QR185.8.I56I575 1999
616.07'9—dc21
DNLM/DLC
For Library of Congress 98-44758
CIP

This book is printed on acid-free paper.

**Headquarters**
Marcel Dekker, Inc.
270 Madison Avenue, New York, NY 10016
tel: 212-696-9000; fax: 212-685-4540

**World Wide Web**
http://www.dekker.com

The publisher offers discounts on this book when ordered in bulk quantities. For more information, write to Special Sales/Professional Marketing at the headquarters address above.



Current printing (last digit):
10 9 8 7 6 5 4 3 2

**PRINTED IN THE UNITED STATES OF AMERICA**

# INTRODUCTION

This volume reports on a scientific voyage that was initiated with much doubt, but is now on the threshold of new application, and benefit, to the patients.

> Without theory, practice is but the routine born of habit. Theory alone can bring forth and develop the spirit of invention. It is to you specially that it will belong not to share the opinion of those narrow minds who disdain everything in science which has no immediate application. You know Franklin's charming saying? He was witnessing the first demonstration of purely scientific discovery, and the people around him said: "But, what is the use of it"? Franklin answered them: "What is the use of a newborn child"?
>
> —Louis Pasteur

This quotation describes the story of the lymphokine, interleukin-5 (IL-5). The role of eosinophils in asthma, now recognized as an inflammatory disease, has been known for decades. But, the discovery that IL-5 is responsible for the differentiation, production, and activation of eosinophils, led to the emergence of new concepts as well as the possibility that if one could block IL-5, a new treatment for asthma and other similar eosinophil-induced inflammatory reactions might be developed.

It appears that debates took place between the doubters and the advocates but the drive for further research prevailed.

Asthma is a complex disease—not caused by a single gene, or a single molecule or compound. In consequence, multiple therapies eventually will be needed to tailor the right therapy to each patient. Inhibitors of IL-5 will undoubtedly be one more step in the search for the right therapy. How important this therapy will be, when found and entered in practice, is yet unknown. But, unless the search goes on, we will never know the answer.

As the editor of this monograph, Dr. Colin J. Sanderson, points out in his Preface, this volume opens the door to new paths and new scientific challenges. The authors, from many countries and nearly all the continents, are to be congratulated for their contributions.

The Lung Biology in Health and Disease series of monographs has presented a number of volumes on asthma, its pathogenesis and its treatment. This work is unique because of its scope and its purpose. I am deeply appreciative to Dr. Colin J. Sanderson and his contributors for the opportunity to add to the series of monographs.

**Claude Lenfant, M.D.**
Bethesda, Maryland

# PREFACE

Il-5 was cloned nearly 10 years ago, and significant research and clinical results have taken place since then. This volume contains a series of reviews by key people in their niche of IL-5 research and clinical application. The timing is important as the molecule moves into an era of pharmaceutical discovery.

Eosinophils have fascinated hematologists for over a century and their association with allergy and helminth infections has been well documented. The significance of the association was given great impetus when Anthony Butterworth, working from Cambridge, but mainly in Africa, showed that eosinophils could kill the schistosomula of *Schistosoma mansoni*. It is remarkable to watch this process under the microscope. Large numbers of eosinophils attach to the parasite, which begins to thrash about like a large animal injured by gunshot wounds. Butterworth went on to show that resistance to reinfection with this parasite was significantly correlated with eosinophilia, providing the first evidence for a role of eosinophils in disease. My own interest in eosinophils was kindled during a sabbatical in Brazil, when we made (to us) the surprising observation that eosinophils could kill the protozoan *Trypanosoma cruzi*. This period began a long association with Angel F. López, from Argentina, who worked with me in Brazil and London and has settled in Australia, and who remains a close colleague. López and colleagues have contributed a chapter on

IL-5 receptor structure (Chapter 11). After moving to the National Institute at Mill Hill in London in 1980, my laboratory began to work on the control of eosinophil production. We sought and found the lymphokine that controls eosinophil production, which in 1985 we called Eosinophil Differentiation Factor (EDF), later called IL-5. In collaboration with Anne O'Garra, we went on to show that EDF was identical to a murine B cell growth factor (BCGFII). While murine IL-5 has this clear-cut activity on B cells in vitro, there is little convincing evidence for a similar activity on human B cells. Furthermore, some doubt has been expressed about the biological relevance of the activity in the mouse, as knockout mice have intact B cell systems (see Chapter 7).

In 1986 Gerald J. Gleich and Cheryl R. Adolphson at the Mayo Clinic reviewed a long series of elegant experiments in animals and with human lung tissue which showed the eosinophil responsible for tissue damage in allergy. For many years Gleich was a lone voice, but this review opened up his work to a wider audience, and was backed up by research from Per Venge in Sweden, Barry Kay in London (reviewed by Douglas S. Robinson in Chapter 3), and many others, and is now almost universally accepted. Gleich and Adolphson review their work in Chapter 1. The role of the eosinophil in the pathology of allergy and the clear link between IL-5 and eosinophilia is the basis for a significant investment from industry to find new agents that will block IL-5 and control the production of eosinophils (Chapters 17 and 18).

Between the discovery of IL-5, an understanding of the role of eosinophils, and the drug discovery programs, lie a number of important contributions. Some of the highlights include: the work from my group and others establishing the unique specificity of IL-5 for eosinophils; the cloning of the gene first by Tasuku Honjo and Kiyoshi Takatsu and their colleagues; and the determination of the structure of IL-5, by Amanda E. I. Proudfoot and colleagues at Glaxo, which is beautifully reviewed by Irwin M. Chaikin and Dr. Proudfoot in Chapter 10.

In summary, this book contains 18 chapters covering all aspects of IL-5, from clinical and experimental research and molecular biology, to insights into new drug discovery programs. It is the first complete overview of IL-5, which was discovered in 1985, and comes at a time when new anti-IL-5 therapeutics are being developed and tested. This book will be important reading for students and clinicians interested in the molecules behind allergy and asthma; to pharmaceutical chemists developing new anti-asthma drugs; to cytokine biologists working on protein structure and gene regulation; and to immunologists interested in the remarkable diversion of the immune response to allergic reactions.

I thank the authors for their contributions, their scientific interactions which I have been privileged to be part of over the last decade, and especially their friendship.

*Colin J. Sanderson*

## CONTRIBUTORS

**Cheryl R. Adolphson, M.S.** Senior Science Writer, Department of Immunology, Mayo Clinic and Mayo Foundation, Rochester, Minnesota

**Diljeet Athwal** CellTech Therapeutics, Slough, Berkshire, United Kingdom

**Christopher J. Bagley, Ph.D.** Senior Research Fellow, Cytokine Receptor Laboratory, Hanson Centre for Cancer Research, Adelaide, Australia

**Martyn Banks, Ph.D.** Senior Research Leader, Department of Lead Discovery, Glaxo Wellcome Research and Development, Stevenage, Hertfordshire, United Kingdom

**Mark W. Bodmer** CellTech Therapeutics, Slough, Berkshire, United Kingdom

**Irwin M. Chaiken, Ph.D.** Research Professor, Department of Medicine, University of Pennsylvania School of Medicine, Philadelphia, Pennsylvania

**Richard W. Chapman, Ph.D.** Senior Research Fellow, Department of Allergy, Schering-Plough Research Institute, Kenilworth, New Jersey

**Chuan-Chu Chou, Ph.D.** Senior Principal Scientist, Department of Immunology, Schering-Plough Research Institute, Kenilworth, New Jersey

**Paul D. Collins, Ph.D.** Lecturer, Leukocyte Biology Section, Biomedical Sciences Division, Imperial College School of Medicine, London, England

**Monica L. De Boer, Ph.D.** Division of Molecular Immunology, TVW Telethon Institute for Child Health Research, West Perth, Western Australia

**Judah A. Denburg, M.D., F.R.C.P.** Professor, Department of Medicine, McMaster University, Hamilton, Ontario, Canada

**Stephen R. Durham, M.D., F.R.C.P.** Reader, Department of Upper Respiratory Medicine, Imperial College School of Medicine at the National Heart and Lung Institute, London, England

**Robert W. Egan, Ph.D.** Senior Director, Department of Allergy, Schering-Plough Research Institute, Kenilworth, New Jersey

**J. Spencer Emtage** CellTech Therapeutics, Slough, Berkshire, United Kingdom

**Juliet A. Fisher** Division of Biochemistry and Molecular Biology, The John Curtin School of Medical Research, Australian National University, Canberra, Australia

**Paul S. Foster, Ph.D.** Doctor, Department of Biochemistry and Molecular Biology, John Curtin School of Medical Research, Australian National University, Canberra, Australia

**Gerald J. Gleich, M.D.** Professor, Mayo Medical School, and Consultant, Department of Immunology, Mayo Clinic and Mayo Foundation, Rochester, Minnesota

**Qutayba Hamid, M.D., Ph.D.** Professor, Department of Medicine, McGill University, Montreal, Quebec, Canada

**Takahiko Hara, Ph.D.** Associate Professor, Institute of Molecular and Cellular Biosciences, University of Tokyo, Tokyo, Japan

**Simon P. Hogan, Ph.D.** Doctor, Department of Biochemistry and Molecular Biology, John Curtin School of Medical Research, Australian National University, Canberra, Australia

**Barbara Holt** Department of Cell Biology, TVW Telethon Institute for Child Health Research, West Perth, Western Australia

**Patrick Holt, D.Sc.** Professor, Department of Cell Biology, TVW Telethon Institute for Child Health Research, West Perth, Western Australia

**Chung-Her Jenh, Ph.D.** Principal Scientist, Department of Immunology, Schering-Plough Research Institute, Kenilworth, New Jersey

**Stéphane Karlen, Ph.D.** Senior Research Officer, Department of Dermatology, University of Berne, Inselspital, Switzerland

**A. Barry Kay** Imperial College School of Medicine at National Heart and Lung Institute, London, United Kingdom

**Taisei Kinoshita, Ph.D.** Assistant Professor, Institute of Molecular and Cellular Biosciences, University of Tokyo, Tokyo, Japan

**Ted T. Kung, Ph.D.** Principal Scientist, Department of Allergy, Schering-Plough Research Institute, Kenilworth, New Jersey

**Kristin M. Leiferman, M.D.** Professor, Mayo Medical School, and Consultant, Department of Dermatology, Mayo Clinic and Mayo Foundation, Rochester, Minnesota

**Angel F. López, M.D., Ph.D., F.R.C.P.A.** Professor, Cytokine Receptor Laboratory, Hanson Centre for Cancer Research, Adelaide, Australia

**Claudia Macaubas, Ph.D.** Research Officer, Department of Cell Biology, TVW Telethon Institute for Child Health Research, West Perth, Western Australia

**Keisuke Masuyama, M.D.** Associate Professor, Department of Otorhinolaryngology, Kumamoto University School of Medicine, Kumamoto, Japan

**Klaus I. Matthaei, Ph.D.** Doctor, Department of Biochemistry and Molecular Biology, John Curtin School of Medical Research, Australian National University, Canberra, Australia

**Peter J. Mauser, Ph.D.** Principal Scientist, Department of Allergy, Schering-Plough Research Institute, Kenilworth, New Jersey

**Andrew N. J. McKenzie, Ph.D.** Staff Scientist, Protein and Nucleic Acid Chemistry Division, MRC Laboratory of Molecular Biology, Cambridge, United Kingdom

**Murray McKinnon, Ph.D.** Group Leader, Cell Biology Unit, Glaxo Wellcome Research and Development, Stevenage, Hertfordshire, United Kingdom

**Atsushi Miyajima, Ph.D.** Professor, Institute of Molecular and Cellular Biosciences, University of Tokyo, Tokyo, Japan

**Viatcheslav A. Mordvinov, Ph.D.** Doctor, Division of Molecular Immunology, TVW Telethon Institute for Child Health Research, West Perth, Western Australia

**Susan L. Prescott, B.Med.Sci., F.R.A.C.P.** Doctor, TVW Telethon Institute for Child Health Research, West Perth, Western Australia

**Amanda E. I. Proudfoot, Ph.D.*** Research Scientist, Department of Biochemistry, Geneva Biomedical Research Institute, Glaxo Wellcome Research and Development, Geneva, Switzerland

**Graeme Robertson, Ph.D.** Principal Research Chemist, Department of Exploratory Chemistry, Glaxo Wellcome Research and Development, Stevenage, Hertfordshire, United Kingdom

**Douglas S. Robinson, M.D., M.R.C.P.** Senior Lecturer and Consultant Physician, Department of Allergy and Clinical Immunology, Imperial College School of Medicine at National Heart and Lung Institute, London, England

**Monica Senna Salerno, M.Sc.** Division of Molecular Immunology, TVW Telethon Institute for Child Health Research, West Perth, Western Australia

**Colin J. Sanderson, Sc.D.** Professor, Division of Molecular Immunology, TVW Telethon Institute for Child Health Research, West Perth, Western Australia

**Gretchen T. F. Schwenger, B.Sc.** Division of Molecular Immunology, TVW Telethon Institute for Child Health Research, West Perth, Western Australia

**Roma Sehmi, Ph.D.** Senior Research Fellow, Department of Medicine, McMaster University, Hamilton, Ontario, Canada

**Peter D. Sly, M.D., F.R.A.C.P.** Associate Professor, Division of Clinical Sciences, TVW Telethon Institute for Child Health Research, West Perth, Western Australia

**Troy Smallacombe, B.Sc.** Research Assistant, Department of Cell Biology, TVW Telethon Institute for Child Health Research, West Perth, Western Australia

**Roberto Solari, Ph.D.** Research Unit Head, Department of Cell Biology, Glaxo Wellcome Research and Development, Stevenage, Hertfordshire, United Kingdom

**Frank C. Stomski, Ph.D.** Research Scientist, Cytokine Receptor Laboratory, Institute of Medical and Veterinary Science, Hanson Centre for Cancer Research, Adelaide, Australia

---

**Current affiliation*: Senior Research Scientist and Protein Biochemistry Group Leader, Serono Pharmaceutical Research Institute, Geneva, Switzerland.

**Kiyoshi Takatsu, Ph.D.** Professor, Department of Immunology, Institute of Medical Science, University of Tokyo, Tokyo, Japan

**Chiok L. Tan** Division of Biochemistry and Molecular Biology, The John Curtin School of Medical Research, Australian National University, Canberra, Australia

**Jan Tavernier, Ph.D.** Professor, Laboratory of Medical Protein Chemistry, University of Ghent, Ghent, Belgium

**Marc Thomas, B.Sc.** Division of Molecular Immunology, TVW Telethon Institute for Child Health Research, West Perth, Western Australia

**Joël Vandekerckhove, Ph.D.** Professor, Laboratory of Medical Protein Chemistry, University of Ghent, Ghent, Belgium

**José Van der Heyden** Roche Research Ghent, Ghent, Belgium

**Barbara H. van Leeuwen** Division of Biochemistry and Molecular Biology, The John Curtin School of Medical Research, Australian National University, Canberra, Australia

**Xaveer Van Ostade, Ph.D.** Laboratory of Medical Protein Chemistry, University of Ghent, Ghent, Belgium

**Thierry Venaille, Ph.D.** Doctor, Department of Cell Biology, TVW Telethon Institute for Child Health Research, West Perth, Western Australia

**Annick Verhee** Laboratory of Medical Protein Chemistry, University of Ghent, Ghent, Belgium

**Timothy J. Williams, Ph.D.** Professor, Leukocyte Biology Centre, Biomedical Science Division, Imperial College School of Medicine, London, England

**Joanna M. Woodcock, Ph.D.** Research Fellow, Cytokine Receptor Laboratory, Institute of Medical and Veterinary Science, Hanson Centre for Cancer Research, Adelaide, Australia

**Akihiro Yabuhara** TVW Telethon Institute for Child Health Research, West Perth, Western Australia

**Ian G. Young, M.Sc., Ph.D.** Doctor, Division of Biochemistry and Molecular Biology, John Curtin School of Medical Research, Australian National University, Canberra, Australia

# CONTENTS


*Introduction* Claude Lenfant *iii*
*Preface* *v*
*Contributors* *vii*

**1. The Eosinophil and Bronchial Asthma: Evidence for a Critical Role of Eosinophils in Pathophysiology** **1**
*Gerald J. Gleich and Cheryl R. Adolphson*

I. Introduction 1
II. Eosinophil Granule Proteins 2
III. Alterations of Respiratory Tissue by Eosinophil Granule Proteins 4
IV. Eosinophil Granule Proteins and Bronchial Hyperreactivity 9
V. In Vitro Models of Bronchial Hyperreactivity 14
VI. Eosinophil Granule Proteins and Vagal Function 15
VII. Effect of Eosinophil Granule Proteins on Other Cells Relevant to Asthma 17
VIII. Evidence for Involvement of Eosinophils and Their Granule Proteins in the Pathophysiology of Bronchial Asthma 21

IX. Summary and Conclusions 26
References 28

**2. Interleukin-5 in Rhinitis: Influence of Treatment 39**
*Stephen R. Durham, Keisuke Masuyama, and Qutayba Hamid*

I. Introduction 39
II. Nasal Late Responses 40
III. Influence of Treatment 41
IV. Seasonal Grass Pollen Exposure 45
V. Perennial Rhinitis 46
VI. Summary 47
References 48

**3. Interleukin-5 and Interleukin-5 Receptor in Asthma 51**
*Douglas S. Robinson*

I. Introduction 51
II. IL-5 in Asthma 53
III. The Cell Source of IL-5 in Asthma 55
IV. Nonatopic Asthma 57
V. The Effect of Corticosteroid Treatment on IL-5 Expression in Asthma 57
VI. IL-5 Receptor Expression in Asthma 60
VII. Conclusion: IL-5 as a Therapeutic Target in Asthma 61
References 61

**4. Bone Marrow in Allergic Disease: The Role of Interleukin-5 as an Eosinophilopoietic Factor 69**
*Roma Sehmi and Judah A. Denburg*

I. Introduction 69
II. Interleukin-5: Background 70
III. IL-5 Receptor: Structure and Function 71
IV. Quantification of Progenitors 71
V. Evidence of Increased Progenitor Activity in Allergic Inflammation 76
VI. Regulation of IL-5R Expression: A Potential Therapeutic Target in Asthma/Allergy 84
VII. Summary 85
References 85

**5. Eosinophils, Interleukin-5, and Cutaneous Disease** **95**
*Kristin M. Leiferman*

I. Introduction 95
II. Atopic Dermatitis 99
III. Bullous Pemphigoid 104
IV. Recurrent Cutaneous Necrotizing Eosinophilic Vasculitis 107
V. Conclusion 111
References 112

**6. Perinatal and Early Childhood Cytokine Responses to Environmental Allergens** **119**
*Claudia Macaubas, Susan L. Prescott, Troy Smallacombe, Akihiro Yabuhara, Thierry Venaille, Barbara Holt, Peter D. Sly, and Patrick Holt*

I. Introduction 119
II. Allergen-Specific Cytokine Responses at Birth 120
III. Allergen-Specific Cytokine Responses in Infancy and Early Childhood 122
IV. Conclusions 124
References 124

**7. The Role of Interleukin-5 in Allergic Airways Disease** **127**
*Paul S. Foster, Simon P. Hogan, Klaus I. Matthaei, and Ian G. Young*

I. Introduction 127
II. Role of IL-5 in Allergic Airways Disease 128
III. Role of IL-4 in Allergic Airways Disease 129
IV. Discussion 130
References 131

**8. Cytokine Control of the Development of a T-Helper 2 Response** **137**
*Andrew N. J. McKenzie*

I. T-Helper Cell Differentiation Pathways 137
II. Factors Affecting T-Cell Differentiation 138
III. Coordinated Cytokine Family Expression 141
References 146

**9. Interactions Between Interleukin-5 and the Eosinophil-Selective Chemokine Eotaxin: Potential Relevance in Allergic Disease 153**
*Paul D. Collins and Timothy J. Williams*

I. Introduction 153
II. Discovery of Eotaxin 154
III. Conclusions 160
References 160

**10. Structure of Interleukin-5 167**
*Irwin M. Chaiken and Amanda E. I. Proudfoot*

I. Introduction 167
II. Primary and Crystallographic Structure 168
III. Dynamics of IL-5 Interaction with Receptor α Chain 170
IV. Alanine Scanning Mutagenesis with wtIL-5 174
V. Asymmetry in Receptor α and $\beta_c$ Recruitment by Symmetrically Dimeric IL-5 176
VI. The Future 183
References 184

**11. The Structural Basis for Interleukin-5 Receptor Assembly 189**
*Christopher J. Bagley, Joanna M. Woodcock, Frank C. Stomski, and Angel F. López*

I. Introduction 189
II. Receptor Structure 190
III. Receptor-Ligand Interactions 191
IV. Mechanism of IL-5 Receptor Activation 196
V. The Future 198
References 200

**12. Analysis of the Expression Pattern of Human Interleukin-5 Receptor α Isoforms In Vitro 205**
*Jan Tavernier, Annick Verhee, Joël Vandekerckhove, Xaveer Van Ostade, and José Van der Heyden*

I. Introduction 205
II. Secreted Receptors in the Cytokine Receptor Family 206
III. Expression Pattern of the IL-5Rα Chain 207
IV. Design of Minigene Constructs 210
V. Expression Pattern of Minigenes in Cos1 and FDC-P1 Cells 211
VI. Design of a Minigene-Based Screening System 213
VII. Conclusion 215
References 219

**13. Role of the Common β Subunit of the Interleukin-3, Interleukin-5, and Granulocyte Macrophage-Colony Stimulating Factor Receptors** **225**
*Atsushi Miyajima, Taisei Kinoshita, and Takahiko Hara*

I. Introduction 225
II. Structure of the IL-3, IL-5, and GM-CSF Receptors 226
III. Expression of the Receptor Subunits 227
IV. Mice Devoid of the IL-3, GM-CSF, and IL-5 Function 228
V. Signal Transduction 229
VI. Signals from the Membrane Proximal Region of the β Subunit 232
VII. Role of Ras in IL-3/GM-CSF/IL-5 Function 234
VIII. Concluding Remarks 235
References 236

**14. Interleukin-5 Receptor and Signal Transduction** **241**
*Kiyoshi Takatsu*

I. Introduction 241
II. Biological Function of IL-5 242
III. Structure of IL-5 Receptor 245
IV. IL-5 Signal Transduction 248
V. Mechanism of IL-5 Receptor Activation 251
VI. Closing Remarks 255
References 256

**15. Regulation of Interleukin-5 Gene Expression** **267**
*Colin J. Sanderson, Monica L. De Boer, Monica Senna Salerno, Gretchen T. F. Schwenger, Marc Thomas, Viatcheslav A. Mordvinov, and Stéphane Karlen*

I. Introduction 267
II. Cell Systems for Analysis of Regulation 268
III. Deletion Analysis 270
IV. Upstream Repressor Elements 275
V. Downstream Repressor Elements 276
VI. Pathways Leading to the Activation of the IL-5 Gene 277
VII. Posttranscriptional Effects 279
VIII. Drug Effects on IL-5 Production 279
IX. Conclusions 282
References 282

**16. Regulation of Interleukin-5 Expression in T Lymphocytes: Repression by Dexamethasone** **289**
*Ian G. Young, Chiok L. Tan, Juliet A. Fisher, Barbara H. van Leeuwen, and Klaus I. Matthaei*

I. Introduction 289
II. Signaling Pathways Involved in IL-5 Regulation 290
III. Localization of the Enhancer Responsive to TCR Stimulation 291
IV. Positive Regulatory Elements in the Promoter 292
V. Repression by Dexamethasone 293
References 295

**17. Interleukin-5 and the Interleukin-5 Receptor: Targets for Drug Discovery in Asthma** **299**
*Murray McKinnon, Martyn Banks, Roberto Solari, and Graeme Robertson*

I. Introduction 299
II. General Strategies for Inhibiting IL-5 Action 300
III. High Throughput Random Screening for Low Molecular Weight Antagonists 302
IV. Low Molecular Weight Antagonists 305
V. Protein Antagonists 313
VI. Summary 316
References 316

**18. Pulmonary Biology of Anti-Interleukin-5 Antibodies** **321**
*Robert W. Egan, Chuan-Chu Chou, Richard W. Chapman, Chung-Her Jenh, Ted T. Kung, Peter J. Mauser, Diljeet Athwal, J. Spencer Emtage, and Mark W. Bodmer*

References 329

*Author Index* *331*
*Subject Index* *377*

# INTERLEUKIN-5

FROM MOLECULE TO DRUG TARGET FOR ASTHMA

# 1

# The Eosinophil and Bronchial Asthma: Evidence for a Critical Role of Eosinophils in Pathophysiology

**GERALD J. GLEICH**

Mayo Medical School, Mayo Clinic and Mayo Foundation
Rochester, Minnesota

**CHERYL R. ADOLPHSON**

Mayo Clinic and Mayo Foundation
Rochester, Minnesota

## I. Introduction

In 1879 P. Ehrlich established procedures to stain peripheral blood cells and discovered the distinctive properties of eosinophilic leukocytes (1). Application of these procedures to disease showed the association of eosinophilia and bronchial asthma (2), including bronchial tissue eosinophilia (3,4). In 1912, striking pulmonary eosinophilia was discovered in guinea pigs surviving anaphylactic shock, and the possibility that eosinophils altered anaphylaxis was suggested (5). This, in turn, led to the view that eosinophils served to protect against anaphylaxis. However, as information about eosinophil granule proteins and their striking biological activities became known, the possibility that eosinophils are effector cells in bronchial asthma has been considered. This review describes the role of eosinophils in bronchial asthma with particular emphasis on the activities of eosinophil granule proteins.

---

Supported by grants from the National Institute of Allergy and Infectious Diseases (AI 09728, AI 34577, and AI 31155) and by the Mayo Foundation.

## II. Eosinophil Granule Proteins

Eosinophils contain a large number of distinctive cytoplasmic granules. The granules of guinea pig (6), human (7), rat (8), and mouse (9) eosinophils have been isolated and granule proteins identified. Four principal eosinophil granule proteins have been identified including major basic protein (MBP), eosinophil cationic protein (ECP), eosinophil-derived neurotoxin (EDN), and eosinophil peroxidase (EPO). The properties of these proteins have been reviewed in detail elsewhere (10) and the characteristics of the granule proteins will only be briefly considered here.

### A. Major Basic Protein

The eosinophil granule MBP was so named because it accounts for more than 50% of the granule protein, its pI is too high to measure, and it is proteinaceous (6,10,11). MBP has been isolated from guinea pig (6,11), human (7), rat (8), and mouse (9) eosinophils. Human MBP consists of a single polypeptide chain of 117 amino acids (12). It is rich in arginine, has an $M_r$ of about $14 \times 10^3$, and has a calculated isoelectric point of 10.9. The MBP cDNA has been sequenced, and it specifies the synthesis of a pre-pro molecule with a 15 amino acid leader sequence and a 90 amino acid pro sequence followed by the 117 amino acid sequence for granule MBP (13,14). Of interest is the observation that the 90 amino acid pro portion is markedly enriched in the acidic amino acids—glutamic acid and aspartic acid. One possible function of the acidic pro portion of proMBP is especially attractive, namely that the pro portion protects the cell from the injurious effects of MBP during the transport of the proMBP from the Golgi apparatus to the eosinophil granule, where proMBP is processed. Also of interest is the finding that two varieties of guinea pig MBP (MBP-1 and MBP-2) have been partially sequenced and their cDNAs cloned (15,16). All of the MBP molecules from the above-mentioned species have been cloned, and they all are comparable in their cDNA organization with a proMBP and a granule MBP portion. The MBPs from the various species (6–9,11) show strong sequence conservation in the *N* terminal secretory signal sequence (67–87%), the mature cationic MBP (53–60%), and all of the reactive half-cysteine residues. However, the sequence similarity does not extend to the pro portion of proMBP (31–42%). Nonetheless, the pro segments share enrichment by acidic amino acids (calculated pI $\sim$ 3.8), which confers a relatively neutral charge on proMBP (calculated pI $\sim$ 6.1). Remarkably, sera from pregnant women contain strikingly elevated concentrations of MBP, and this has now been shown to be largely proMBP (17,18).

MBP is a potent toxin to parasites and mammalian cells (10) and, as noted above, has been implicated in the tissue damage seen in bronchial asthma. MBP is also a potent cytostimulatory molecule and is able to stimulate histamine re-

lease from basophils and rat mast cells (19,20) and to activate neutrophils (21) and platelets (22). Curiously, MBP appears to inhibit alveolar macrophage function (23). Finally, as will be noted later, MBP can be linked to the acquisition of bronchial hyperreactivity (BHR) in animal models.

### B. Eosinophil Cationic Protein

ECP is comparable to MBP with a pI of approximately 10.8, consists of a single polypeptide chain (24,25), and displays striking molecular weight heterogeneity (26). The nucleotide sequence of ECP cDNA codes for a pre-pro protein of 160 amino acids and a protein of 133 amino acids with an $M_r$ of 15,600 (27,28). The deduced ECP amino acid sequence reveals 66% identity to EDN and 31% identity to human pancreatic RNase. Thus ECP is a member of the RNase gene superfamily, the other members being EDN, pancreatic RNase, and human angiogenin (29). The RNase activity of ECP is approximately 50 to 100 times less than that of EDN (30). The ECP gene has been localized to the q24-q31 region of human chromosome 14.

ECP is a potent toxin for many targets, especially parasites and bacteria. Surprisingly, ECP does not cause histamine release from basophils (20). Finally, ECP appears to damage target cell membranes through the formation of pores or transmembrane channels (31).

### C. Eosinophil-Derived Neurotoxin (EDN)

Neurotoxic reactions in experimental animals were first investigated by M. H. Gordon (32) and are referred to as the Gordon phenomenon. Ultimately the reactions were traced to eosinophils and then to EDN (33). EDN has an $M_r$ of approximately 18,600 and is remarkably homologous to ECP (25). Both EDN and ECP are homologous to pancreatic RNase (25), but EDN has about 100 times more RNase activity than ECP (30). EDN cDNA has been cloned (34,35), and the deduced amino acid sequence specifies a 134 amino acid polypeptide with an $M_r$ of 15,500 and a 27 residue amino terminal hydrophobic leader. This sequence is identical to that of human urinary RNase (36) and to the amino terminal sequence of human liver RNase (37). EDN, like ECP, belongs to the RNase gene superfamily. The human genomic DNAs for ECP and EDN have been cloned and sequenced (38). Analyses of these data suggest that the genes for EDN and ECP arose as a consequence of a gene duplication event that took place approximately 25 to 40 million years ago. The eosinophil protein referred to as EPX appears to be identical to EDN (39).

EDN is a potent neurotoxin causing the Gordon phenomenon (33,40); in rabbits, EDN and ECP showed comparable neurotoxic reactions (25). Concerning toxicity, EDN is considerably less potent as a toxin for parasites and other targets than the other eosinophil granule proteins (10).

### D. Eosinophil Peroxidase (EPO)

Human EPO has been purified and consists of two subunits, a heavy chain with an $M_r$ of 50,000 to 58,000 and a light chain with an $M_r$ of 10,500 to 15,000 in 1:1 stoichiometry (41,42). EPO cDNA has been cloned and has an open reading frame of 2106 nucleotides coding for a 381 base pair pro sequence, a 333 base pair sequence corresponding to the coding region of the light chain, a 1392 base pair sequence coding for the EPO heavy chain, and a 452 base pair untranslated 3′ region (43). The human EPO gene has been cloned, and it is similar to the human MPO gene consisting of 12 axons and 11 introns spanning approximately 12 kDa (44).

EPO is able to oxidize halides to form reactive hypohalous acids (45). For example, chloride is oxidized to form hypochlorous acid: $H_2O_2 + Cl^- + H^+ \rightarrow HOCl + H_2O$. Analyses of the EPO's halide preference showed that eosinophils preferentially use bromide over chloride (46); however, more recent studies showed that the pseudohalide thiocyanate, at a concentration of 1 μM is a potent inhibitor of the reactivity of EPO with bromide and or iodide, both present at 100 μM (47). Thus the peroxidatic product of an EPO-thiocyanate reaction is hypothiocyanous acid, a weak, primarily sulfhydryl-reactive oxidant, and this appears to be the major oxidant produced by EPO in physiological fluids. The EPO/$H_2O_2$/halide system is able to generate potent oxidants when the halide is chloride or bromide, and these have the capacity to kill a large number of targets (reviewed in ref. 10). EPO is also toxic to some targets in the absence of halide or $H_2O_2$, although it is considerably less potent than when it is a part of the EPO/$H_2O_2$/halide system. As will be noted later, EPO, either by itself or when acting as a peroxidase, is able to damage respiratory epithelium.

### E. Localization of Granule Proteins

As shown in Figure 1.1, EPO, ECP, and EDN are all localized to the matrix of the eosinophil granule (48,49), whereas MBP is localized to the crystalline core (49,50). The properties of the human eosinophil granule proteins and the encoding cDNAs and genes are summarized in Table 1.

## III. Alterations of Respiratory Tissue by Eosinophil Granule Proteins

### A. Damage to Respiratory Epithelium by Eosinophil Granule Proteins

Initially we tested whether MBP was toxic for respiratory epithelium. When MBP was tested with cultures of guinea pig respiratory epithelium, concentrations as

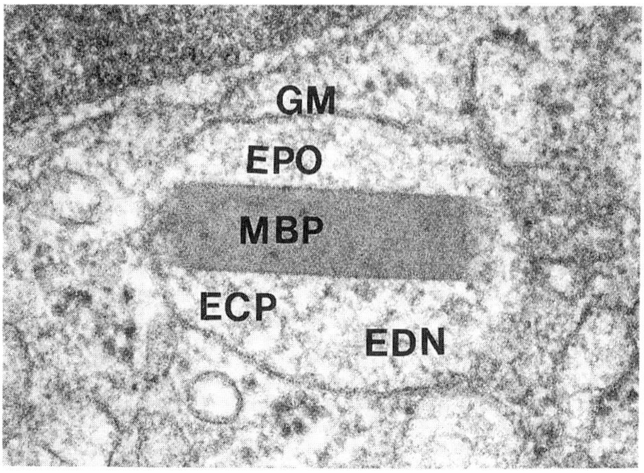


**Figure 1** Electron photomicrograph showing an eosinophil granule from rat bone marrow. The secondary eosinophil granule is bounded by a membrane designated GM. The matrix contains three proteins: ECP, EDN, and EPO. The core of the granule contains MBP; this photomicrograph shows a regular longitudinal array of dense bands in the core. The original photomicrograph has been modified to show the locations of the proteins. Original magnification 40,000×. Courtesy of Dr. E. DeHarven, Sloan-Kettering Institute for Cancer Research, New York, NY.

low as 10 μg/ml produced ciliostasis at 48 hr, and 100 μg/ml slowed ciliary beating within 3 hr and stopped ciliary motion within 23 hr (51–53). By microscopy, varying degrees of epithelial damage were present; this damage could be directly related to the dose and length of exposure to MBP. The lowest concentration of MBP tested, 10 μg/ml, caused disruption of the epithelium and damaged cells were free in the lumen of the guinea pig tracheal rings. Higher MBP concentrations, 50 μg/ml and 100 μg/ml, caused extensive damage to the epithelium. Furthermore, brush cells and ciliated cells were detached and individual cells were destroyed, leaving behind only basal cells. Both human and guinea pig MBP had these effects on respiratory epithelium, and the levels of MBP detected in sputum specimens of patients with asthma approximated or exceeded those needed for biologic activity in vitro (53). Comparisons of all of the eosinophil granule proteins incubated with guinea pig tracheal epithelium revealed that MBP and EPO were active, whereas ECP was considerably less potent and EDN failed to damage respiratory epithelium (54). Surprisingly, EPO damaged respiratory epithelium either by itself or in the presence of $H_2O_2$ and a halide. Furthermore, other experiments showed that MBP caused lysis of human A549 and rat type II pneumocytes (55), and that the EPO/$H_2O_2$/halide system is particularly effective in causing lytic injury to these cells (56). Finally,

**Table 1** Properties of Human Eosinophil Granule Protein and their Encoding cDNA and Genes

| Protein | Site | $M_r$ ($\times 10^{-3}$) | Isoelectric point[a] | Cell content (μg/$10^6$) | Molecular biology activities | cDNA | Gene |
|---|---|---|---|---|---|---|---|
| MBP | Core | 14 | 10.9 | 9 | Potent helminthotoxin and cytotoxin<br>Bactericidal<br>Inhibits C3b<br>Histamine release from basophils and rat mast cells<br>Unique, strong platelet agonist<br>Activates neutrophils and alveolar macrophages<br>Promotes bronchospasm<br>Increases bronchial reactivity to methacholine<br>Blocks muscarinic $M_2$ receptors | ~900 nt[b] (pre-proMBP) | 3.3 kb<br>5 introns<br>6 exons |
| ECP | Matrix | 18–21 | 10.8 | 5 | Potent helminthotoxin and cytotoxin<br>Bactericidal<br>Potent neurotoxin<br>Causes histamine release from rat mast cells<br>Weak RNase activity | ~725 nt (preECP) in UTR | ~1.2 kb<br>1 intron |

| | | | | | | | |
|---|---|---|---|---|---|---|---|
| EDN | Matrix | 18–19 | 8.9 | 3 | Potent neurotoxin<br>Potent RNase activity<br>Weak helminthotoxin | ~725 nt (preEDN) in UTR | ~1.2 kb<br><br>1 intron |
| EPO | Matrix | 66 | 10.8 | 12 | In the presence of $H_2O_2$ + $I^-$ or $Br^-$:<br>Kills microorganisms and tumor cells<br>Causes histamine release from rat mast cells<br>Inactivates leukotrienes<br>Kills *Brugia microfilariae* and damages respiratory epithelium<br>In the absence of $H_2O_2$:<br>Damages respiratory epithelium<br>Causes bronchospasm<br>Kills helminths | ~2500 nt (2106 nt (ORF) | 12 kb<br>11 introns |

[a]Calculated from amino acid sequence deduced from the cDNA.
[b]nt = nucleotides; kb = kilobases; ORF = open reading frame; UTR = untranslated region.
*Source*: modified and used with permission from Gleich GJ, Kita H, Adolphson CR. Samter's Immunologic Diseases, 1994:205–245 (10).

human nasal epithelium showed these same toxic effects after in vitro treatment with the EPO/$H_2O_2$/halide system or MBP (57).

As noted above, MBP abolished the ciliary activity of respiratory epithelium (51–53). Using rabbit tracheal rings and analyses of their ciliary beat frequency, the effect of MBP was subsequently investigated in more detail (58). While MBP reduced the ciliary beat frequency, it more strikingly abolished the zones of ciliary activity in the tracheal ring. After treatment with MBP, the beating of axonemes was completely inhibited; in the case of the isolated axonemes, a moderate concentration of MBP—28 μg/ml—had a clear-cut effect on their activity. Finally, the MBP effect appeared to be caused by inhibition of axonemal ATPase activity.

### B. Effects on Epithelial Secretion

The MBP effect on the electrical properties of tracheal tissue was studied with canine tracheal membranes mounted in Ussing chambers (59). Addition of MBP to the mucosal side (but not the submucosal side) of the membrane increased the short-circuit current and increased the net chloride secretion; net sodium movement was unaffected. Surprisingly, cationic proteins such as polyarginine, polylysine, and histone did not cause significant short-circuit (or potential) differences. However, at higher concentrations, all of these proteins were toxic and caused a marked drop in short-circuit current and potential differences. These effects on epithelial secretions suggested that MBP, by stimulating airway epithelial chloride and water secretion, could contribute to abnormalities in airway secretions in patients with asthma.

### C. Vascular Permeability

The effect of eosinophil granule proteins on vascular permeability has been analyzed in the hamster cheek pouch (60). MBP applied topically at 0.1 nM and 0.5 nM increased the clearance of fluoresceinated dextran (FITC-dx) and caused muscle fasciculation and prominent arteriolar dilatation. ECP was as potent as MBP, whereas EPO was less potent. Supplementation of EPO with $H_2O_2$ resulted in a considerable increase in the plasma clearance of FITC-dx. EDN required a 2000-fold higher concentration (1 μM) to elicit a significant increase of FITC-dx clearance compared with MBP, ECP, and EPO. The effects of the eosinophil granule proteins on vascular permeability were not mediated by histamine because histamine could not be detected in perfusate fluids. These results demonstrate that MBP, ECP, EPO, and EDN all increase microvascular transport in the hamster cheek pouch, and that this increase is independent of endogenous histamine release. As will be discussed later, the concentrations of eosinophil granule proteins causing increased vascular permeability are achieved in many pathologic conditions, suggesting that they play an important role not only in asthma, but in other diseases associated with the occurrence of edema (61).

## IV. Eosinophil Granule Proteins and Bronchial Hyperreactivity

The information discussed above indicates that eosinophil granule proteins are active on the bronchi and on various components of bronchial tissue. Further, these effects can be related to the pathophysiology of bronchial asthma. A critical feature of bronchial asthma is airway hyperreactivity, and this has been related to the eosinophil (62).

### A. Relationship of Hyperreactivity and Blood Eosinophilia

The relationship between peripheral blood eosinophilia and bronchial hyperreactivity has been documented in three separate studies (63–65). These reports came to comparable conclusions. They showed that the degree of bronchial hyperreactivity to histamine or methacholine was inversely related to the number of peripheral blood eosinophils. Observations were made both in individuals with allergic asthma and in individuals with nonatopic asthma (65). In one experiment, 23 asthmatic subjects, 14 of whom were atopic and 9 who were nonatopic, were studied and an inverse relationship was found between baseline eosinophil counts and $PC_{20}$ ($r = -0.71$, $p < 0.001$). In subjects with atopy, peripheral blood eosinophil counts and the histamine $PC_{20}$ were inversely related ($r = -0.74$, $p < 0.01$). In nonatopic subjects, the peripheral blood eosinophil count and histamine sensitivity were also inversely related ($r = -0.68$, $p < 0.05$) (65). Analysis of the relationship between airway reactivity and various atopic factors was conducted utilizing methacholine challenge in 87 patients with asthma (64). No significant correlations were observed between airway reactivity and the threshold of intracutaneous reaction with house dust, serum IgE concentration, or the level of IgE antibody to mites; in contrast, a significant correlation was found between airway reactivity and peripheral blood eosinophil counts (64).

### B. Bronchial Hyperreactivity and Pulmonary Eosinophilia

The relationship between bronchial eosinophils and bronchial hyperreactivity was subsequently analyzed utilizing bronchoalveolar lavage (BAL) fluids. Seventeen patients with mild atopic asthma (9 were symptomatic and 8 were asymptomatic) and 14 nonasthmatic control subjects were invested (66). A significant difference ($p < 0.01$) existed between the percentages of eosinophils in the BAL fluids of patients with reactive airways (methacholine $PC_{20} < 4$ mg/ml) and those without reactive airways (methacholine $PC_{20} > 4$ mg/ml). Further, the quantity of MBP recovered in the BAL fluids was lowest in nonatopic normal individuals and increased in patients with hay fever, asymptomatic asthma, and symptomatic asthma. The latter group had the highest MBP levels ($p < 0.01$ for the difference between symptomatic asthma patients and normal controls, and $p < 0.05$ for the difference between symptomatic asthma patients and hay fever patients). In addition, the levels of MBP recovered in the BAL fluids were related to the percentages of eosinophils in the BAL fluids ($r = 0.64$, $p < 0.001$). The MBP levels in the BAL fluids were inversely related to the degree of airway reactivity ($r = -0.59$, $p < 0.01$). In addition, the degree of airway reactivity was inversely related to the percentage of eosinophils in the BAL fluids ($r = -0.53$, $p < 0.05$) and the percentage of epithelial cells in the BAL fluids ($r = -0.41$, $p < 0.05$). These results show that MBP levels are inversely related to the degree of bronchial hyperreactivity and suggest that asthma, even mild asthma, and bronchial hyperreactivity are caused by eosinophil-mediated inflammation.

### C. Relationship Between BAL Eosinophilia and Hyperreactivity

Experiments using cynomolgus monkeys showed a relationship between eosinophils and airway reactivity (67,68). Therefore the effect of repeated inhalation of *Ascaris suum* extract on airway composition and airway responsiveness was tested (69). Over a 10 week period, periodic BAL was conducted and airway responsiveness to methacholine administration was measured. Control animals were exposed to inhalation of vehicle and were compared to the animals repeatedly inhaling *A. suum* extracts. A prolonged inflammatory reaction characterized by a striking increase in airway eosinophils (from $3 \pm 1\%$ to $59 \pm 15\%$; $p < 0.01$) occurred in the *A. suum* treated animals. The association between airway eosinophilia and an increase in airway responsiveness was shown by a leftward shift of the methacholine dose response curve, an increased slope of the methacholine dose response curve, and a decrease in the methacholine $PC_{100}$ values (the dose of methacholine required to cause a 100% increase in lung resistance). Both eosinophil numbers and MBP concentrations in the BAL fluids correlated with the methacholine $PC_{100}$ values ($r = 0.61$, $p < 0.01$ and $r = 0.64$, $p < 0.01$, respectively). Lung biopsies of these animals at week 10 showed striking eosinophil infiltration in the antigen-challenged animals. Furthermore, at week 2 no increased responsiveness to methacholine was evident, in spite of striking BAL eosinophilia; BAL fluid MBP levels were not significantly different from control levels. At week 4 bronchial hyperreactivity increased strikingly and BAL fluid eosinophilia and MBP levels were maximal. Thus the numbers of BAL eosinophils are likely not as critical as the levels of BAL MBP. This observation, in turn, supports the hypothesis that release of toxic eosinophil granule proteins is a better correlate of bronchial hyperreactivity than the number of eosinophils per se (69).

## D. Provocation of Hyperreactivity by Cationic Molecules

As noted above, MBP levels are related to bronchial hyperreactivity in humans and primates, suggesting that MBP might cause hyperreactivity. To directly test this possibility, purified eosinophil granule proteins were administered to primates and their effects on pulmonary function and airway responsiveness were measured (70). In these analyses MBP, EPO, ECP, and EDN were directly instilled into the monkey's trachea above the carina and the effects of this instillation on both respiratory resistance and airway reactivity were measured. As shown in Figure 2, the administration of MBP and EPO significantly increased airway resistance within 5 min, which decreased to baseline levels in 60 min. In five animals, a randomized crossover study design tested the effect of direct instillation of purified eosinophil granule proteins on airway responsiveness compared to the effect of column buffer instillation. Instillation of MBP resulted in a dose-related increase in $PC_{100}$ values for each animal (Table 2). For MBP, the mean change in log $PC_{100}$ values for 0.5 mg and 1.0 mg were – –0.39 ± 13 and –1.02 ± 0.36, respectively. Instillation of MBP caused a parallel shift to the left in the cumulative methacholine dose response curves (Fig. 3), and only MBP significantly changed the log methacholine $PC_{100}$ result. Somewhat surprising was the finding that EPO did not cause such changes even though a considerably higher dose, 2.0 mg, was administered in an effort to seek a dose response relationship between EPO administration and airway reactivity. Furthermore, administration of EPO/$H_2O_2$/KI was not associated with a change in airway reactivity. Overall these results suggest that MBP has an effector role

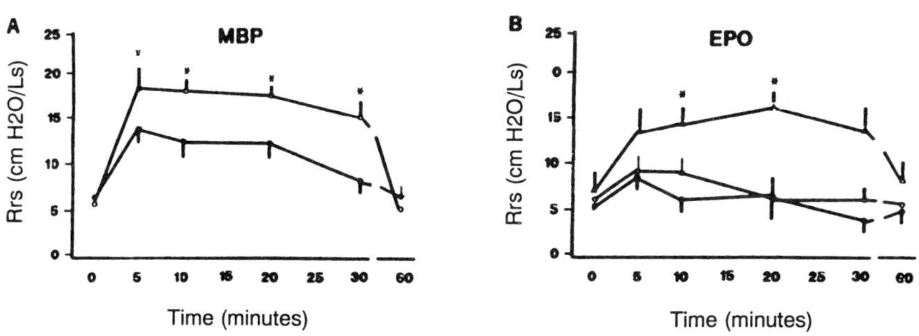


**Figure 2** The effect of intratracheal instillation of purified MBP and EPO on Rrs in cynomolgus monkeys. (**A**) MBP (0.5 and 1.0 mg) administration resulted in a transient increase in Rrs (a measure of respiratory system impedance derived from forced oscillations superimposed on tidal breathing) which occurred immediately after instillation and resolved by 60 min. (**B**) EPO (0.5, 1.0, and 2.0 mg) administration resulted in a non-dose-related increase in Rrs occurring immediately and resolving by 60 min. (Figure has been modified and is used with permission from Gundel RH, Letts LG, Gleich GJ. J Clin Invest 1991;87:1470–1473, copyright permission of The Rockefeller University Press) (70).

**Table 2** Effects of Eosinophil Granule Proteins on Airway Responsiveness

| Substance | Dose (mg) | Change in log methacholine $PC_{100}$ (mean ± SD) |
|---|---|---|
| MBP | 0.5 | -0.39 ± 0.13[a] |
| | 1.0 | -1.02 ± 0.36[a] |
| ECP | 0.5 | 0.18 ± 0.49 |
| | 1.0 | 0.37 ± 0.17 |
| EPO | 0.5 | -0.03 ± 0.27 |
| | 1.0 | -0.15 ± 0.21 |
| | 2.0 | -0.09 ± 0.20 |
| EPO + $H_2O_2$ + KI[b] | 1.0 | -0.18 ± 0.14 |
| EDN | 1.0 | 0.04 ± 0.06 |
| Buffer | | 0.02 ± 0.08 |

[a] $p < 0.05$, n = 5.
[b] $H_2O_2$ ($2 \times 10^{-5}$ mol/L), KI ($10^{-4}$ mol/L).
*Source*: table used with permission of Gundel RH, Letts LG, Gleich GJ. J Clin Invest 1991; 87:1470–1473, copyright permission of The Rockefeller University Press (70).

on the pathogenesis of airway responsiveness and that this may involve interaction with resident airway tissue cells (70).

The effects of eosinophil granule proteins on airway responsiveness have also been analyzed in rodents, with particular attention to the role of MBP. In

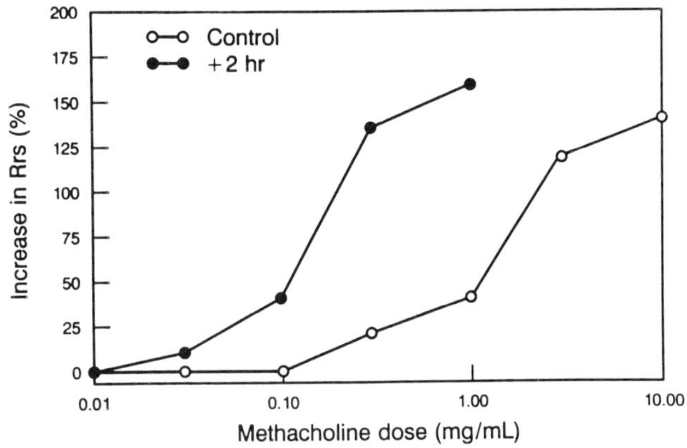


**Figure 3** Methacholine concentration response curve from an adult male cynomolgus monkey that received an intratracheal instillation of 1.0 mg MBP. The open circles show the responses to column buffer and the closed circles show the responses to 1.0 mg MBP after 2 hr. The administration of column buffer had no effect on airway responsiveness. Rrs is as defined in Figure 2. (Figure has been modified and is used with permission from Gundel RH, Letts LG, Gleich GJ. J Clin Invest 1991;87:1470–1473, copyright permission of The Rockefeller University Press) (70).

a rat model, cationic proteins were directly instilled into the trachea and the response to inhaled methacholine was determined (71). MBP caused a marked immediate increase in airway responsiveness to methacholine, and this subsided within 48 hr. Poly-L-arginine and poly-L-lysine also increased methacholine sensitivity; acetylation of the charged groups on poly-L-lysine abolished this effect. Histologic examination of the airway failed to reveal epithelial shedding 1 hr after polycation or MBP instillation. These results indicate that airway MBP instillation causes a short-lived increase in airway responsiveness, that the high density of surface cationic charge of MBP may be responsible for this effect, and that airway epithelial shedding is not a necessary requirement for the MBP effect. Subsequently the effect of a series of cationic proteins was investigated, including MBP, platelet factor 4 (PF4), poly-L-lysine, and cathepsin G (72). All of these molecules stimulated a two- to threefold increase in airway responsiveness 1 hr after administration; heparin inhibited the effects of the cationic proteins on bronchial hyperreactivity.

The mechanism of the MBP effect was studied further, using poly-L-lysine as the agonist (73). Instillation of poly-L-lysine caused a fivefold increase in airway responsiveness, and this was inhibited by neonatal capsaicin treatment and potentiated by phosphoramidon. Pretreatment of the animals with a selective NK-1 receptor antagonist inhibited the poly-L-lysine-induced airway responsiveness and plasma protein extravasation. Thus cationic proteins likely activate C fibers in the airways, and there may be a link between inflammatory cell accumulation and sensory nerve activation. Another analysis of the effect of MBP and synthetic polycations on the induction of airway responsiveness has pointed to the conclusion that bradykinin generation is critical (74). In these experiments, BAL was performed after intratracheal administration of MBP or poly-L-lysine, and the levels of kinin and kallikrein-like activity were determined. MBP and poly-L-lysine induced three- and eightfold increases in the levels of kallikrein-like activity and immunoreactive kinins, respectively. Analyses of dose response curves to methacholine before and after MBP or poly-L-lysine administration showed increases in airway responsiveness; these increases were inhibited by pretreatment with a selective bradykinin-2 receptor antagonist (NPC 17713). Therefore MBP and poly-L-lysine may activate kallikrein and thereby stimulate the generation of immunoreactive kinins in vivo. Furthermore, this effect is related to the cationic charge of these proteins. Thus these results suggest that MBP instillation causes an increase in airway responsiveness and that this is due to the generation of kinin activity. These results are interesting and provocative. It would be of interest to know whether the charge effect seen in the rat model of bronchial hyperreactivity is also present in the cynomolgus monkey model; the results in Table 2 suggest that charge is not critical in the primate model. It would also be interesting to know whether ECP and EPO are active in the rat model of hyperreactivity; one would predict that these are active. If so, the result would distinguish the primate from the rat model and identify two mechanisms for induction of hyperreactivity.

## V. In Vitro Models of Bronchial Hyperreactivity

To explore the mechanism by which eosinophil granule proteins alter bronchial hyperreactivity, an in vitro model would be most useful. Therefore experiments have been conducted exploring the ability of eosinophil granule proteins to cause hyperreactivity of respiratory smooth muscle in vitro (75). Rings of guinea pig trachea, some with the epithelium gently removed by rubbing, were incubated with buffer or with MBP. The tracheal rings were then analyzed for their reactivity to acetylcholine and histamine. MBP did not affect the reactivity of rings where epithelium had been removed, but it significantly augmented the reactivity of rings (with intact epithelium) to acetylcholine and histamine. Thus MBP likely interacted with the epithelium and indirectly caused increased reactivity in respiratory smooth muscle (75). Next a series of experiments using an in vivo in situ tracheal preparation from which epithelium could be excised explored the effects of MBP on hyperreactivity in the presence and absence of respiratory epithelium. The first experiments in dogs showed that the response to intra-arterial acetylcholine was substantially augmented in animals receiving MBP by intraepithelial instillation (76). In contrast, MBP instillation directly into the subepithelial tracheal smooth muscle did not alter contractility. When performed in guinea pigs, these same experiments using direct application of MBP to the respiratory epithelium showed active force generation within 1 min of contact (77). Denatured MBP (by boiling) did not elicit active tension. MBP also augmented contraction to intravenous acetylcholine. Thus MBP likely causes direct contraction of airway smooth muscle in an epithelial-dependent manner with an increase in responsiveness to acetylcholine (presumably analogous to bronchial hyperreactivity). Lastly, the ability of MBP to cause contraction of guinea pig trachealis muscle is blocked by atropine, whereas the ability of polylysine or polyarginine to cause contraction of guinea pig trachealis muscle is not affected by atropine (78). In contrast, tracheal smooth muscle contraction elicited by MBP or polylysine is inhibited by pretreatment with indomethacin. Thus MBP-induced muscle contraction is likely mediated through both stimulation of the parasympathetic nervous system (because it is inhibited by atropine) and by secretion of a product of the cyclooxygenase pathway (because it is blocked by indomethachin), while neither polylysine nor polyarginine causes tracheal smooth muscle contraction via the parasympathetic nervous system. The finding that indomethacin inhibits MBP-induced muscle contraction is in keeping with prior observations that MBP stimulates prostaglandin $E_2$ ($PGE_2$) and $PGF_{2\alpha}$ secretion from tracheal epithelial cells (79). In turn, these findings distinguish different pathways to influence muscles in which charge effects are important, but are not solely responsible for the MBP effect on tracheal smooth muscle in the guinea pig (78).

## VI. Eosinophil Granule Proteins and Vagal Function

### A. Evidence for Decreased Lung M2 Muscarinic Receptor Function in Sensitized Animals

The possibility that increased reactivity of the vagus nerve is involved in the pathophysiology of asthma has long been suspected. Recently a series of experiments have directed attention to increased vagal responsiveness in a guinea pig model of asthma, and findings in patients suggest that this also happens in disease. For example, antigen inhalation in guinea pigs is associated with increased release of acetylcholine from the vagus nerve (80). In the lung, acetylcholine from the vagus nerve is under control of inhibitory receptors on postganglionic nerves (81). Inhibitory muscarinic receptors are classified as M2 receptors, whereas the stimulatory muscarinic receptors on airway smooth muscle are classified as M3 receptors (82). As shown in Figure 4, acetylcholine released from the vagus nerve stimulates both muscarinic M3 receptors on airway smooth muscle, causing contraction, and muscarinic M2 receptors on nerves, decreasing further release of acetylcholine. The negative feedback control of acetylcholine on M2 receptors can be blocked by gallamine, which potentiates vagal-induced bronchoconstriction as much as tenfold (83). In an opposite manner, pilocarpine stimulates M2 receptors and decreases vagally induced bronchospasm (81). Investigations of vagal function following antigen challenge of sensitized animals, including guinea pigs and mice, have shown that the function of the M2 inhibitory receptors is impaired (83–85). Of interest is the prior

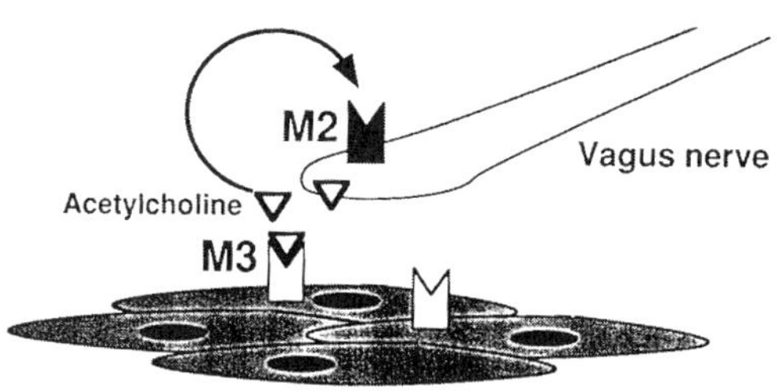


**Figure 4** In the airways, release of acetylcholine from the vagus nerve contracts smooth muscle by stimulating muscarinic M3 receptors. At the same time, the acetylcholine feeds back onto inhibitory muscarinic M2 receptors on the nerve endings and thereby limits further release of acetylcholine. (Used with permission from Jacoby DB, Gleich GJ, Fryer AD. J Clin Invest 1993;91:1314–1318, copyright permission of The Rockefeller University Press) (89).

finding that positively charged molecules, such as polyarginine, polylysine, basic histones, and protamine, are antagonists for the M2 receptor (86). Therefore the possibility that, as a consequence of antigen challenge, positively charged eosinophil granule proteins, such as MBP, could be released and then block M2 receptor function was considered. Knowledge that negatively charged substances, such as heparin and polyglutamate, are able to neutralize the effect of MBP (52,87,88) suggested a test of this hypothesis. Therefore guinea pigs were anesthetized, tracheotomized, vagotomized, paralyzed, and ventilated (84). Stimulation of the vagus nerve of these animals caused bronchospasm and bradycardia; in control animals, pilocarpine attenuated vagally induced bronchospasm by stimulating neuronal M2 muscarinic receptors and gallamine potentiated vagally stimulated bronchospasm by blocking M2 receptors. In contrast, in the sensitized and challenged animals, the effects of both drugs were markedly reduced in keeping with the hypothesis that the M2 receptor function is impaired. Administration of heparin or polyglutamic acid intravenously restored the effects of both pilocarpine and gallamine on vagally induced bronchospasm, indicating a recovery of M2 receptor function.

Therefore these experiments suggested that a polycationic substance, such as MBP, EPO, or ECP, might be responsible for the antigen-induced pulmonary M2 receptor dysfunction. A direct test of this hypothesis was conducted by analyzing the ability of purified eosinophil granule proteins to bind to M2 and M3 receptors (89). MBP inhibited the binding of N-[$^3$H]methylscopolamine to M2 but not to M3 receptors; MBP also inhibited the atropine-induced dissociation of the N-[$^3$H]methylscopolamine receptor complex in a dose-dependent fashion, showing that interaction of MBP with the M2 receptor is allosteric. Thus MBP likely functions as an endogenous allosteric inhibitor of agonist binding to the M2 muscarinic receptor.

Subsequently, treatment with an antibody to interleukin-5 (IL-5) was employed to inhibit tissue eosinophilia and thus determine whether eosinophils are critical for production of the M2 muscarinic receptor blockade (90). Pretreatment of guinea pigs with the monoclonal antibody to IL-5—TRFK-5—prevented the loss of the muscarinic M2 receptor function induced by sensitization and challenge. Furthermore, treatment with TRFK-5 selectively inhibited the migration of eosinophils into the lungs, as measured by lung lavage. Thus IL-5 appears to be a key molecule in the pulmonary eosinophil infiltration in sensitized and antigen-challenged guinea pigs.

The adhesion molecules critical for eosinophil infiltration in the sensitized and challenged guinea pigs have also been investigated. Prior experiments showed that antibody to VLA-4 blocks eosinophil infiltration, eosinophil degranulation, and the development of bronchial hyperreactivity (91). Similarly, antibody to VLA-4 also protected M2 muscarinic receptor function in the antigen-challenged animals; in confirmation of prior results, the antibody inhibited development of hyperresponsiveness and selectively inhibited eosinophil accumulation into the lung (92). In contrast, antibody to L-selectin had no effect on the increased infiltration into the lungs, the development of bronchial hyperresponsiveness, or M2 receptor function.

Considerable evidence suggests that the mere presence of eosinophils in the lung is not critical for the development of bronchial hyperresponsiveness, but rather their degranulation (53,66,69,70). Tests of the requirement for eosinophil degranulation in animal models have shown that it is associated with the development of bronchial hyperreactivity (69,70,91), and the intensity of the bronchial response to methacholine is correlated with the levels of eosinophil granule proteins in BAL fluids (93). Moreover, antibody to MBP blocks the development of bronchial hyperreactivity (94) and protects the M2 muscarinic receptor (95).

Finally, eosinophils localize to airway nerves (90,92,96) in the guinea pig asthma model, and densities of eosinophils around nerves are greater than around normal blood vessels or in the airway wall (96). Preliminary analysis of tissue from patients dying of asthma also showed an association of eosinophils with nerves and release of MBP in the vicinity of nerves (96). Altogether, these observations suggest that bronchial hyperreactivity in the guinea pig model of asthma is due to eosinophil degranulation with MBP deposition onto M2 receptors. Two tests of this model in man have shown results in keeping with the hypothesis (97,98). Clearly, additional clinical investigation of this point is required.

## VII. Effect of Eosinophil Granule Proteins on Other Cells Relevant to Asthma

### A. Effects on Basophils and Mast Cells

Basophils, mast cells, and eosinophils have been implicated in the pathophysiology of bronchial asthma. Because eosinophil granule proteins are elevated in sputa from patients with asthma (see below), the hypothesis that the granule proteins might activate basophils was tested (19). Incubation of blood cells enriched for basophils with MBP produced a dose-related increase in histamine release, which reached a maximum in 1 hr and was calcium, energy, and temperature dependent (19). Purified peritoneal rat mast cells behaved in a similar manner, although, in this case, histamine release was largely complete in 1 min (20). Thus MBP causes a noncytolytic histamine release from leukocytes, and it can activate both mast cells and basophils. Subsequently the other eosinophil granule proteins were tested for their capacity to activate human basophils and rat mast cells and cause histamine release. With basophils, only MBP caused leukocyte histamine release, whereas with rat peritoneal mast cells, both MBP and ECP were active (20). Analysis of responsiveness of leukocytes from individual selected donors revealed a considerable range of MBP responsiveness from baseline levels of approximately 5% histamine release to over 50% histamine release (99). Although it is known that the leukocytes of atopic individuals are often activated, it was not possible to distinguish leukocytes of atopic individuals from normal individuals in their response to MBP. As noted above, the MBP-stimulated histamine release from basophils was calcium, energy, and temperature dependent (19); it was blocked by both a calmodulin antagonist and by theophylline and partially blocked by an inhibitor of phospholipase $A_2$ (100). The MBP-stimulated histamine release was unaffected by inhibition of protein kinase C, whereas pretreatment with pertussis toxin caused a concentration-dependent inhibition of histamine release. More recently the ability of eosinophil granule proteins to alter histamine release from human mast cells has been tested. Analysis of the ability of eosinophil granule proteins to release histamine from human skin mast cells indicated that the four cationic proteins did not induce histamine release over a concentration range of 10 to 200 μg/ml (101). Further, they did not promote anti-IgE-induced histamine release from human skin mast cells significantly over the same concentration range. Curiously, however, incubation of MBP and EPO with the mast cells significantly inhibited histamine release induced by substance P and by compound 48/80™. Similarly, eosinophil granule proteins did not induce histamine release from human lung mast cells (L. M. Lichtenstein, unpublished observations). In contrast, analysis of the effects of the four eosinophil granule proteins on human heart mast cells indicated that ECP, and to a lesser extent MBP, but not EDN or EPO, stimulated the release of preformed mediators, including histamine and tryptase, and the de novo synthesis of vasoactive and proinflammatory mediators, such as PGD2, from human heart mast cells. Activation of the heart mast cells by ECP and MBP was calcium and temperature-dependent and was abolished by preincubation with 2-deoxy-D-glucose and antimycin A (102).

The possible interaction of cytokines and MBP in the release of mediators by basophils has been investigated (103). Preincubation of mononuclear cells containing basophils with IL-3 or IL-5 caused a concentration-dependent enhancement of MBP-dependent histamine release. Likewise, preincubation with granulocyte macrophage colony-stimulating factor (GM-CSF) also enhanced MBP-induced histamine release. Incubation with cytokines reduced the threshold MBP concentrations needed for histamine release and also enhanced the rate of histamine release. Using purified basophils, 84 to 99% pure, MBP stimulated low levels of leukotriene (LT)$C_4$ release; this $LTC_4$ release was enhanced by preincubation with IL-3, IL-5, and GM-CSF. Thus IL-3, IL-5, and GM-CSF may contribute to the pathogenesis of allergic and other disorders characterized by eosinophilia, not only by stimulating eosinophil proliferation and activating eosinophils, but also by potentiating basophil mediator release stimulated by MBP (103).

Mast cell granules bind EPO, and the resulting granule-EPO complexes catalyze the iodination of proteins during killing of microorganisms (104). EPO/$H_2O_2/I^-$ also induces rat mast cell degranulation and histamine release (105). The EPO/$H_2O_2/I^-$ system was noncytotoxic at low EPO concentrations, but at higher concentrations ultrastructural analysis showed damaged mast cells. Interestingly the EPO-mast cell granule complex was more effective than free EPO for stimulating mast cell secretion.

### B. Effects on Neutrophils

Eosinophils and neutrophils are commonly present in certain allergic reactions, particularly late-phase reactions in skin (106). Therefore the ability of MBP to activate neutrophils was tested (21). Neutrophils incubated with MBP produced concentration-dependent chemiluminescence that peaked after 50 to 70 min, whereas ECP and EDN did not. This MBP chemiluminescence was calcium dependent and was absent in neutrophils from two individuals with chronic granulomatous disease. MBP also stimulated the release of superoxide anion and lysozyme, but not the release of β-glucuronidase or lactate dehydrogenase. In addition, MBP and platelet activating factor (PAF) synergistically induced superoxide release. Thus MBP activates neutrophils in a noncytolytic manner, and an interaction between eosinophils and neutrophils seems likely, particularly in allergic late-phase reactions.

Subsequently the activities of MBP on basophils and neutrophils were compared. MBP activated both cell types with many common characteristics, but these cells differed in their calcium signaling and sensitivity to priming by cytokines (107). In neutrophils, the MBP-induced superoxide anion release was independent of calcium elevation and was not enhanced by exposure to GM-CSF. In contrast, in basophils calcium elevation appeared to be essential for MBP activation. Furthermore, as noted previously, in basophils mediator release stimulated by MBP is enhanced by IL-3, IL-5, and GM-CSF (103).

### C. Effects on Platelets

Platelets are associated with bronchial asthma and therefore could be stimulated by eosinophil granule proteins (108,109). When the eosinophil granule proteins were incubated with unstirred purified platelets, MBP and EPO induced a concentration-dependent nonlytic secretion of platelet 5-hydroxytryptamine even in the presence of indomethacin (22). MBP also caused secretion of platelet-α granule and lysosome components. $PGE_1$ inhibited the platelet secretion caused by MBP and EPO, but the characteristics of the inhibition differed from those of thrombin. Because EPO promoted secretion in the absence of $H_2O_2$ and in the presence of sufficient catalase to degrade any endogenously produced $H_2O_2$, EPO-mediated secretion was not due to its enzymatic activity. Furthermore, although heparin has no effect on the catalytic activity of EPO, it did inhibit EPO-dependent secretion, probably by binding to EPO. Therefore MBP and EPO can likely be classified as strong platelet active agonists with distinctive mechanisms. These results contrast with earlier reports where the EPO-mediated mast cell secretion absolutely depended on the enzymatic activity of EPO and required exogenously added $H_2O_2$ and halide (105).

### D. Effects on Mucous Secreting Cells

A prominent feature of an asthma attack is hypersecretion of mucus from the airway mucosa. The effect of eosinophil granule proteins on mucous secretion has been tested; eosinophil lysates and crude eosinophil granule extracts caused concentration-dependent release of respiratory glycoconjugates from cultured feline tracheal explants (110). Purified MBP, ECP, and EDN also were tested, and ECP increased respiratory glycoconjugates from both feline and human airway explants and stimulated the release of the serous cell marker lactoferrin from human bronchial explants. EDN failed to affect respiratory glycoconjugate release, whereas MBP inhibited release from feline explants. Thus ECP stimulates mucous and lactoferrin release, while MBP inhibits mucous release.

### E. Effects on Eosinophils

Because eosinophils are bathed by their granule proteins during the course of degranulation, the effects of the granule proteins on eosinophils themselves have been tested. Both MBP and EPO at concentrations easily achieved in vivo induce eosinophil degranulation, as measured by release of EDN; in contrast, ECP was inactive (111). The quantities of EDN stimulated by MBP and EPO were comparable to those released by one of the strongest agonists for eosinophils, secretory IgA (sIgA). Degranulation of eosinophils induced by MBP was only partially dependent on calcium, and no elevation of intracellular calcium concentration was observed in MBP-stimulated eosinophils. Interestingly, MBP stimulated the production of IL-8 by eosinophils, up to eightfold, in a concentration-dependent manner; the eosinophils' expression of IL-8 mRNA was confirmed by the reverse transcription polymerase chain reaction (111). These results suggest MBP and EPO act as autocrine mediators in the pathophysiology of eosinophil-associated diseases, especially bronchial asthma, by creating a vicious cycle of eosinophil infiltration, eosinophil degranulation, and continued eosinophil activation.

### F. Effects on Lung Macrophages

Because pulmonary secretions from patients with asthma contain MBP, the effects of MBP on superoxide anion release from alveolar macrophages were tested

(23). Guinea pig alveolar macrophages were harvested, incubated with MBP, and stimulated by phorbol myristate acetate (PMA); the immediate release of superoxide from these macrophages was reduced. Similarly, in macrophages incubated with MBP for 48 hr, PMA-induced superoxide anion release was also reduced. While the immediate decrease in superoxide anion release was not caused by cytotoxic effects, at 48 hr the decrease was due to a direct toxic effect of MBP on the alveolar macrophages. Thus MBP can likely adversely affect macrophage function, and the cytotoxic effects of MBP are partly responsible. These effects may be relevant to the pathophysiology of asthma because the alveolar macrophage is likely responsible for ingestion of both apoptotic cells and eosinophil granule proteins and for their orderly degradation. Interference by eosinophils with the degradation processes of macrophages would presumably increase the intensity of eosinophil-associated inflammation (112).

## VIII. Evidence for Involvement of Eosinophils and Their Granule Proteins in the Pathophysiology of Bronchial Asthma

The information listed above indicates that eosinophil granule proteins have potent activities on a variety of cells by activating or inhibiting cell functions. Furthermore, many of these actions are relevant to bronchial asthma. Experimental results illustrating eosinophil degranulation in human asthma and in experimental models of asthma are summarized below.

### A. The Pathology of Asthma

The in vitro findings that eosinophil granule proteins cause ciliostasis and desquamation of respiratory epithelium were impressive because these abnormalities are very similar to the pathological changes observed in bronchial asthma. In bronchial asthma, an exudate of eosinophils, normal and degenerating bronchial epithelial cells, Creola bodies, and Charcot-Leyden crystals are present in the bronchial lumen (3,4,113–127). The Creola body is a cluster of cells found in the sputa from patients with asthma and is believed to be derived by desquamation from bronchial epithelium (121,122). An example of a Creola body is shown in Figure 5, which also shows evidence of desquamated epithelial cells and Charcot-Leyden crystals in sputum. In the bronchial mucosa and submucosa, edema, separation, and shedding of ciliated cells and eosinophil infiltration are present. In the subepithelial region, thickening of the basement membrane and eosinophil infiltration, enlargement of the glands, and smooth muscle hypertrophy are present. Many of these same findings have recently been confirmed by

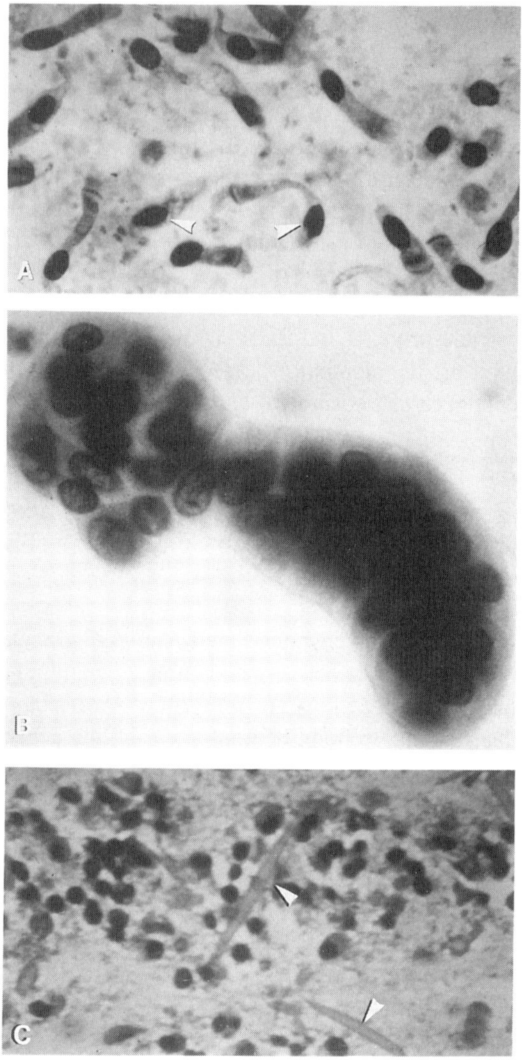

**Figure 5** Sputum samples from patients with asthma. (**A**) Elongated ciliated cells (arrowheads) desquamated from bronchial epithelium. When cells are viewed in a wet preparation, the cilia frequently are extremely motile, propelling themselves in a circular path (Papanicolaou stain; original magnification 300×). (**B**) Creola body, a compact cluster of epithelial cells shed from the bronchial epithelium (Papanicolaou stain) (reproduced with permission from Bernard Naylor, M.D.). (**C**) CLC (arrowheads) and eosinophils identified by their large refractile granules and bilobed nuclei (H&E; original magnification 400×). (Used with permission from Frigas E, Gleich GJ. J Allergy Clin Immunol 1986;77:527–537) (127).

biopsy specimens from patients with relatively mild asthma, either before or after antigen challenge.

### B. MBP Levels in Sputa from Patients with Bronchial Asthma

Because exposure of respiratory epithelium to MBP caused damage that mimicked the pathology of asthma, MBP levels in sputa from patients with asthma were measured to determine whether they are elevated and to what degree (53,128). Figure 6 shows the MBP levels in consecutive sputum samples from 206 patients with various respiratory diseases. These samples were sputum samples sent for microbiological assay and were screened to exclude samples containing saliva (as judged by the number of squamous epithelial cells). In 165 patients without measurable MBP or with concentrations of sputum MBP of less than 0.1 μg/ml (Figure 6, groups A and B), only one patient was diagnosed by the attending physicians as having asthma. Among 41 patients with sputum concentrations of MBP of greater than 0.1 μg/ml (Figure 6, group C), 28 had asthma. In the remaining 13 patients, the diagnoses were bronchopneumonia in seven, pulmonary neoplasm in three, acute bronchitis in two, and lympocytic leukemia in one. Six of the 13 had had previous diagnoses of chronic obstructive lung disease. The MBP geometric mean concentrations for the 28 patients with asthma differed significantly from patients without a diagnosis ($p < 0.001$) (Figure 6). These results show that an increased sputum concentration of MBP is a useful marker for asthma.

The association between increased sputum MBP levels and asthma prompted analysis of the levels of MBP in 15 consecutive patients hospitalized for treatment of acute exacerbations of asthma (53,128). Figure 7 shows that the hospitalized patients with asthma had significantly ($p < 0.001$) increased sputum MBP concentrations compared to the outpatients with asthma, suggesting that during an acute attack of asthma, the sputum MBP increases. Note that 7 of the 25 hospitalized patients with asthma had MBP sputum levels of less than 10 μg/ml ($1.1 \times 10^{-6}$ M), the lowest MBP level found toxic to respiratory epithelium in vitro (52). After treatment the patients' sputum MBP concentrations decreased significantly ($p < 0.005$) from admission to release.

More recently sputum MBP has been measured in patients with asthma using sputum induction by hypertonic saline (129). In this study, not only total eosinophils and MBP in the sputum but also ECP, EDN, fibrinogen, and tryptase were analyzed. Sputum induction provides samples, which are reproducible, both in terms of the numbers of eosinophils present in the sample and the levels of inflammatory mediators. As expected, patients with asthma had a higher proportion of sputum eosinophils and elevated levels of ECP, MBP, and EDN when compared to healthy subjects and smokers with bronchitis. The proportion of sputum eosinophils correlated positively with sputum levels of ECP, MBP, EDN,

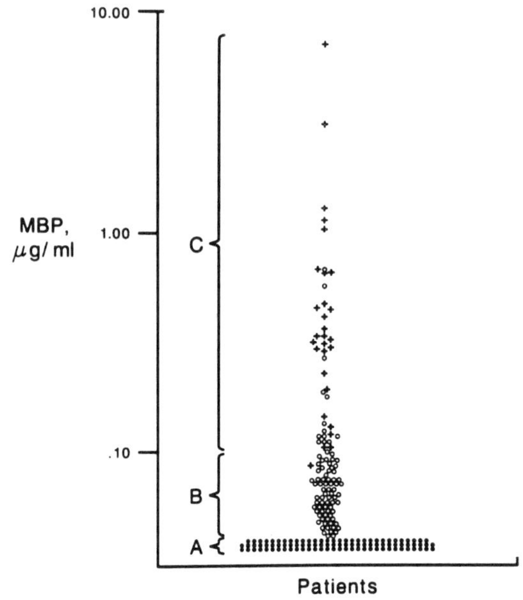


**Figure 6** Sputum MBP levels in 206 patients with various respiratory diseases including asthma. Each symbol represents one patient. The crosses identify the patients with asthma; patients without measurable MBP and without asthma (●); patients with measurable MBP but without asthma (○). (Used with permission from Frigas E, Gleich GJ. J Allergy Clin Immunol 1986;77:527–537) (127).

albumin, and fibrinogen levels. Interestingly, in the asthma patients, IL-5 correlated with eosinophil counts. Furthermore, there was a significant negative correlation between the sputum indices and the expiratory flows in methacholine $PC_{20}$. Thus this study showed that methods for measuring cell and fluid phase markers of induced sputum are reproducible and that they reflect reliably the severity of airway inflammation. These studies also validate the prior observations of sputum made in the early 1980s (53,128).

### C. MBP Localization in Lung Tissues of Patients with Bronchial Asthma

The findings that levels of MBP and other eosinophil granule proteins are elevated in sputum stimulated efforts to localize these molecules in the lungs of patients with asthma. We developed an immunofluorescent procedure for analysis of formalin-fixed, paraffin-embedded tissues to study lung tissues from patients who died of asthma and from control patients who died of other causes (130).

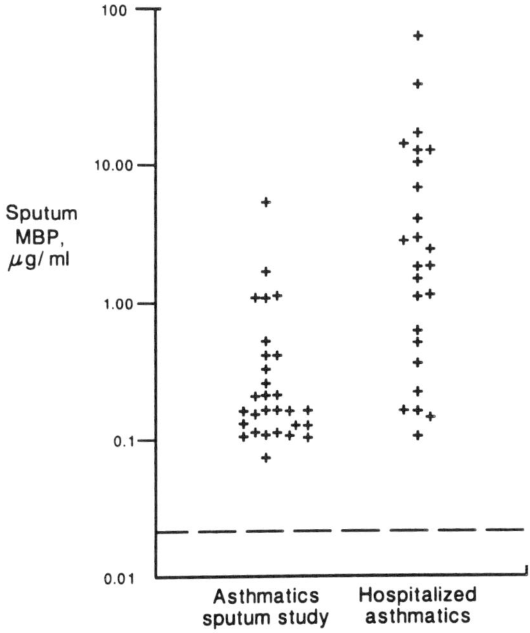


**Figure 7** Sputum MBP levels from outpatients with asthma (Figure 6) and hospitalized patients with an acute flare of asthma. Each cross represents one patient. Dashed line designates the limit of sensitivity of the RIA for sputum MBP. (Used with permission from Frigas E, Gleich GJ. J Allergy Clin Immunol 1986;77:527–537) (127).

Lung tissue samples from 22 autopsy cases at the Mayo Clinic between 1967 and 1979 were studied. Examination of sections stained with hematoxylin and eosin (H&E) demonstrated that all patients with asthma had a thickened basement membrane zone, goblet cell hyperplasia, and peribronchial inflammatory infiltrates with eosinophils in the submucosa. Examination of the same sections by immunofluorescence demonstrated MBP staining that was cell associated, as well as outside of cells (extracellular staining). Some eosinophils were intact, whereas others were partially degranulated and surrounded by their extruded granules, and still others were totally disrupted and unrecognizable by H&E stain. Patients whose deaths were not due to asthma demonstrated neither epithelial damage nor extracellular MBP immunofluorescence; intact eosinophils, as judged by the occurrence of intracellular MBP, were noted. Figures 8 and 9 show examples of patterns of MBP deposition in patients whose deaths were due to asthma. Figure 8 shows diffuse staining of a mucous plug with streaks and whorls of brilliant fluorescence, as well as staining of the epithelial surface of this bronchiole in a patchy, scalloped manner. Figure 9 shows diffuse extra-

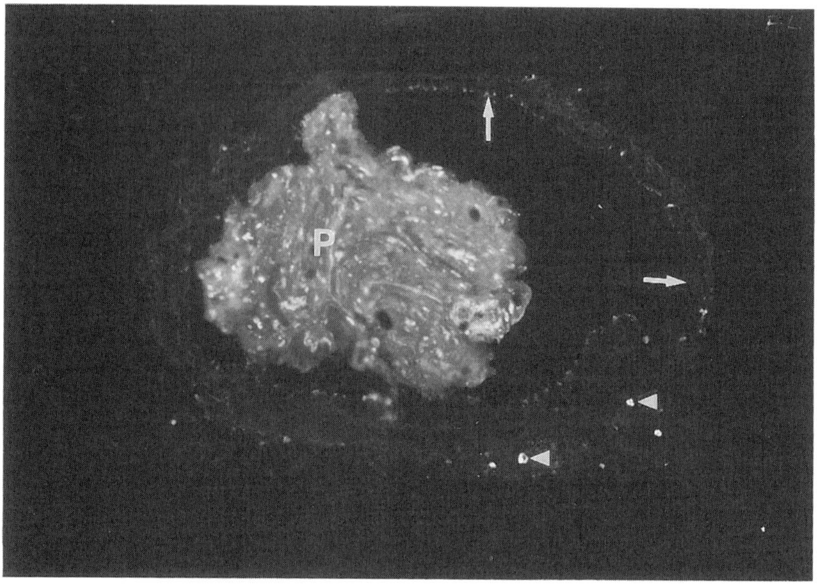


**Figure 8** Section of bronchiole from a patient with asthma stained with anti-MBP. Note the diffuse staining of the mucous plug (P) with brilliant swirls and the patchy, scalloped, less intense staining of the luminal surface of the respiratory epithelium (arrows). There are also discrete eosinophils in the peribronchiolar area (arrowheads) (original magnification 100×). (Used with permission from Filley WV, Holley KE, Kephart GM, Gleich GJ. Lancet 1982;2:11–16, copyright permission the Lancet Ltd.) (130).

cellular MBP fluorescence in the submucosa corresponding to the presence of necrotic, amorphous, eosinophilic material on the H&E stained section.

## IX. Summary and Conclusions

Information relating to eosinophil granule proteins with particular reference to their characteristics and properties, as well as their activities in bronchial asthma, has been reviewed. In addition, information supporting a role for these molecules in bronchial asthma has been summarized. Overall these findings strongly support a role for eosinophils in the pathophysiology of bronchial asthma. Furthermore, recent investigations have studied the predominant cytokine controlling eosinophil development, namely IL-5, in the pathophysiology of asthma. These studies have shown that anti-IL-5 causes a loss of eosinophils from the

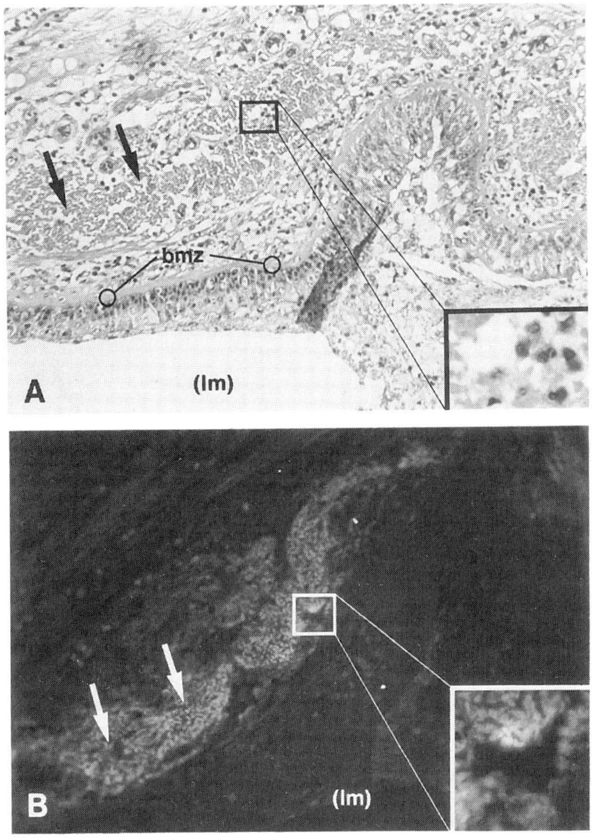


**Figure 9** Section of a bronchus from a patient with asthma. (**A**) Light microscopy reveals inflammatory cell infiltrate in the lamina propria with large patches of amorphous necrotic eosinophilic material (arrows) and a thick hyaline layer below the basement membrane (bmz); lm, bronchial lumen (H&E; original magnification 100× and 400×). (**B**) Immunofluorescence staining for MBP. Areas below the basement membrane in the lamina propria stain intensely for extracellular MBP. Although some discrete eosinophils could be observed with H&E (insert A), the entire area was diffusely positive when area was stained with anti-MBP (insert B) (original magnification 100× and 400×). (Modified and reproduced with permission from Filley WV, Holley KE, Kephart GM, Gleich GJ. Lancet 1982;2:11–16, copyright the Lancet Ltd.) (130).

lung in animals in keeping with the hypothesis that IL-5 is a major determinant of eosinophil inflammation (131–137). Figure 10 summarizes the eosinophil hypothesis and shows schematically how the eosinophil might alter lung tissue; present findings support this hypothesis. Once therapies are available to spe-

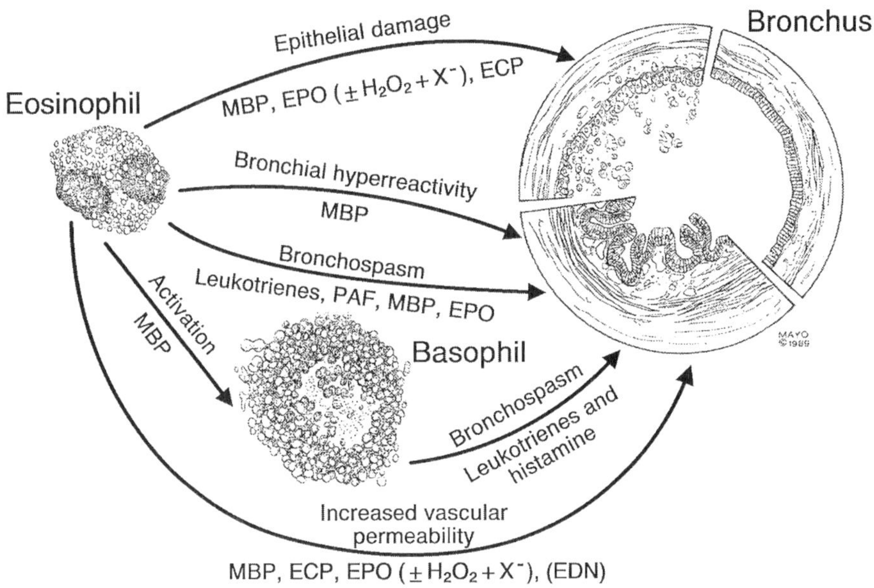


**Figure 10** Schematic summary of the proposed role of eosinophils in bronchial asthma. The effects on the bronchus are shown by comparing a section of normal bronchus (top right) with a portion damaged by MBP, EPO, or ECP (top left) showing epithelial desquamation with a section (bottom) showing smooth muscle hypertrophy, constriction, and edema of the lamina propria, resulting in a reduction in the caliber of the airway.

cifically block IL-5 activity in patients, we will be able to test the eosinophil hypothesis in patients with asthma.

## References

1. Gleich GJ. The eosinophilic leukocyte: past, present and future. In: Makino S, Fukuda T, eds. Eosinophils: Biological and Clinical Aspects. Boca Raton: CRC Press, 1993:1–10.
2. Gollasch. Zur kenntniss dur asthmatischen sputums. Fortschr Med (Berlin) 1889;7:361–365.
3. Ellis AG. The pathological anatomy of bronchial asthma. Am J Med Sci 1908;136:407–429.
4. Huber HL, Koessler KK. The pathology of bronchial asthma. Arch Intern Med 1922;30:687–760.
5. Schlecht H, Schwenker G. Über lokale eosinophilie in den bronchien und in der lunge anaphylaktischen meerschweinchen. Arch Exp Pathol Pharmakol 1912;68:163–170.

6. Gleich GJ, Loegering DA, Maldonado JE. Identification of a major basic protein in guinea pig eosinophil granules. J Exp Med 1973;137:1459–1471.
7. Gleich GJ, Loegering DA, Mann KG, Maldonado JE. Comparative properties of the Charcot-Leyden crystal protein and the major basic protein from human eosinophils. J Clin Invest 1976;57:633–640.
8. Lewis DM, Loegering DA, Gleich GJ. Isolation and partial characterization of a major basic protein from rat eosinophil granules. Proc Soc Exp Biol Med 1976;152:512–515.
9. Larson KA, Horton MA, Madden BJ, Gleich GJ, Lee NA, Lee JJ. The identification and cloning of a murine major basic protein gene expressed in eosinophils. J Immunol 1995;155:3002–3012.
10. Gleich GJ, Kita H, Adolphson CR. Eosinophils. In: Frank MM, Austen KF, Claman HN, Unanue ER, eds. Samter's Immunologic Diseases. Boston: Little, Brown, 1994:205–245.
11. Gleich GJ, Loegering DA, Kueppers F, Bajaj SP, Mann KG. Physiochemical and biological properties of the major basic protein from guinea pig eosinophil granules. J Exp Med 1974;140:313–332.
12. Wasmoen TL, Bell MP, Loegering DA, Gleich GJ, Prendergast FG, McKean DJ. Biochemical and amino acid sequence analysis of human eosinophil granule major basic protein. J Biol Chem 1988;263:12559–12563.
13. Barker RL, Loegering DA, Arakawa KC, Pease LR, Gleich GJ. Cloning and sequence analysis of the human gene encoding eosinophil major basic protein. Gene 1990;86:285–289.
14. McGrogan M, Simonsen C, Scott R, Griffith J, Ellis N, Kennedy J, Campanelli D, Nathan C, Gabay J. Isolation of a complementary DNA clone encoding a precursor to human eosinophil major basic protein. J Exp Med 1988;168:2295–2308.
15. Aoki I, Shindoh Y, Nishida T, Nakai S, Hong YM, Mio M, Saito T, Tasaka K. Comparison of the amino acid and nucleotide sequences between human and two guinea pig major basic proteins. FEBS Lett 1991;282:56–60.
16. Aoki I, Shindoh Y, Nishida T, Nakai S, Hong YM, Mio M, Saito T, Tasaka K. Sequencing and cloning of the cDNA of guinea pig eosinophil major basic protein. FEBS Lett 1991;279:330–334.
17. Maddox DE, Butterfield JH, Ackerman SJ, Coulam CB, Gleich GJ. Elevated serum levels in human pregnancy of a molecule immunochemically similar to eosinophil granule major basic protein. J Exp Med 1983;158:1211–1226.
18. Oxvig C, Sand O, Kristensen T, Gleich GJ, Sottrup-Jensen L. Circulating human pregnancy-associated plasma protein-A is disulfide-bridged to the proform of eosinophil major basic protein. J Biol Chem 1993;268:12243–12246.
19. O'Donnell MC, Ackerman SJ, Gleich GJ, Thomas LL. Activation of basophil and mast cell histamine release by eosinophil granule major basic protein. J Exp Med 1983;157:1981–1991.
20. Zheutlin LM, Ackerman SJ, Gleich GJ, Thomas LL. Stimulation of basophil and rat mast cell histamine release by eosinophil granule-derived cationic proteins. J Immunol 1984;133:2180–2185.
21. Moy JN, Gleich GJ, Thomas LL. Noncytotoxic activation of neutrophils by eosin-

ophil granule major basic protein: effect on superoxide anion generation and lysosomal enzyme release. J Immunol 1990;145:2626–2632.
22. Rohrbach MS, Wheatley CL, Slifman NR, Gleich GJ. Activation of platelets by eosinophil granule proteins. J Exp Med 1990;172:1271–1274.
23. Rankin JA, Harris P, Ackerman SJ. The effects of eosinophil-granule major basic protein on lung-macrophage superoxide anion generation. J Allergy Clin Immunol 1992;89:746–752.
24. Venge P, Dahl R, Hallgren R, Olsson I. Cationic proteins of human eosinophils and their role in the inflammatory reaction. In: Mahmoud AAF, Austen KF, eds. The Eosinophil in Health and Disease. New York: Grune & Stratton, 1980:131–146.
25. Gleich GJ, Loegering DA, Bell MP, Checkel JL, Ackerman SJ, McKean DJ. Biochemical and functional similarities between human eosinophil-derived neurotoxin and eosinophil cationic protein: homology with ribonuclease. Proc Natl Acad Sci USA 1986:83:3146–3150.
26. Olsson I, Persson A-M, Winqvist I. Biochemical properties of the eosinophil cationic protein and demonstration of its biosynthesis in vitro in marrow cells from patients with an eosinophilia. Blood 1986;67:498–503.
27. Barker RL, Loegering DA, Ten RM, Hamann KJ, Pease LR, Gleich GJ. Eosinophil cationic protein cDNA. Comparison with other toxic cationic proteins and ribonucleases. J Immunol 1989;143:952–955.
28. Rosenberg HF, Ackerman SJ, Tenen DG. Human eosinophil cationic protein: molecular cloning of a cytotoxin and helminthotoxin with RNase activity. J Exp Med 1989;170:163–176.
29. Snyder MR, Gleich GJ. Eosinophil-associated ribonucleases. In: D'Alessio G, Riordan JF, eds. Ribonucleases: Structure and Function. New York: Academic Press, 1997:425–444.
30. Slifman NR, Loegering DA, McKean DJ, Gleich GJ. Ribonuclease activity associated with human eosinophil-derived neurotoxin and eosinophil cationic protein. J Immunol 1986;137:2913–2917.
31. Young JD-E, Peterson CG, Venge P, Cohn ZA. Mechanism of membrane damage mediated by human eosinophil cationic protein. Nature 1986;321:613–616.
32. Gordon MH. Remarks on Hodgkin's disease. A pathogenic agent in the glands, and its application in diagnosis. Br Med J 1933;1:641–644.
33. Durack DT, Ackerman SJ, Loegering DA, Gleich GJ. Purification of human eosinophil-derived neurotoxin. Proc Natl Acad Sci USA 1981;78:5165–5169.
34. Hamann KJ, Barker RL, Loegering DA, Pease LR, Gleich GJ. Sequence of human eosinophil-derived neurotoxin cDNA: identity of deduced amino acid sequence with human nonsecretory ribonucleases. Gene 1989;83:161–167.
35. Rosenberg HF, Tenen DG, Ackerman SJ. Molecular cloning of the human eosinophil-derived neurotoxin: a member of the RNase gene family. Proc Natl Acad Sci USA 1989;86:4460–4464.
36. Beintema JJ, Hofsteenge J, Iwama M, Morita T, Ohgi K, Irie M, Sugiyama RH, Schieven GL, Dekker CA, Glitz DG. Amino acid sequence of the nonsecretory ribonuclease of human urine. Biochemistry 1988;27:4530–4538.

37. Sorrentino S, Tucker GK, Glitz DG. Purification and characterization of a ribonuclease from human liver. J Biol Chem 1988;263:16125–16131.
38. Hamann KJ, Ten RM, Loegering DA, Jenkins RB, Heise MT, Schad CR, Pease LR, Gleich GJ, Barker RL. Structure and chromosome localization of the human eosinophil-derived neurotoxin and eosinophil cationic protein genes: evidence for intronless coding sequences in the ribonuclease gene superfamily. Genomics 1990;7:535–546.
39. Slifman NR, Venge P, Peterson CGB, McKean DJ, Gleich GJ. Human eosinophil-derived neurotoxin and eosinophil protein X are likely the same protein. J Immunol 1989;143:2317–2322.
40. Durack DT, Sumi SM, and Klebanoff SJ. Neurotoxicity of human eosinophils. Proc Natl Acad Sci USA 1979;76:1443–1447.
41. Olsen RL, Little C. Purification and some properties of myeloperoxidase and eosinophil peroxidase from human blood. Biochem J 1983;209:781–787.
42. Carlson MGCh, Peterson CGB, Venge P. Human eosinophil peroxidase: purification and characterization. J Immunol 1985;134:1875–1879.
43. Ten RM, Pease LR, McKean DJ, Bell MP, Gleich GJ. Molecular cloning of the human eosinophil peroxidase. Evidence for the existence of a peroxidase multigene family. J Exp Med 1989;169:1757–1769.
44. Sakamaki K, Tomonaga M, Tsukui K, Nagata S. Molecular cloning and characterization of a chromosomal gene for human eosinophil peroxidase. J Biol Chem 1989;264:16828–16836.
45. Klebanoff SJ, Jong EC, Henderson WR Jr. The eosinophil peroxidase: purification and biological properties. In: Mahmoud AAF, Austen KF, eds. The Eosinophil in Health and Disease. New York: Grune & Stratton, 1980:99–114.
46. Weiss SJ, Test ST, Eckmann CM, Roos D, Regiani S. Brominating oxidants generated by human eosinophils. Science 1986;234:200–203.
47. Slungaard A, Mahoney JR Jr. Thiocyanate is the major substrate for eosinophil peroxidase in physiologic fluids: implications for cytotoxicity. J Biol Chem 1991;266:4903–4910.
48. Egesten A, Alumets J, von Mecklenburg C, Palmegren M, Olsson I. Localization of eosinophil cationic protein, major basic protein, and eosinophil peroxidase in human eosinophils by immunoelectron microscopic technique. J Histochem Cytochem 1986;34:1399–1404.
49. Peters MS, Rodriguez M, Gleich GJ. Localization of human eosinophil granule major basic protein, eosinophil cationic protein, and eosinophil-derived neurotoxin by immunoelectron microscopy. Lab Invest 1986;54:656–662.
50. Lewis DM, Lewis JC, Loegering DA, Gleich GJ. Localization of the guinea pig eosinophil major basic protein to the core of the granule. J Cell Biol 1978;77:702–713.
51. Gleich GJ, Frigas E, Loegering DA, Wassom DL, Steinmuller D. Cytotoxic properties of the eosinophil major basic protein. J Immunol 1979;123:2925–2927.
52. Frigas E, Loegering DA, Gleich GJ. Cytotoxic effects of the guinea pig eosinophil major basic protein on tracheal epithelium. Lab Invest 1980;42:35–43.
53. Frigas E, Loegering DA, Solley GO, Farrow GM, Gleich GJ. Elevated levels of

the eosinophil granule major basic protein in the sputum of patients with bronchial asthma. Mayo Clin Proc 1981;56:345–353.

54. Motojima S, Frigas E, Loegering DA, Gleich GJ. Toxicity of eosinophil cationic proteins for guinea pig tracheal epithelium in vitro. Am Rev Respir Dis 1989;139:801–805.
55. Ayars GH, Altman LC, Gleich GJ, Loegering DA, Baker CB. Eosinophil- and eosinophil granule-mediated pneumocyte injury. J Allergy Clin Immunol 1985;76:595–604.
56. Agosti JM, Altman LC, Ayars GH, Loegering DA, Gleich GJ, Klebanoff SJ. The injurious effect of eosinophil peroxidase, hydrogen peroxide, and halides on pneumocytes in vitro. J Allergy Clin Immunol 1987;79:496–504.
57. Ayars GH, Altman LC, McManus MM, Agosti JM, Baker C, Luchtel DL, Loegering DA, Gleich GJ. Injurious effect of the eosinophil peroxide-hydrogen peroxide-halide system and major basic protein on human nasal epithelium in vitro. Am Rev Respir Dis 1989;140:125–131.
58. Hastie AT, Loegering DA, Gleich GJ, Kueppers F. The effect of purified human eosinophil major basic protein on mammalian ciliary activity. Am Rev Respir Dis 1987;135:848–853.
59. Jacoby DB, Ueki IF, Widdicombe JH, Loegering DA, Gleich GJ, Nadel JA. Effect of human eosinophil major basic protein on ion transport in dog tracheal epithelium. Am Rev Respir Dis 1988;137:13–16.
60. Minnicozzi M, Durán WN, Gleich GJ, Egan RW. Eosinophil granule proteins increase microvascular macromolecular transport in the hamster cheek pouch. J Immunol 1994;153:2664–2670.
61. Gleich GJ, Schroeter AL, Marcoux JP, Sachs MI, O'Connell EJ, Kohler PF. Episodic angioedema associated with eosinophilia. N Engl J Med 1984;310:1621–1626.
62. Gleich GJ, Fryer AD, Jacoby DB. Eosinophil granule proteins and bronchial hyperreactivity. In: Holgate ST, Austen KF, Lichtenstein LM, Kay AB, eds. Asthma: Physiology, Immunopharmacology, and Treatment. London: Academic Press, 1993:119–129.
63. Durham SR, Kay AB. Eosinophils, bronchial hyperactivity and late-phase asthmatic reactions. Clin Allergy 1985;15:411–418.
64. Iijima M, Adachi M, Kobayashi H, Takahashi T. Relationship between airway hyperreactivity and various atopic factors in bronchial asthma. Jpn J Allergol 1985;34:226–233.
65. Taylor KJ, Luksza AR. Peripheral blood eosinophil counts and bronchial responsiveness. Thorax 1987;42:452–456.
66. Wardlaw AJ, Dunnette S, Gleich GJ, Collins JV, Kay AB. Eosinophils and mast cells in bronchoalveolar lavage in subjects with mild asthma: relationship to bronchial hyperreactivity. Am Rev Respir Dis 1988;137:62–69.
67. Wegner CD, Koker PJ, Gundel RH. Relationship between eosinophils and airway reactivity in monkeys (abstract). Am Rev Respir Dis 1987;135:A222.
68. Gundel RH, Gerritsen ME, Wegner CD. Increase in airway eosinophils is associated with an increase in airways reactivity. Am Rev Respir Dis 1989;140:629–633.

69. Gundel RH, Gerritsen ME, Gleich GJ, Wegner CD. Repeated antigen inhalation results in a prolonged airway eosinophilia and airway hyperresponsiveness in primates. J Appl Physiol 1990;68:779–786.
70. Gundel RH, Letts LG, Gleich GJ. Human eosinophil major basic protein induces airway constriction and airway hyperresponsiveness in primates. J Clin Invest 1991;87:1470–1473.
71. Uchida DA, Ackerman SJ, Coyle AJ, Larsen GL, Weller PF, Freed J, Irvin CG. The effect of human eosinophil granule major basic protein on airway responsiveness on the rat in vivo: comparison with polycations. Am Rev Respir Dis 1993;147:982–988.
72. Coyle AJ, Ackerman SJ, Irvin CG. Cationic proteins induce airway hyperresponsiveness dependent on charge interactions. Am Rev Respir Dis 1993;147:896–900.
73. Coyle AJ, Perretti F, Manzini S, Irvin CG. Cationic protein-induced sensory nerve activation: role of substance P in airway hyperresponsiveness and plasma protein extravasation. J Clin Invest 1994;94:2301–2306.
74. Coyle AJ, Ackerman SJ, Burch R, Proud D, Irvin CG. Human eosinophil-granule major basic protein and synthetic polycations induce airway responsiveness in vivo dependent upon bradykinin generation. J Clin Invest 1995;95:1735–1740.
75. Flavahan NA, Slifman NR, Gleich GJ, Vanhoutte PM. Human eosinophil major basic protein causes hyperreactivity of respiratory smooth muscle. Role of the epithelium. Am Rev Respir Dis 1988;138:685–688.
76. Brofman JD, White SR, Blake JS, Munoz NM, Gleich GJ, Leff AR. Epithelial augmentation of trachealis contraction caused by major basic protein of eosinophils. J Appl Physiol 1989;66:1867–1873.
77. White SR, Ohno S, Munoz NM, Gleich GJ, Abrahams C, Solway J, Leff AR. Epithelium-dependent contraction of airway smooth muscle caused by eosinophil MBP. Am J Physiol (Lung Mol Cell Physiol 3) 1990;259:L294–L303.
78. Strek ME, Williams FS, Gleich GJ, Leff AR, White SR. Mechanisms of smooth muscle contraction elicited by cationic proteins in guinea pig trachealis. Am J Physiol (Lung Cell Mol Physiol 14) 1996;270:L133–L140.
79. White SR, Sigrist KS, Spaethe SM. Prostaglandin secretion by guinea pig tracheal epithelial cells caused by eosinophil major basic protein. Am J Physiol (Lung Cell Mol Physiol 9) 1993;265:L234–L242.
80. McCaig DJ. Comparison of autonomic responses in the trachea isolated from normal and albumin-sensitive guinea-pigs. Br J Pharmacol 1987;92:809–816.
81. Fryer AD, Maclagan J. Muscarinic inhibitory receptors in pulmonary parasympathetic nerves in the guinea-pig. Br J Pharmacol 1984;83:973–978.
82. Barnes PJ, Minette P, Maclagan J. Muscarinic receptor subtypes in airways. TIPS 1988;9:412–416.
83. Fryer AD, Wills-Karp M. Dysfunction of M2 muscarinic receptors in pulmonary parasympathetic nerves after antigen challenge. J Appl Physiol 1991;71:2255–2261.
84. Fryer AD, Jacoby DB. The function of pulmonary M2 muscarinic receptors in antigen challenged guinea-pigs is restored by heparin and poly-L-glutamate. J Clin Invest 1992;90:2292–2298.

85. Larsen GL, Fame TM, Renz H, Loader JE, Graves J, Hill M, Gelfand EW. Increased acetylcholine release in tracheas from allergen-exposed IgE-immune mice. Am J Physiol 1994;266:L263–L270.
86. Hu J, Wang SZ, Forray C, El-Fakahany EE. Complex allosteric modulation of cardiac muscarinic receptors by protamine: a potential model for putative endogenous ligands. Mol Pharmacol 1992;42:311–324.
87. Barker RL, Gleich GJ, Pease LR. Acidic precursor revealed in human eosinophil granule major basic protein cDNA. J Exp Med 1988;168:1493–1498.
88. Barker RL, Gundel RH, Gleich GJ, Checkel JL, Loegering DA, Pease LR, Hamann KJ. Acidic polyamino acids inhibit human eosinophil granule major basic protein toxicity: Evidence of a functional role for proMBP. J Clin Invest 1991;88:798–805.
89. Jacoby DB, Gleich GJ, Fryer AD. Human eosinophil major basic protein is an endogenous allosteric antagonist at the inhibitory muscarinic M2 receptor. J Clin Invest 1993;91:1314–1318.
90. Elbon CL, Jacoby DB, Fryer AD. Pretreatment with an antibody to interleukin-5 prevents loss of pulmonary M2 muscarinic receptor function in antigen-challenged guinea pigs. Am J Respir Cell Mol Biol 1995;12:320–328.
91. Pretolani M, Ruffie C, Lapa e Silva JR, Joseph D, Lobb RR, Vargaftig BB. Antibody to very late activation antigen 4 prevents antigen-induced bronchial hyperreactivity and cellular infiltration in the guinea pig airways. J Exp Med 1994;180:795–805.
92. Fryer AD, Costello RW, Yost BL, Lobb RR, Tedder TF, Steeber DA, Bochner BS. Antibody to VLA-4, but not to L-selectin, protects neuronal M2 muscarinic receptors in antigen-challenged guinea pig airways. J Clin Invest 1997;99:2036–2044.
93. Pretolani M, Ruffie C, Joseph D, Campos MG, Church MK, Lefort J, Vargaftig BB. Role of eosinophil activation in the bronchial reactivity of allergic guinea pigs. Am J Respir Crit Care Med 1994;149:1167–1174.
94. Lefort J, Nahori MA, Ruffie C, Vargaftig BB, Pretolani M. In vivo neutralization of eosinophil-derived major basic protein inhibits antigen-induced bronchial hyperreactivity in sensitized guinea pigs. J Clin Invest 1996;97:1117–1121.
95. Evans CM, Fryer AD, Jacoby DB, Gleich GJ, Costello RW. Pretreatment with antibody to eosinophil major basic protein prevents hyperresponsiveness by protecting neuronal M2 muscarinic receptors in antigen-challenged guinea pigs. J Clin Invest 1997; 100:2254–2262.
96. Costello RW, Schofield BH, Kephart GM, Gleich GJ, Jacoby DB, Fryer AD. Localization of eosinophils to airway nerves and the effect on neuronal M2 muscarinic receptor function. Am J Physiol (Lung Cell Mol Physiol), 1997; 273:L93–L103.
97. Ayala LE, Ahmed T. Is there loss of protective muscarinic receptor mechanism in asthma? Chest 1989;96:1285–1291.
98. Minette PA, Lammers JW, Dixon CM, McCusker MT, Barnes PJ. A muscarinic agonist inhibits reflex bronchoconstriction in normal but not in asthmatic subjects. J Appl Physiol 1989;67:2461–2465.
99. Zheutlin LM, Ackerman SJ, Gleich GJ, Thomas LL. Donor sensitivity to baso-

phil activation by eosinophil granule major basic protein. Int Arch Allergy Appl Immun 1985;77:216–217.

100. Thomas LL, Zheutlin LM, Gleich GJ. Pharmacological control of human basophil histamine release stimulated by eosinophil granule major basic protein. Immunology 1989;66:611–615.

101. Okayama Y, el-Lati SG, Leiferman KM, Church MK. Eosinophil granule proteins inhibit substance P-induced histamine release from human skin mast cells. J Allergy Clin Immunol 1994;93:900–909.

102. Patella V, de Crescenzo G, Marinò I, Genovese A, Adt M, Gleich GJ, Marone G. Eosinophil granule proteins activate human heart mast cells. J Immunol 1996;157:1219–1225.

103. Sarmiento EU, Espiritu BR, Gleich GJ, Thomas LL. IL-3, IL-5, and granulocyte-macrophage colony-stimulating factor potentiate basophil mediator release stimulated by eosinophil granule major basic protein. J Immunol 1995;155:2211–2221.

104. Henderson WR, Jong EC, Klebanoff SJ. Binding of eosinophil peroxidase to mast cell granules with retention of peroxidatic activity. J Immunol 1980;124:1383–1388.

105. Henderson WR, Chi EY, Klebanoff SJ. Eosinophil peroxidase-induced mast cell secretion. J Exp Med 1980;152:265–279.

106. Leiferman KM, Fujisawa T, Gray BH, Gleich GJ. Extracellular deposition of eosinophil and neutrophil granule proteins in the IgE-mediated cutaneous late phase reaction. Lab Invest 1990;62:579–589.

107. Thomas LL, Haskell MD, Sarmiento EU, Bilimoria Y. Distinguishing features of basophil and neutrophil activation by major basic protein. J Allergy Clin Immunol 1994;94:1171–1176.

108. Metzger WJ, Sjoerdsma K, Richerson HB, Moseley P, Zvala D, Monick M, Hunninghake GW. Platelets in bronchoalveolar lavage from asthmatic patients and allergic rabbits with allergin-induced late phase responses. Agents Actions 1987;21(suppl):151–159.

109. Page CP. The involvement of platelets in non-thrombotic processes. TIPS 1988;9:66–71.

110. Lundgren JD, Davey RT Jr, Lundgren B, Mullol J, Marom Z, Logun C, Baraniuk J, Kaliner MA, Shelhamer JH. Eosinophil cationic protein stimulates and major basic protein inhibits airway mucous secretion. J Allergy Clin Immunol 1991;87:689–698.

111. Kita H, Abu-Ghazaleh RI, Sur S, Gleich GJ. Eosinophil major basic protein induces degranulation and IL-8 production by human eosinophils. J Immunol 1995;154:4749–4758.

112. Tsuyuki S, Bertrand C, Erard F, Trifilieff A, Tsuyuki J, Wesp M, Anderson GP, Coyle AJ. Activation of the Fas receptor on lung eosinophils leads to apoptosis and the resolution of eosinophilic inflammation of the airways. J Clin Invest 1995;96:2924–2931.

113. Cardell BS, Pearson RSB. Death in asthmatics. Thorax 1959;14:341–352.

114. Houston JC, De Nevasquez S, Trounce JR. A clinical and pathological study of fatal cases of status asthmaticus. Thorax 1953;8:207–213.
115. Dunnill MS. The pathology of asthma with special reference to changes in the bronchial mucosa. J Clin Pathol 1960;13:27–33.
116. Glynn AA, Michaels L. Bronchial biopsy in chronic bronchitis and asthma. Thorax 1960;15:142–153.
117. Gough J. Post-mortem differences in "asthma" and in chronic bronchitis. Acta Allergol 1961;16:391–399.
118. Carabelli AA. Cytologic patterns in bronchopulmonary disease. Am Rev Tuberculosis 1958;77:22–31.
119. Leyden zu Königsberg E. Zur kenntniss des bronchial asthma. Arch Pathol Anat Physiol 1872;54:324–352.
120. Von Hoesslin H. Das sputum. Berlin: Springer, 1921.
121. Naylor B. The shedding of the mucosa of the bronchial tree in asthma. Thorax 1962;17:69–72.
122. Naylor B. Creola bodies: their "discovery" and significance. Cytotechnol Bull 1985;22:33–34.
123. Jeffery PK. Pathology of asthma. Br Med Bull 1992;48:23–39.
124. Kay AB. Pathology of mild, severe, and fatal asthma. Am J Respir Crit Care Med 1996;154:S66–S69.
125. Laitinen A, Laitinen LA. Pathology of asthma. Allergy Proc 1994;15:323–328.
126. Beasley R, Burgess C, Crane J, Pearce N, Roche W. Pathology of asthma and its clinical implications. J Allergy Clin Immunol 1993;92:148–154.
127. Frigas E, Gleich GJ. The eosinophil and the pathophysiology of asthma. J Allergy Clin Immunol 1986;77:527–537.
128. Dor PJ, Ackerman SJ, Gleich GJ. Charcot-Leyden crystal protein and eosinophil granule major basic protein in sputum of patients with respiratory diseases. Am Rev Respir Dis 1984;130:1072–1077.
129. Pizzichini E, Pizzichini MMM, Efthimiadis A, Evans S, Morris MM, Squillace D, Gleich GJ, Dolovich J, Hargreave FE. Indices of airway inflammation in induced sputum: reproducibility and validity of cell and fluid phase measurements. Am J Respir Crit Care Med 1996;154:308–317.
130. Filley WV, Holley KE, Kephart GM, Gleich GJ. Identification by immunofluorescence of eosinophil granule major basic protein in lung tissues of patients with bronchial asthma. Lancet 1982;2:11–16.
131. Kita H, Gleich GJ. The eosinophil: structure and functions. In: Kaplan AP, ed. Allergy, 2nd ed. Philadelphia: W. B. Saunders, 1997:148–178.
132. van Oosterhout AJ, Ladenius AR, Savelkoul HF, van Ark I, Delsman KC, Nijkamp FP. Effect of anti-IL-5 and IL-5 on airway hyperreactivity and eosinophils in guinea pigs. Am Rev Respir Dis 1993;147:548–552.
133. Mauser PJ, Pitman A, Witt A, Fernandez X, Zurcher J, Kung J, Jones H, Watnick AS, Egan RW, Kreutner W, Adams GK. Inhibitory effect of the TRFK-5 anti-IL-5 antibody in a guinea pig model of asthma. Am Rev Respir Dis 1993;148:1623–1627.
134. van Oosterhout AJ, van Ark I, Folkerts G, van der Linde HJ, Savelkoul HF,

Verheyen AK, Nijkamp FP. Antibody to interleukin-5 inhibits virus-induced airway hyperresponsiveness to histamine in guinea pigs. Am J Respir Crit Care Med 1995;151:177–183.
135. Mauser PJ, Pitman AM, Fernandez X, Foran SK, Adams GK III, Kreutner W, Egan RW, Chapman RW. Effects of an antibody to interleukin-5 in a monkey model of asthma. Am J Respir Crit Care Med 1995;152:467–472.
136. Foster PS, Hogan SP, Ramsay AJ, Matthaei KI, Young IG. Interleukin 5 deficiency abolishes eosinophils, airways hyperreactivity, and lung damage in a mouse asthma model. J Exp Med 1996;183:195–201.
137. Hamelmann E, Oshiba A, Loader J, Larsen GL, Gleich G, Lee J, Gelfand EW. Anti-interleukin-5 antibody prevents airway hyperresponsiveness in a murine model of airway sensitization. Am J Respir Crit Care Med 1997;155:819–825.

# 2

# Interleukin-5 in Rhinitis: Influence of Treatment

**STEPHEN R. DURHAM**

Imperial College School of Medicine at
the National Heart and Lung Institute
London, England

**KEISUKE MASUYAMA**

Kumamoto University School of Medicine
Kumamoto, Japan

**QUTAYBA HAMID**

McGill University
Montreal, Quebec, Canada

## I. Introduction

Eosinophilia is characteristic of human allergic inflammation and interleukin-5 (IL-5) is a major pro-inflammatory cytokine with distinct eosinophil modifying properties (1–4). It seems likely therefore that IL-5 may play a major role in the recruitment, activation, and persistence of eosinophils at allergic tissue sites and, presumably, the clinical expression of allergic disease. However, certain criteria need to be fulfilled before we can assume that these associations are "casual" in man:

- IL-5 should have biological properties that are relevant to either naturally occurring or experimentally induced allergic disease.
- Administration of IL-5 should result in eosinophilia and symptoms/signs of allergic disease.
- IL-5 should be demonstrable in allergic tissue responses.
- IL-5 should correlate with eosinophils in a time- and dose-dependent fashion at allergic sites.

Specific antagonists should abrogate eosinophils and associated diseases. Alternatively, treatment of the disease should be associated with a decrease in both IL-5 and eosinophilia which correlates with clinical improvement.

We have used the human nasal mucosa as a "window" to the lower respiratory tract and an accessible model of allergic inflammation in order to address some of the questions in man. We have performed allergen provocation and observed the effects of natural exposure to grass pollen. We have examined the influence of treatment including topical corticosteroid therapy and allergen injection immunotherapy. Taken together these studies support IL-5 as a major target for therapeutic attack. However, the key question remains, what is the influence of specific strategies against IL-5 such as monoclonal anti-IL-5 on natural disease in controlled clinical trials?

## II. Nasal Late Responses

Allergen provocation of the nose results in immediate symptoms of itching/sneezing followed by watery nasal discharge and nasal congestion within minutes, maximal at 15 to 30 min after challenge. In a proportion of subjects there follows late nasal symptoms with occasional sneezing/discharge but mainly evidenced as late nasal obstruction. In contrast to late allergic responses in the skin and lung, these late clinical manifestations occurring hours after challenge are less prominent and quantifiable in the nose. Naclerio et al. showed that both early and late nasal responses were associated with the release of pharmacologic mediators, detectable in nasal lavage fluid, including histamine, kinins, and TAME esterase during both early and late responses (5). In contrast, prostaglandin $D_2$ (specific for mast cells) was detectable only during early response, which implied that the cell source of the delayed increases in histamine was the basophil. The same group demonstrated that the late nasal response was associated with an influx of eosinophils and basophils in nasal fluid (6). Both mediator release and inflammatory cells detected in nasal lavage were inhibited by pretreatment with oral and topical corticosteroids (6,7).

Our own studies have involved the application of 4 mm circular filter paper discs to the undersurface of the nasal inferior turbinate (8). The disc, including 7 ml of allergen solution and an allergen diluent (control), is left in place for 10 min and removed. Symptoms are recorded as a sneeze count, volume of nasal secretions, and obstruction (subjective severity scale 0–4), and more recently, use of acoustic rhinometry to quantify nasal volume and cross-sectional area of the nasal cavity. Following nasal provocation a 2.5 mm biopsy is taken at 24 hr from the site of allergen challenge using cup and ring (Gerritsma) forceps (or the control site, usually with an interval of 2 weeks between challenges).

Biopsies are divided into halves which are processed separately for immunohistology and in situ hybridization. Immunohistology is performed on 6 μm cryostat sections using a modified alkaline phosphatase antialkaline phosphatase technique. Monoclonal antibodies employed include those directed against T-cell markers (CD4, CD8, CD25) and eosinophils. BMK13 (supplied by Dr. Redwan Moqbel) detects the eosinophil granule protein, major basic protein (MBP), whereas EG2 detects the cleaved, secreted form of eosinophil cationic protein (ECP) consistent with eosinophil "activation" (8). In situ hybridization was employed using genetic probes directed against specific cytokines. The IL-5 probe was prepared from a cDNA (supplied by Dr. Colin Sanderson). Controls in these experiments included use of a sense probe (with an identical sequence to native mRNA) and pretreatment of nasal biopsy sections with RNAse to confirm specificity of hybridization (9).

By use of these techniques we showed that the late nasal response was associated with an increase in total and "activated" eosinophils at 24 hr. We also detected an increase in neutrophils. T-lymphocyte numbers ($CD4^+$) were also increased and the ratio of CD4/CD8 T cells increased in nasal tissue, but not peripheral blood CD4/CD8 ratios, suggesting that T-cell recruitment was occurring selectively to the nasal mucosa (9). Numbers of $CD25^+$ cells also increased, mainly activated T lymphocytes (confirmed by dual immunostaining techniques), although possibly a contribution from macrophages and/or eosinophils which also express CD25 (10).

In situ hybridization demonstrated increases in cytokine mRNA positive cells for IL-3, IL-4, IL-5, and GM-CSF. Only occasional positive hybridization signals for IL-2 and interferon-γ (IFN-γ) were observed and no change after allergen exposure (9). There was a highly significant correlation between $IL\text{-}5^+$ cells and the number of EG2 eosinophils ($r = 0.95$, $p < 0.001$) (Fig. 1). Taken together these studies confirm that allergen-induced late nasal responses are associated with the recruitment and activation of eosinophils and that this may occur as a consequence of IL-5 and possibly IL-3 and GM-CSF expressed locally within the nasal mucosa (Fig. 2).

In order to investigate the cell source of "Th2-type" cytokines during late nasal responses the technique of double immunohistochemistry/in situ hybridization was employed using the alkaline phosphatase anti-alkaline phosphatase (APAAP) technique for phenotypic markers, followed by hybridization using digoxigenin-labeled riboprobes for cytokines. Seventy to eighty percent of IL-4 and IL-5 $mRNA^+$ cells could be accounted for by $CD3^+$ T lymphocytes, with lesser contributions from mast cells (particularly IL-4) and eosinophils (particularly IL-5) (Fig. 3) (11,12).

## III. Influence of Treatment

We tested the hypothesis that topical steroids inhibit late responses by inhibiting cells expressing mRNA for TH2-type cytokines. We performed a random-

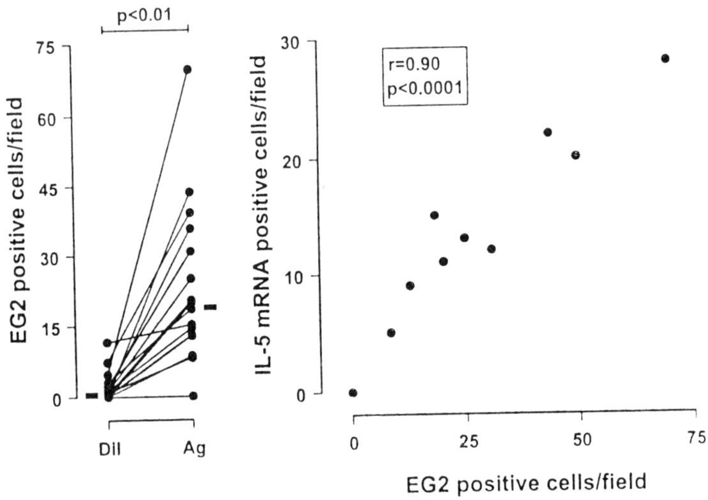


**Figure 1** In situ hybridization of nasal biopsies before and 24 hr after nasal provocation with a grass pollen extract. Increases in IL-5 mRNA$^+$ cells correlated closely with tissue eosinophilia represented by number of EG2$^+$ (ECP secreting) eosinophils.

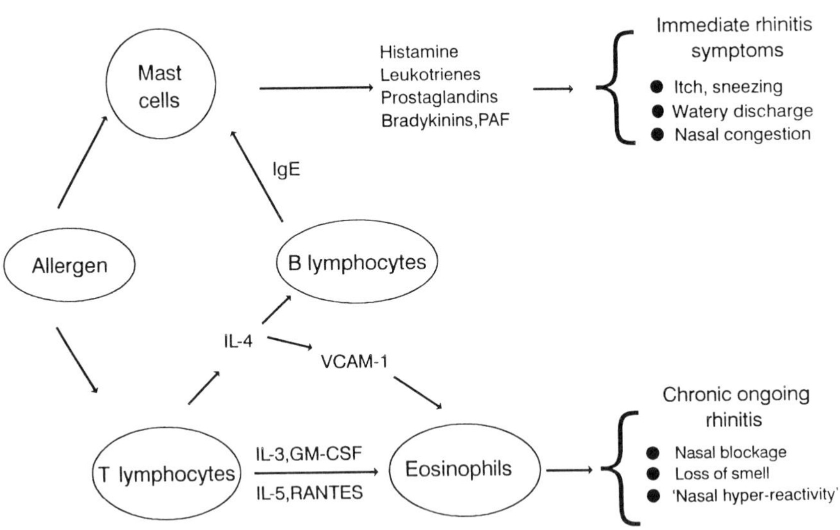


**Figure 2** Hypothesis on mechanisms of allergen-induced rhinitis. Early symptoms depend on mediator release from mast cells, whereas late symptoms are associated with tissue eosinophilia. Both IgE synthesis and eosinophilia are dependent on "TH2-type" cytokines produced mainly by T lymphocytes but also mast cells and eosinophils. Reproduced with permission from Allergy 1994; 49(Suppl 19).

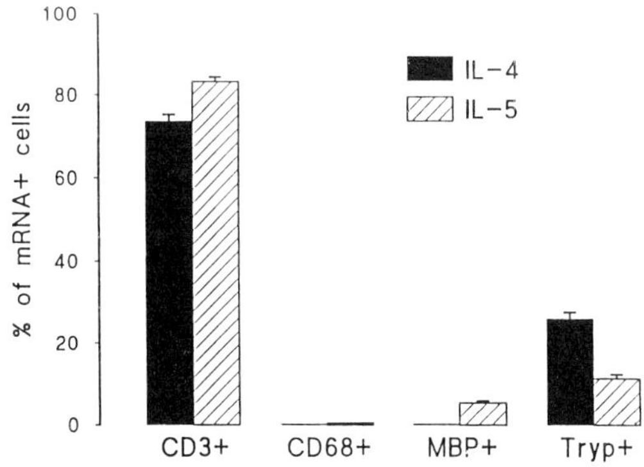


**Figure 3** Double-immunohistochemistry/in situ hybridization of nasal biopsies during late responses (n = 6). Immunohistochemistry for phenotypic markers for T cells (CD3), macrophages (CD68), eosinophils (MBP), and mast cells (tryptase) was followed by hybridization of sections using digoxigenin-labeled antisense riboprobes directed against IL-4 and IL-5.

ized double-blind, placebo-controlled trial of 6 weeks treatment with topical aqueous fluticasone propionate nasal spray 200 mg twice daily in 48 patients with grass pollen allergy and severe summer hay fever (13). Steroid treatment resulted in an approximate 50% reduction in the early nasal response after grass pollen challenge and almost complete inhibition of late nasal symptoms (Fig. 4). This was associated with a marked reduction in IL-4 mRNA$^+$ cells but had no influence on allergen-induced increase in IL-5$^+$ cells, although a marked reduction in tissue eosinophilia was observed (14). It is possible that inhibition of IL-5 mRNA$^+$ cells would have been observed had we sampled at different time points or in response to a different allergen dose. An alternative explanation is that corticosteroid-induced inhibition of eosinophil recruitment (persistence during late responses) is dependent on an IL-4-dependent mechanism such as upregulation of VCAM-1 on endothelial cells (15) or possibly an effect on IL-3 GM-CSF or IL-13 expression.

A more recent study measured cytokine concentrations in nasal fluid collected on filter paper strips applied to the nasal mucosa following allergen challenge (16). Increases in IL-1 and GM-CSF were observed which were time dependent, paralleled the late response, correlated with the late response (area under curve), and were inhibited by topical corticosteroids. The effect of steroids on IL-5 was not reported in this study.

Other recent studies (17,18) examined the effect of allergin injection immunotherapy on nasal early and late responses and mucosal expressions of cells and the cytokines produced, including IL-5. Forty patients with severe summer

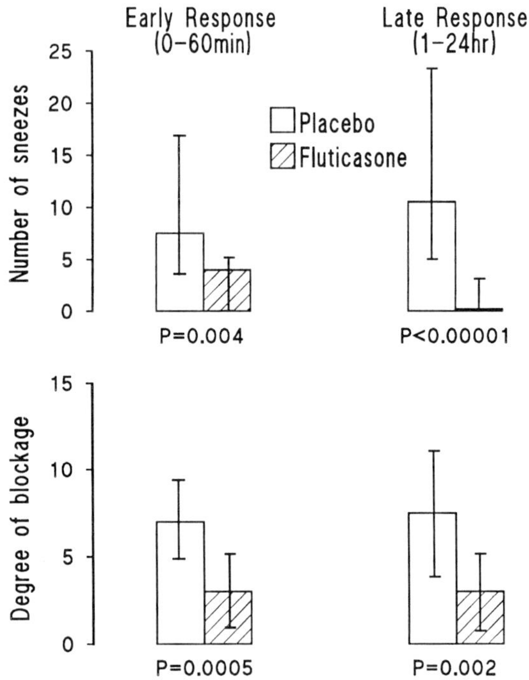


**Figure 4** Effect of 6 weeks treatment with topical nasal corticosteroid (fluticasone propionate 200 mg twice daily) on early and late nasal symptoms after challenge with a grass pollen extract.

hay fever received 12 months treatment with a depot grass pollen extract (Alutard SQ, ALK, Denmark) by subcutaneous injections. Immunotherapy in these selected patients was highly effective and resulted in inhibition of both early and late nasal responses following provocation with a grass pollen extract (Fig. 4). Nasal biopsy studies demonstrated increases in $CD4^+$ T lymphocytes and eosinophils. Although there was a trend for a reduction in IL-$5^+$ cells ($p = 0.1$), this was not statistically significant. In contrast, a significant increase in the number of IFN-$\gamma$ $mRNA^+$ cells after allergen challenge was observed. Furthermore, these allergen-induced increases in IFN-$\gamma$ correlated closely with the patients seasonal hay fever symptoms and requirements for rescue medication. These results suggested that one way in which immunotherapy might act is by inducing immune deviation with a shift in the balance of Th2/Th1 cytokines in favor of Th1, with increases in "protective" IFN-$\gamma$ rather than a reduction in IL-4/IL-5 (19). However, other studies performed in vitro on human T cells cultured before and during immunotherapy suggest this "switch" in favor of Th1 responses occurs also as a consequence of a decrease in IL-4 and IL-5 production (20,21). It is not clear at the present time whether these immunotherapy-induced changes result from allergen-specific immune unresponsiveness ("anergy" of Th2/Th0 cells) or an increase in Th1/Th0 cells.

## IV. Seasonal Grass Pollen Exposure

The limitations of studies of nasal allergen provocation are that large doses of allergen are given over a short period in soluble form, which is in contrast to the natural exposure to low doses of allergen in particle form over prolonged periods. Studies of nasal lavage, brushings, imprints on plastic strips (22) applied to the mucosa, and nasal biopsy have confirmed the characteristic immunocytochemical findings of increases in eosinophils and eosinophil activation [with increases in eosinophil cationic protein (ECP) concentration] and a transepithelial migration of mast cells of the so-called mucosal or tryptase-only phenotype (23,24).

In order to study the effects of corticosteroids on the nasal mucosa during the pollen season we performed a double-blind, placebo-controlled trial on 47 patients with moderate to severe summer hay fever treated with topical fluticasone propionate for 6 weeks (25–27). Nasal biopsies were performed before the season (baseline) and following the peak of the pollen counts (Fig. 5). Immunohistological studies demonstrated highly significant decreases in

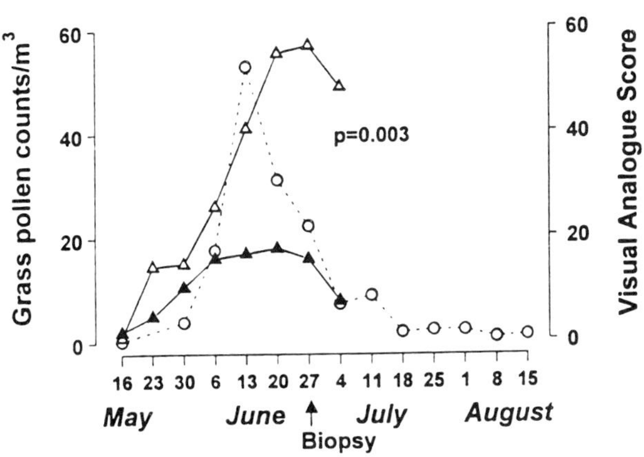


**Figure 5** Effect of 6 weeks treatment with topical steroids on seasonal symptoms (visual analog scale) during the pollen season. Timing of nasal biopsy in relation to pollen counts and symptoms is shown.

CD4$^+$ T lymphocytes (Fig. 6), MBP-containing and ECP-containing eosinophils, and a decrease in both mucosal (tryptase only) and connective tissue-type (tryptase + chymase containing) mast cells. In placebo-treated patients seasonal increases in cells expressing IL-5, and GM-CSF mRNA were observed. However, in contrast to the findings following allergen challenge, a highly significant decrease in IL-5$^+$ cells (Fig. 7) was observed in the steroid-treated group, whereas seasonal increases in GM-CSF cells remained unchanged. Studies from Holland have shown increases in a population of Fc$\varepsilon$R1$^+$ CD1a$^+$ Langerhans' cells during the pollen season, an effect which is also inhibited by topical steroids.

## V. Perennial Rhinitis

Perennial rhinitis represents a more heterogeneous disease when compared to clear-cut seasonal rhinitis, where the dominant etiology is allergy to pollen.

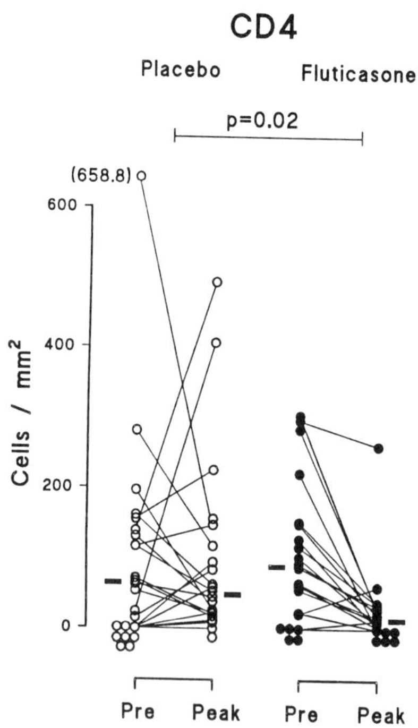


**Figure 6** Effect of 6 weeks topical steroid (fluticasone propionate) on CD4$^+$ T cells in the nasal epithelium before (pre) and during the peak pollen season (peak).

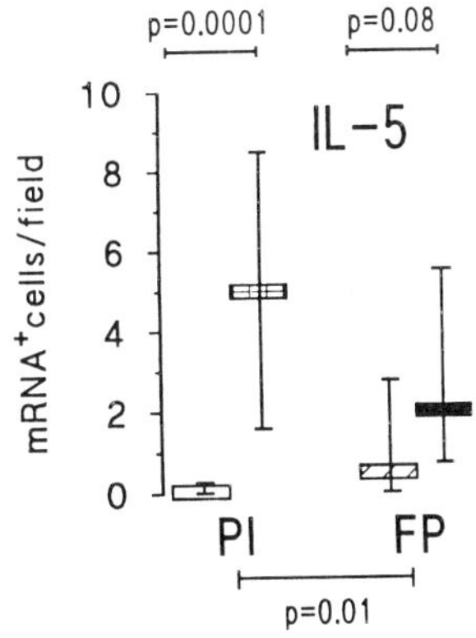


**Figure 7** Effect of topical corticosteroid (fluticasone propionate) on nasal mucosal IL-5 mRNA$^+$ cells.

Perennial rhinitis includes several conditions including allergy to perennial allergens such as house dust mite and domestic pets, chronic rhinosinusitis where an infective component exists, structural problems such as deflected septum and nasal polyposis, and so-called vasomotor rhinitis (28). In patients with perennial allergic rhinitis, IL-4 and IL-5 protein-containing cells are present (29). The striking findings in patients with nasal polyps were intense eosinophilia and increases in GM-CSF immunostained cells (30).

## VI. Summary

Interleukin-5 has been detected at mRNA and protein levels in symptomatic patients with allergic rhinitis either following allergen provocation or during natural seasonal exposure. There is a correlation between IL-5 expression and eosinophil numbers, suggesting that IL-5 may promote terminal maturation and "activation" or eosinophils, prolong eosinophil survival, and possibly inhibit apoptosis of eosinophils, all of which may account for persistence of eosinophils and ongoing allergic inflammation. Topical steroids are highly effective in suppressing both symptoms and eosinophil numbers during both late responses and natural grass exposure. However, our findings of the effect of steroids on cytokine production differ, with preferential inhibition of IL-4 during late responses and IL-5 during natural exposure. These results suggest that different mechanisms may be dominant in regulating tissue eosinophilia depending on the time course. Eosinophil recruitment during late responses may be rate limited by IL-4-dependent upregulation of the eosinophil selective adhesion molecule VCAM-1 on vascular endothelium. Prolonged eosinophil survival and protection from apoptosis during seasonal grass exposure may be IL-5 dependent, whereas GM-CSF may possibly be the principle cytokine responsible for the intense eosinophil infiltration of nasal polyps. These observations suggest that there may be considerable redundancy in the factors responsible for promoting and sustaining eosinophilia during allergic inflammation, such that targeting a single cytokine may not be effective. Only one study examined the direct effects of IL-5 on the nasal mucosa (31). Topical recombinant human IL-5 was observed to increase histamine-induced nasal symptoms and associated eosinophilia. However, further studies are required, especially on the effects of strategies directed specifically against IL-5 on experimentally provoked and natural allergic diseases including allergic rhinitis.

## References

1. Clutterbuck EJ, Hirst EMA, Sanderson CJ. Human interleukin-5 (IL-5) regulates the production of eosinophils in human bone marrow cultures: comparison and interaction with IL-1, IL-3, IL-6, and GM-CSF. Blood 1989;73:1504–1512.
2. Lopez IG, Vadas MA. Recombinant human interleukin-5 is a selective activator of human eosinophiil function. J Exp Med 1988;167:129–224.
3. Walsh GM, Hartnell A, Wardlaw AJ, Kurihara K, Sanderson CJ, Kay AB. IL-5 enhances the in vitro adhesion of human eosinophils but not neutrophils in a leucocyte integrin (CD11/18)-dependent manner. Immunology 1990;71:258–265.
4. Rothenberg ME, Petersen J, Stevens RJ, Silberstein DS, McKenzie DT, Austen KF, Owen WF. IL-5-dependent conversion of normodense human eosinophils to the hypodense phenotype uses 3T3 fibroblasts for enhanced viability, accelerated hypodensity, and sustained antibody-dependent cytotoxicity. J Immunol 1989;143:2311–2316.
5. Naclerio RM, Proud D, Togias AG, Adkinson NF, Meyers DA, Kagley-Sobotka A, Plaut M, Normal PS, Lichtenstein LM. Inflammatory mediators in late antigen-induced rhinitis. N Engl J Med 1985;313:65–70.
6. Bascom R, Pipkorn U, Lichtenstein LM, Naclerio RM. The influx of inflammatory cells into nasal washings during the late response to antigen challenge effect of systemic steroid pretreatment. Am Rev Respir Dis 1988;138:406–412.
7. Pipkorn U, Proud D, Lichtenstein LM, Kagey-Sobotka A, Normal PS, Naclerio RM. Inhibition of mediator release in allergic rhinitis by pretreatment with topical glucocorticosteroids. N Engl J Med 1987;316:1506–1510.
8. Varney VA, Jacobson MR, Sudderick RM, Robinson DS, Irani A-MA, Schwartz LB, Mackay IS, Kay AB, Durham SR. Immunohistology of the nasal mucosa following allergen-induced rhinitis. Identification of activated T lymphocytes, eosinophils and neutrophils. Am Rev Respir Dis 1992;145:170–176.
9. Durham SR, Ying S, Varney VA, Jacobson MR, Sudderick RM, Mackay IS, Kay AB, Hamid QA. Cytokine messenger RNA expression for IL-3, IL-4, IL-5 and GM-CSF in the nasal mucosa after local allergen provocation: relationship to tissue eosinophilia. J Immunol 1992;148:2390–2394.

10. Hamid Q, Barkans J, Robinson DS, Durham SR, Kay AB. Co-expression of CD25 and CD3 in atopic allergy and asthma. Immunology 1992;75:659–663.
11. Ying S, Durham SR, Jacobson MR, Rak S, Lowhagen O, Kay AB, Hamid QA. T lymphocytes and mast cells express messenger for the interleukin-4 in the nasal mucosa in allergen-induced rhinitis. Immunology 1994;82:200–206.
12. Ying S, Durham SR, Barkans J, Masuyama K, Jacobson M, Rak S, Löwhagen O, Moqbel R, Kay AB, Hamid QA. T cells are the principal source of interleukin-5 mRNA in allergen-induced rhinitis. Am J Resp Cell Mol Biol 1993;9:356–360.
13. Rak S, Jacobson MR, Sudderick RM, Masuyama K, Kay AB, Hamid Q, Lowhagen O, Durham SR. Influence of prolonged treatment with topical corticosteroid (fluticasone propionate) on early and late phase nasal responses and cellular infiltration in the nasal mucosa after allergen challenge. Clin Exp Allergy 1994;24:930–939.
14. Masuyama K, Jacobson MR, Rak S, Meng Q, Sudderick RM, Kay AB, Lowhagen O, Hamid Q, Durham SR. Topical glucocorticosteroid (fluticasone propionate) inhibits cytokine mRNA expression for interleukin-4 (IL-4) in the nasal mucosa in allergic rhinitis. Immunology 1994;82:192–199.
15. Schleimer RP, Sterdinsky SA, Kaiser J, Bickel CA, Kleng DA, Tomioka K, et al. IL-4 induces adherence of human eosinophils and basophils but not neutrophils to endothelium associated with expression of VCAM-1. J Immunol 1992;148:1086.
16. Sim T, Alum R, Grant TA. Secretion of chemokines and other cytokines in allergen-induced nasal responses: inhibition by topical steroid treatment. Am J Resp Crit Care Med 1995; 152(3):927–933.
17. Varney VA, Hamid QA, Gaga M, Ying S, Jacobson M, Frew AJ, Kay AB, Durham SR. Influence of grass pollen immunotherapy on cellular infiltration and cytokine mRNA expression during allergen-induced late-phase cutaneous responses. J Clin Invest 1993;92:644–651.
18. Durham SR, Ying S, Varney VA, Jacobson MR, Sudderick RM, Mackay IS, Kay AB, Hamid QA. Grass pollen immunotherapy inhibits allergen-induced infiltration of CD4+ T lymphocytes and eosinophils in the nasal mucosa and increases the number of cells expressing messenger RNA for interferon-gamma. J Allergy Clin Immunol 1996;97:1356–1365.
19. Durham SR. New insights into mechanisms of immunotherapy. Eur Arch Oto-Rhino-Laryngol 1995;252(suppl 1):564–567.
20. Secrist H, Chelea CJ, Wen Y, Marshall JD, Umetsu DT. Allergen immunotherapy decreases interleukin-4 production in CD4 T cells from allergic individuals. J Exp Med 178:2123–2130.
21. Jutel M, Pichler WJ, Skrbric D, Urwyler A, Dahinden C, Muller UR. 1995. Bee venom immunotherapy results in decrease of IL-4 and IL-5 and increase of IFN-γ secretion in specific allergen stimulated T cells cultures. J Immunol 1995; 154:4181–4194.
22. Pipkorn U, Karlsson G, Enerback L. The cellular response of the human allergic mucosa to natural allergen exposure. J Allergy Clin Immunol 1988; Dec; 82(6): 1046–1054.
23. Viegas M, Gomez E, Brooks J, Gatland D, Davies RJ. Effect of the pollen season on nasal mast cells. Br Med J 1987; 294:414.

24. Bentley AM, Jacobson MR, Cumberworth V, Barkans JA, Moqbel R, Schwartz LB, Irani A-MA, Kay AB, Durham SR. Immunohistology of the nasal mucosa in seasonal allergic rhinitis: increases in activated eosinophils and epithelial mast cells. J Allergy Clin Immunol 1992;89:821–829.
25. Jacobson MR, Juliusson S, Lowhagen R, Durham SR. Influence of topical corticosteroids (fluticasone propionate) on seasonal symptoms and nasal epithelial T lymphocytes in patients with summer hayfever [abstract]. J Allergy Clin Immunol 1995; 95:256.
26. Juliusson S, Karlsson G, Jacobson MR, Durham SR. Topic fluticasone propionate reduces symptoms in hayfever after nasal allergen challenge [abstract]. J Allergy Clin Immunol 1995;95:194.
27. Masuyama K, Jacobson M, Julisson S. Lowhagen O, Kay AB, Hamid Q, Durham SR. Topical corticosteroid (fluticasone propionate) inhibits seasonal increases in IL-5 messenger RNA+ cells in the nasal mucosa [abstract]. J Allergy Clin Immunol 1995;95:300.
28. Lund V. International consensus report on the diagnosis and management of rhinitis. Allergy 1994; 49:(suppl 19).
29. Bradding P, Feather IH, Howarth PH, Mueller R, roberts JA, Britten K, bews JP, Hunt TC, Okayama Y, Heusser CH. Interleukin 4 is localized to and released by human mast cells. J Exp Med 1992 Nov 1; 176(5):1381–1386.
30. Ohno I, Lea R, Finotto S, Marshall J, Denburg J, Dolovich J, Gauldie J, Jordana M. Am J Respir Cell Mol Biol 1991 Dec; 5(6):505–510.
31. Terada N, Konno, A, Tada H, Shirotori K, Ishikawa K, and Togawa K. (1992). The effect of recombinant human interleukin-5 on eosinophil accumulation and degranulation in human nasal mucosa. J Allergy Clin Immunol 90; 160–168.

# 3

# Interleukin-5 and the Interleukin-5 Receptor in Asthma

**DOUGLAS S. ROBINSON**

Imperial College School of Medicine at the National Heart and Lung Institute
London, England

## I. Introduction

An association between the eosinophil and asthma has long been recognized (1,2). Current asthma definitions include the presence of an eosinophil-rich inflammatory infiltrate in the bronchial mucosa (3). Eosinophils have unique basic granule proteins: major basic protein (MBP), eosinophil cationic protein (ECP), eosinophil peroxidase (EPO), and eosinophil protein X (EPX) (4). Major basic protein was shown to damage respiratory epithelium in vitro, in concentrations present in sputa from asthmatic subjects (5), and will induce bronchial hyperresponsiveness when introduced into the airways of monkeys (6). Similarly, ECP is toxic to airway epithelium, and increased concentrations of ECP can be detected in blood, sputa, and bronchoalveolar lavage fluid from asthmatic subjects (7–9). These mechanisms thus likely contribute to the airway hyperresponsiveness that characterises asthma, and eosinophil synthesis of lipid mediators such as platelet activating factor (PAF) and leukotriene $C_4$ may also play a role in acute bronchospasm in response to allergen, infection or irritants (4). Eosinophil infiltration of both bronchial biopsies and bronchoalveolar lavage fluid from atopic asthmatics was noted in early bronchoscopic studies of asthma (10–12), and correlations with epithelial damage were noted in some studies (12).

The dependence of eosinophil responses on T lymphocytes was described in the 1970s (13,14), and the cloning of interleukin-5 (IL-5) as a T-cell-derived eosinophil-specific cytokine in 1986 provided the link between T-cell activation and eosinophilic disease (15,16). IL-5 promotes eosinophil differentiation from hematopoietic precursors (17). Whilst IL-3 and granulocyte macrophage colony stimulating factor (GM-CSF) act in early development from CD34+ progenitors, IL-5 acts in eosinophil maturation, although IL-5 alone appears sufficient for eosinophil development, as shown in mice transgenic for IL-5 under the CD2 promoter (18). IL-5 promotes tissue survival of eosinophils by mechanisms that include antagonism of programmed cell death (19,20). In vitro studies show weak agonist activity of IL-5 in terms of chemotaxis (21,22), and degranulation (23). Most data suggest that IL-5 acts as a priming factor for chemotaxis (21), adhesion (24), degranulation (23), lipid synthesis (25), and cytotoxicity (26).

IL-5 was initially shown to be derived from $CD4^+$ T cells and is one of the defining cytokines of the Th2 T-cell subset as initially described for murine T-cell clones by Mosmann et al. (27). There is now a considerable body of evidence for a human equivalent of Th2-like T cells and that this is the predominant pattern seen in allergen-specific T-cell clones derived both from blood and tissues of atopic donors (27–31). Th2 T cells also produce IL-4, but not interferon-γ (IFN-γ), and thus provide B-cell help for IgE switching (32). It is therefore an attractive hypothesis that activation of a Th2-like allergen-specific T-cell population drives atopic allergic inflammation in asthma.

### A. T-Cell Activation in Asthma

In support of the hypothesis that T lymphocytes produce IL-5 and drive airway inflammation in asthma, the numbers of activated T-cells in peripheral blood was markedly elevated in patients admitted to hospital with acute severe asthma ("status asthmaticus") when compared with control subjects (34). Cells expressing CD25 (the IL-2 receptor), HLA-DR, and very late antigen-1 (VLA-1). CD25 and VLA-1 markers were confined almost exclusively to the $CD4^+$ population of cells and the numbers of $CD4/CD25^+$ cells decreased after successful treatment with corticosteroids. Furthermore, there was a direct correlation between the numbers of activated peripheral blood T-cells and airway narrowing as measured by the peak expiratory flow rate (PEFR). Serum concentrations of the soluble IL-2R were also elevated in patients with acute severe asthma as compared to controls and the values decreased in association with corticosteroid therapy producing clinical improvement.

Bronchoscopy of asthmatic subjects demonstrated marked epithelial fragility even in mild asthmatics, which was closely linked to airway hyperreactivty (12). In the same study (in which cell counts were performed on transmission electron microscopy sections) a striking increase in the number of "irregularly shaped" lymphocytes in the lamina propria and submucosa of symptomatic asthmatics was noted. Immunohistochemical studies demonstrated a significant increase in the numbers of $CD25^+$ cells in bronchial biopsies from asthmatics compared with nonasthmatic atopic and normal control subjects (35). At the same time an increase in the numbers of eosinophils in asthma compared to controls was confirmed. Bradley et al. (10) extended these observations by demonstrating positive correlations between the total numbers of T cells ($CD3^+$) and activated $EG2^+$ eosinophils, between $CD3^+$ and $CD25^+$ cells and between $CD25^+$ and $EG2^+$ cells. Furthermore, the ratio of $EG2^+$ to $CD45^+$ cells (total leucocytes) cells correlated with the methacholine PC20. Therefore this study supported the hypothesis that activated (CD25) T-cells released products which regulated recruitment of eosinophils into the airway wall, and therby disease severity. By double immunofluorescence it was possible to establish that the majority (>85%) of $CD25^+$ cells were indeed T-cells (36).

The increase in activated airway T cells in atopic asthma, as compared to normal controls, was also confirmed by flow cytometric analysis of BAL cells, and a correlation was shown between $CD4^+/CD25^+$ lymphocytes and eosinophils in BAL (37–39).

These studies, in relatively mild asthmatics, had failed to reveal increases in the local numbers of total ($CD3^+$) T cells or either $CD4^+$ or $CD8^+$ subsets. Azzawai et al. (40) measured T-cell and B-cells in post-mortem cases of fatal asthma and compared with cystic fibrosis (CF) and nonasthmatic cases of sudden death matches for age and sex. Tissue eosinophilia was significantly greater in asthma compared to CF or the nonasthmatic controls. The mean numbers of T-cells ($MT\text{-}1^+$) in the asthma and CF groups were approximately twice those in the controls. B-cell ($MB2^+$) numbers were similar in the asthma and sudden death groups, but were increased in CF. Thus the immunopathology of death from asthma was characterized by a high T:B-cell ratio and the presence of relatively large numbers of activated ($EG2^+$) eosinophils. This suggested that increases in the total numbers of $CD3^+$ cells, as opposed to activated T lymphocytes, may only become apparent in severe disease.

## II. IL-5 in Asthma

Measurement of IL-5 in serum and airway samples from asthmatics was hampered by the lack of sensitive immunoassays, but eosinophil survival activity was demonstrated in serum from asthmatic subjects, and in supernatant from cultured blood CD4 cells, that was inhibited by neutralizing antibodies to IL-5 and GM-CSF (41). More recently IL-5 was detected by ELISA in serum from subjects with symptomatic exacerbations of asthma (42) and in children with asthma (43). IL-5 was also detected in the serum of chronic severe asthma patients with persistent airway narrowing, even when they were receiving oral corticosteroid therapy (44). Measurement of inflammatory mediators in blood in asthma is clearly easier than examining airway samples directly. It may be an indrect assessment of "spill over" into the circulation for airways inflammation, as in detecting activated CD4 lymphocytes, or eosinophil granule proteins (8,34). However, recent animal work suggests that detecting circulating IL-5 asthmatics may be of much greater significance. Collins et al. (45) showed evidence for synergy between local eotaxin acting as to attract eosinophils from the circulation to the site of inflammation, and intravenous IL-5 which mobilized eosinophils from the bone marrow. This raises the possibility that IL-5 acts almost as a hormone, with IL-5 released from the inflamed airway circulating to mobilize eosinophils from the bone marrow and prime for subsequent activation at the sites of allergic inflammation (Fig. 1). The presence of IL-5 in the circulation of asthmatic subjects lends support to such a hypothesis.

Investigation of IL-5 expression in the airway in asthma initially focused on the identification of mRNA transcripts. By in situ hybridization, Hamid et al. demonstrated increased numbers of cells expressing mRNA for IL-5 in bronchial biopsies obtained from asthmatic subjects when compared to normal controls (46). Furthermore, there was a correlation between numbers of cells expressing IL-5 mRNA and eosinophil numbers detected by EG2 immunostaining.

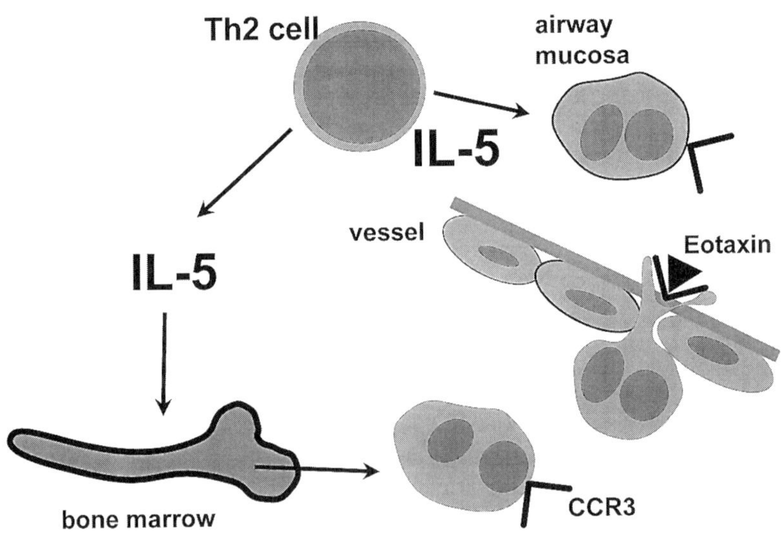


**Figure 1** Proposed actions of IL-5 in eosinophil recruitment to asthmatic airways. IL-5 is released from airway cells in response to allergen and acts distantly to promote eosinophilopoiesis and to prime eosinophils for chemotactic actions of chemokines such as eotaxin. At the site of inflammation IL-5 primes for adherence and activation and prolongs tissue survival of eosinophils.

This finding was confirmed by study of bronchoalveolar lavage cells where an increased proportion of cells expressed IL-5, together with IL-4, IL-3, GM-CSF, and IL-2, but not IFN-γ mRNA, when compared to healthy nonatopic control subjects (47). IL-5 mRNA expression in BAL cells from asthmatic subjects was related to clinical severity of asthma as assessed by symptom score, lung function measures, and bronchial responsiveness to methacholine (48). More recently we have extended these findings using RT-PCR to provide a semiquantitative assessment of IL-5 mRNA copy number in bronchial biopsies and to confirm increased expression in atopic asthma compared to control subjects (49). In addition, immunohistochemistry using a monoclonal antibody to IL-5 showed increased numbers of cells expressing IL-5 protein when compared to control subjects (50) (Fig. 2). IL-5 protein was also detected in concentrated BAL fluid from asthmatic subjects, but not controls (51).

## III. The Cell Source of IL-5 in Asthma

Although IL-5 was described as a T-cell product (52), it is now clear that a number of other cell types have the potential to produce this cytokine and others relevant to allergic inflammation. In particular, human mast cells and eosino-

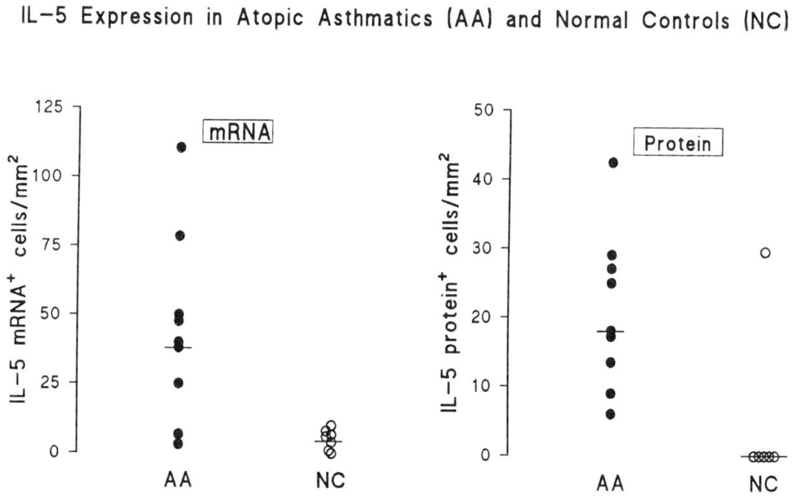


**Figure 2** IL-5 mRNA and protein expression in bronchial biopsies from atopic asthmatic and control subjects. IL-5 mRNA expression was assessed by in situ hybridization using $^{35}$S-labeled riboprobes, and positive cells per square millimeter bronchial biopsy were counted. Monoclonal antibody to IL-5 was used for immunohistochemistry and positive cells enumerated in the same way.

phils were shown to have the potential for IL-5 production (53,54). When BAL T cells were enriched by immunomagnetic separation the majority of IL-5 mRNA was shown to be associated with T cells (47). This result was confirmed with combined immunohistochemistry and in situ hybridization, which showed that 70 to 80% of the mRNA signal in both BAL and bronchial biopsies from asthmatic subjects originated from CD3 T lymphocytes with a minor contribution from mast cells and eosinophils (55). However, in contrast to these findings, Bradding et al. reported that most of the IL-5 protein detected in bronchial biopsies by immunohistology was associated with mast cells (53). The reason for this apparent discrepancy may lie in the finding that both mast cells and eosinophils store cytokines in their granules (56,57), whereas T cells secrete cytokine rapidly and may do so in a directed manner to cells they contact (58). This may lead to detection of cytokine protein in the granules of mast cells and eosinophils by immunohistochemistry but a failure to detect T-cell associated cytokine by this technique. We have recently examined this possibility and confirmed that substantially fewer IL-5 protein positive cells were detected by immunohistochemistry than were those expressing IL-5 mRNA by in situ hybridization in the same bronchial biopsies. Furthermore, IL-5 protein was not detected in T cells in the biopsies by immunohistochemistry, but could be visualized in T cells that had been stimulated in vitro in the presence of monensin, which blocks the Golgi apparatus thus preventing secretion of cytokines (50). Thus, on balance, current evidence suggests that the major source of IL-5 in the airway in asthma is the T lymphocyte, although there are contributions from both mast cells and eosinophils which may serve as important amplifying signals in the inflammatory cascade.

In addition to CD4 T cells IL-5 production by CD8 T cells has been described (59) and a Tc2-subtype of CD8 T cell analogous to Th2 has been designated (60). Production of IL-5 by BAL CD8 T cells was detected in a mouse model of virus-induced airway hyperreactivity (61). Till et al. raised allergen-specific T cell lines from CD4 and CD8 human BAL cells and demonstrated IL-5 production from both (62). More recently we have examined the contribution of CD8 T cells to the IL-5 mRNA expressing population in the bronchial mucosa in asthma. Combined immunohistology and in situ hybridization showed that 10 to 50% of IL-5 mRNA signal was associated with CD8 cells (50). Whether these CD8 T cells are HLA class I restricted and what antigens they respond to remains to be determined.

### A. Allergen Challenge

Inhalation challenge of sensitised asthmatic subjects with allergen extract leads to immediate airway narrowing within 15 min which may persist for 1–2 hours and is termed the early asthmatic response. This may be followed at 3–8 hours by further airway narrowing which accompanied by increased airway responsiveness to nonspecific stimuli and may be folllowed by increased symptoms for several days (63,64). This late asthamtic response is also associated with airway hyperexpansion (65). Allergen challenge has been used as a model for airway inflammation in asthma, and is widely used in drug testing. With the advent of bronchoscopic study of asthma, this has been complemented by direct instillation of allergen extract into the segmental airways in a local allergen challenge.

Examination of cytokine gene expression at 24 hours after allergen challenge showed increased mRNA$^+$ cells for IL-4, IL-5, and GM-CSF in both BAL and biopsies from atopic asthmatic subjects (66,67). These changes were predominantly localized to T lymphocytes, and GM-CSF mRNA was demonstrated in lymphocytes and macrophages after allergen challenge in a separate study (68). IL-5 was measured by ELISA in lavage fluid following local allergen challenge (69). Correlations amongst IL-5 mRNA expression, T-cell activation and eosinophil numbers in BAL 24 hours after challenge and the preceding fall in $FEV_1$ during the late response supported a link between T cell activation of eosinophils and clinical effects of allergen inhalation (67). Furthermore Virchow et al. (70), using segmental allergen challenge found a correlation between IL-5 concentrations, eosinophil numbers, and activated T-cells.

## IV. Nonatopic Asthma

Eosinophil infiltration of the bronchial mucosa and T-cell activation were present in both occupational (toluene di-isocyanate induced) and intrinsic asthmatics (71,72). Recently we have compared IL-5 mRNA expression by in situ hybridization and RT-PCR and IL-5 protein by immunohistochemistry in bronchial biopsies from atopic asthmatics, nonatopic (intrinsic) asthmatics, and atopic and nonatopic control subjects (49). IL-5 mRNA and protein expression was elevated to a similar degree in both atopic and nonatopic asthmatics when compared to the control groups. Furthermore, the cell phenotype expressing IL-5 mRNA was also similar in atopic and nonatopic asthmatics, with the majority signal localized to CD4$^+$ T cells, with minor contributions from CD8 cells, mast cells, and eosinophils. Walker et al. also reported detectable IL-5 in concentrated BAL fluid from both atopic and nonatopic asthmatics (51). The antigen responsible for initiating IL-5 production in nonatopic asthma remains to be established.

## V. The Effect of Corticosteroid Treatment on IL-5 Expression in Asthma

Several studies have shown that successful treatment of asthma by inhaled corticosteroids or allergen avoidance was associated with decreased eosinophil infiltration and activation and reduction in bronchial mucosal T-cell activation (73–77). In an open study Djukanovic et al. (73) demonstrated a significant decrease in mucosal T-cell, eosinophil, and mast cell numbers after six weeks of therapy with inhaled beclomethasone dipropionate (BDP). This was accompanied by clinical improvement. Using a similar experimental design Wilson et al. (74) demonstrated decreases in $CD25^+$ and $HLA\text{-}DR^+$ cells but not in the total numbers of $CD3^+$, $CD4^+$, or $CD8^+$ cells after treatment with BDP. Similarly, high altitude climate therapy reduced both the numbers of activated T-cells in peripheral blood as well as the degree of airway obstruction in children with house dust mite allergic asthma (75). We examined cytokine mRNA expression in BAL and bronchial biopsies obtained before and after a two week course of oral prednisolone or placebo in a double blind parallel group study of symptomatic asthmatics. Patients receiving prednisolone showed reduced bronchial responsiveness to methacholine and a signficant reduction in eosinophil numbers in BAL and biopsies. In addition by in situ hybridization, there were significant reductions in numbers of cells expression mRNA for IL-4, IL-5 and GM-CSF in both BAL and bronchial biopsies in those randomised to prednisolone, but not subjects receiving placebo (78). Similar findings were reported by Leung et al. (79) in a group of asthmatic subjects showing symptomatic and spirometric improvement after prednisolone treatment.

Glucocorticorticosteroids are remarkably effective in the majority of asthmatics in controlling symptoms. In vitro, very low doses inhibit T-cell proliferative responses to mitogens; concentrations of methylprednisolone as low as $10^{-10}$ M being effective in inhibiting human T-cell expansion (80). A small proportion of asthmatic subjeccts do not show clinical improvement with glucocorticoid treatment (81). Formal definitions vary, but most would encompass failure to show a 10% or more increase in forced expiratory volume in one second ($FEV_1$) after two weeks treatment with 40 mg per day prednisolone or equivalent in subjects with asthma symptoms and demonstrated reversibility of airflow obstruction of at least 15% to inhaled β agonists. Small alterations in glucocorticoid pharmacokinetics and ligand binding affinity are seen in these subjects, but are probably insufficient to account for the clinical features. Peripheral blood mononuclear cells from patients with corticosteroid-resistant asthma proliferated to phytohaemagglutinin in the presence of relatively high doses of methylprednisolone (82,83). A clear relationship was shown between clinical responsiveness to steroids and the in vitro effect of steroids on mitogen-driven colony counts. It has been suggested that steroid-resistance might arise from the cytokine environment of the T-cell. Sher et al. (84) found that the majority of patients with steroid-resistant (SR) asthma had a reversible defect in GR binding affinity which could be sustained in vitro by the addition of the combination of IL-2 and IL-4 but not the individual cytokines. Furthermore, in vitro incubation of normal T-cells with the combination of IL-2 and IL-4, in the absence of $IFN_\gamma$, reduced their GR binding affinity to the levels seen in SR asthma (85). On this basis they suggested two types of glucocorticosteroid resistance: a reduced affinity of GR binding confined to T lymphocytes which reverted to normal after 48 hours in culture, and a much less common reduction in GR density (in only two of 17 SR patients) which did not normalize with prolonged incubation (85). This supported the concept that there may be different types of steroid resistance in asthma. These in vitro data suggested that pattern of cytokine gene expression may play a role in determining steroid resistance. For this reason Leung et al. (79) used the technique of in situ hybridization to examine whether airway cells from SR asthmatics versus steroid-sensitive (SS) asthmatics expressed different patterns of mRNA for cytokines, particularly after treatment with oral steroids. Steroid sensitive asthmatics responded well to glucocorticoids and this was accompanied by decrease in the numbers of cells expressing mRNA for IL-4 and IL-5 and an increase in $IFN_{\gamma}$ transcripts. In contrast, after prednisolone therapy, SR asthmatics had no significant changes in either the number of BAL cells expressing mRNA for IL-4 or IL-5. Furthermore instead of a decrease there was an increase in the numbers of $IFN_{\gamma}$ $mRNA^{+}$ cells. These findings suggested that SR asthma is associated with dysregulation of expression of the genes encoding Th2/Th1 cytokines in airway cells and is compatible with the concept that a combination of IL-2 and IL-4 induce GR binding affinity and T-cell responsiveness to glucocorticoids. Alexander et al. (44) were able to detect IL-5 in the serum of patients with continued severe chronic asthma despite oral prednisolone treatment. These findings further support a link between airways expression of IL-5 and clinical manifestations of asthma.

Studies by Adcock et al. (86) have suggested dysregulation of transcription factors in glucocorticoid-resistant asthma, with increase expression of the pro-inflammatory AP-1 interfering with steroid actions by cytoplasmic binding to the glucocorticoid receptor. Whether there are alterations in the IL-5 promoter/emhancer in such subjects is unknown, but warrants investigation.

### A. Cyclosporin A

It is generally accepted that the primary mode of action of cyclosporin A is through inhibition of T-cell activation secondary to blocking of early calcium-dependent transcription of messenger RNA encoding several cytokines (87). Experience with the use of cyclosporin A is chronic steroid-dependent asthma supports the T-cell hypothesis, although it is accepted that this agent also has effects on cytokine synthesis and release from granulocytes, including basophils, mast cells, and eosinophils.

In a group of severe steroid-dependent asthamtics treatment over a 12-week period with cyclosporin A at low dosage (5 mg/kg/day) was associated with improvement in lung function and a reduction in the numbers of disease exacerbations requiring an increase in corticosteroid dosage (88). Cyclosporin A also has a corticosteroid-sparing effect in steroid-dependent asthmatics (89). In both studies lung function concurrently improved despite the reduction in corticosteroid dose, although in one study this improvement was small.

Since cyclosporin A inhibits both cytokine mRNA transcription by T-cells and mast cell degranulation in vitro it might be expected to inhibit both the EAR and LAR as well as the associated elevation in blood eosinophils. Sihra et al. (90) have recently demonstrated in a double-blind, placebo-controlled, randomized crossover trial that, compared to placebo treatment, CsA reduced the magnitude of the LAR but not the EAR following allergen challenge. This provides strong indirect evidence that CsA is effective in this model of asthmatic allergic inflammation through its effects on the T-cell as opposed to mast cell and basophils.

## VI. IL-5 Receptor Expression in Asthma

The receptors for IL-5, IL-3, and GM-CSF were cloned by Tavernier et al. (91) and Kitamura et al. (92) in 1991. This revealed a common β subunit for all three cytokine receptors which is associated with JAK kinases in receptor signaling, and a cytokine specific α chain which binds the cytokine. Lopez and others used ligand binding studies demonstrated that IL-5Rα subunit expression was confined to eosinophils (93), and we have recently used monoclonal antibodies to confirm these findings and to show that IL-5Rα expression was also seen on peripheral blood basophils, although the major receptor expressed by basophils was the IL-3Rα (94). It is possible that this explains relative differences in cytokine sensitivity, with eosinophils primarily responsive to IL-5 and GM-CSF, and basophils to IL-3.

Tavernier demonstrated alternate splicing of the IL-5Rα gene to yield membrane associated (m) and soluble (s) isoforms of the receptor (95). With in vitro culture systems, the sIL-5Rα antagonized the effects of IL-5, presumably by direct competition for binding. Whether a similar system operates in vivo remains to be established.

We have recently examined expression of the two IL-5Rα isoforms in bronchial mucosal biopsies from asthmatic subjects (96). There were increased numbers of cells expressing both mIL-5Rα and sIL-5Rα in bronchial biopsies from atopic and nonatopic asthmatic subjects when compared to nonasthmatic control subjects, and over 90% of cells expressing IL-5R were eosinophils. Furthermore there was an inverse correlation between mIL-5Rα positive cell numbers and $FEV_1$ (a measure of airways obstruction), whereas sIL-5Rα was directly correlated with $FEV_1$. This raised the possibility that the more severe the asthma, the more mIL-5Rα was expressed and the less sIL-5Rα was encoded. Such a switch from sIL-5Rα to mIL-5Rα might lead to increased IL-5 sensitivity of eosinophils in the airway, increasing survivial, and functional priming. These interesting results need confirmation and further study.

## VII. Conclusion: IL-5 as a Therapeutic Target in Asthma

Taken together, there is now compelling evidence that IL-5 is a major player in the eosinophilic inflammation of the bronchial mucosa in asthma. It is worth raising a note of caution in that although as a whole, airway eosinophilia correlates with clinical measures of asthma severity, there are patients with severe asthma with relatively mild eosinophil infiltration (8,9), and a subset of patients dying of asthma without evidence of eosinophil degranulation is described (97). However, in most animal models targeting IL-5 has been spectactularly successful in ablating late phase bronchial hyperresponsiveness and eosinophil influx in allergen challenge models in rodents (98,99; see also Chap. 7). In a monkey model of allergen challenge, a single dose of humanized anti-IL-5 antibody blocked hyperresponsiveness for up to three months (100). The application of such reagents in human studies, first of allergen challenge, but more importantly in clinical asthma will be the ultimate test of the IL-5 hypothesis of asthma: these experiments are eagerly awaited. Development of IL-5-specific therapy based on increased understanding of IL-5 gene regulation should also yield exciting therapeutic agents (see Chap. 15).

## References

1. Horn BR, Robin ED, Theodore J, Van Kessel A. Total eosinophil counts in the management of bronchial asthma. N Engl J Med 1975;292:2252–2255.
2. Durham SR, Kay AB. Eosinophils, bronchial hyperreactivity and late-phase reactions. Clin Allergy 1985;15:411–418.
3. American Thoracic Society. Standards for the diagnosis and care of patients with chronic obstructive pulmonary disease (COPD) and asthma. Am Rev Resp Dis 1987;136:225–244.
4. Gleich GJ. The eosinophil and bronchial asthma: current understanding. J Allergy Clin Immunol 1990;85:422–436.
5. Frigas E, Loergering DA, Solley G, Farrow G, Gleich GJ. Elevated levels of the eosinophil major basic protein in the sputum of patients with bronchial asthma. Mayo Clin Proc 1981;56:345–353.
6. Gundel RH, Letts LG, Gleich GJ. Human eosinophil major basic protein induces airway constriction and airway hyperresponsiveness in primates. J Clin Invest 1991;87:1470–1473.
7. Bousquet J, Chanez P, Lacoste JY, Barneon G, Ghavanian N, Enander I, Venge

P, Ahlstedt S, Simony-Lafontaine J, Godard P, Michel FB. Eosinophilic inflammation in asthma. N Engl J Med 1990;323:1033–1039.

8. Robinson DS, Assoufi B, Durham SR, Kay AB. Eosinophil cationic protein (ECP) and eosinophil protein X (EPX) concentrations in serum and bronchial lavage fluid in asthma. Effect of prednisolone treatment. Clin Exp Allergy 1995;25:1118–1127.
9. Wardlaw AJ, Dunnette S, Gleich GH, Collins JV, Kay AB. Eosinophils and mast cells in bronchoalveolar lavage in mild asthma: relaionship to bronchial reactivity. Am Rev Respir Dis 1988;137:62–69.
10. Bradley BL, Azzawai M, Jacobson M, Assoufi B, Collins JV, Irani A-MA, Schwartz LB, Durham SR, Jeffery PK, Kay AB. Eosinophils, T-lymphocytes, mast cells, neutrophils and macrophages in bronchial biopsy specimens from atopic subjects with asthma: Comparison with biopsy specimens from atopic subjects without asthma and normal control subjects and relationship to bronchial hyperresponsiveness. J Allergy Clin Immunol 1990;88:661–674.
11. Beasley R, Roche WR, Roberts JA, Holgate ST. Cellular events in the bronchi before and after bronchial provocation. Am Rev Respir Dis 1989;139:806–817.
12. Jeffery PK, Wardlaw AJ, Nelson FC, Collins JV, Kay AB. Bronchial biopsies in asthma: an ultrastructural, quantitative study and correlation with hyperreactivity. Am Rev Respir Dis 1989;140:1745–1753.
13. Basten A, Beeson PB. Mechanism of eosinophlia. II. The role of the lymphocyte. J Exp Med 1970;131:1288–1305.
14. Raghavachar A, Fleischer S, Frickhofen N, Heimpel H, Fleischer B. T lymphocyte control of human eosinophil granulopoiesis. J Immunol 1987;139:3753–3758.
15. Campbell HD, Tucker WQJ, Hort Y, Martinson ME, Mayo G, Clutterbuck EJ, Sanderson CJ, Young IG. Molecular cloning, nucleotide sequence and expression of the gene encoding human eosinophil differentiation factor (interleukin 5). Proc Natl Acad Sci USA 1987;84:6629–6633.
16. Kinashi T, Harada N, Severinson E, Tanabe T, Sideras P, Konishi M, Azuma C, Tominaga A, Bergstedt-Lindqvist S, Takahashi M, Matsuda F, Yaoita Y, Takatsu K, Honjo T. Cloning of complementary DNA encoding T cell replacement factor and identity with B cell factor II. Nature 1986;324:70–72.
17. Clutterbuck EJ, Hirst EM, Sanderson CJ. Human interleukin 5 (IL-5) regulates the production of eosinophils in human bone marrow cultures: comparison and interaction with IL-1, IL-3, IL-6, and GM-CSF. Blood 1989;73:1504–1512.
18. Dent LA, Strath M, Mellor AL, Sanderson CJ. Eosinophilia in transgenic mice expressing interleukin 5. J Exp Med 1990;172:1425–1431.
19. Stern M, Meagher L, Savill J, Haslett C. Apoptosis in human eosinophils: programmed cell death in the eosinophil leads to phagocytosis by macrophages and is modulated by IL-5. J Immunol 1992;148:3543.
20. Her E, Frazer J, Austen KF, Owen WF Jr. Eosinophil hematopoietins antagonize the programmed cell death of eosinophils. J Clin Invest 1991;88:1982–1987.
21. Sehmi R, Wardlaw AJ, Cromwell O, Kurihara K, Waltmann P, Kay AB. Interleukin 5 selectively enhances the chemotactic response of eosinophils obtained from normal but not eosinophilic donors. Blood 1992;79:2952–2959.
22. Warringa RAJ, Koenderman L, Kok PTM, Krekniet J, Bruijnzeel PLB. Modu-

lation and induction of eosinophil chemotaxis by granulocyte-macrophage colony stimulating factor and interleukin-3. Blood 1991;77:2694–2700.
23. Fujisawa T, Abu-Ghazaleh R, Kita H, Sanderson CJ, Gleich GJ. Regulatory effect of cytokines on eosinophil degranulation. J Immunol 1990;144:642–646.
24. Walsh GM, Hartnell A, Wardlaw AJ, Kurihara K, Sanderson CJ, Kay AB. IL-5 enhances the in vitro adhesion of human eosinophils, but not neutrophils in a leucocyte integrin (CD11/CD18)-depenent manner. Immunology 1990;71:258–265.
25. Takafuji S, Bischoff SC, De Weck AL, Dahinden CA. IL-3 and IL-5 prime normal human eosinophils to produce leukotriene C4 in response to soluble agonists. J Immunol 1991;147:3855–3861.
26. Lopez AF, Sanderson CJ, Gamble JR, Campbell HD, Young IG, Vadas MA. Recombinant human interleukin 5 is a selective activator of human eosinophil function. J Exp Med 1988;167:219–224.
27. Mosmann TR, Cherwinski H, Bond MW, Gieldin MA, Coffman RL. Two types of murine helper T cell clones. J Immunol 1986;136:2348–2357.
28. Wierenga EA, Snoek M, deGroot C, Chretien I, de Bos J, Jansen HM, Kapsenberg ML. Evidence for compartmentalization of functional subsets of CD4+ T lymphocytes in atopic patients. J Immunol 1990;144:4651–4656.
29. Del Prete GF, De Carli M, Mastromauro C, Macchia D, Biagiotti R, Ricci M, Romagnani S. Purified protein derivative of mycobacterium tuberculosis and excreteory antigens of *Toxocara canis* expand in vitro human T cells with stable and opposite (type 1 T helper or type 2 T helper) profile of cytokine production. J Clin Invest 1991;88:346–350.
30. Romagnani S. Human Th1 and Th2: doubt no more. Immunol Today 1991;12:256–257.
31. Maggi E, Biswas P, Del Prete G, Parronchi P, Macchia D, Simonelli C, Emmi L, De Carli M, Tiri A, Ricci M, Romagnani S. Accumulation of Th2-like helper T cell in the conjunctiva of patients with vernal conjunctivitis. J Immunol 1991;146:1169–1174.
32. van Reijsen FC, Bruijnzeel-Koomen CAFM, Kalthoff FS, Maggi E, Romagnani S, Westland JKT, Mudde GC. Skin-derived aeroallergen-specific T cell clones of Th2 phenotype in patients with atopic dermatitis. J Allergy Clin Immunol 1992;90:184–92.
33. Del Prete GF, Maggi E, Parronchi P, Chretien I, Tiri A, Macchia D, Ricci M, Banchereau J, de Vries J, Romagnani S. IL-4 is an essential factor for the IgE synthesis induced in vitro by human T cell clones and their supernatants. J Immunol 1988;140:4193–4198.
34. Corrigan CJ, Hartnell AH, Kay AB. CD4 T lymphocyte activation in acute severe asthma. Lancet 1988;I:1129–1132.
35. Azzawi M, Bradley B, Jeffery PK, Frew AJ, Wardlaw AJ, Knowles GK, Assoufi B, Collins JV, Durham SR, Kay AB. Idenification of activated T lymphocytes and eosinophils in bronchial biopsies in stable atopic asthma. Am Rev Respir Dis 1990;142:1407–1413.
36. Hamid Q, Barkans J, Robinson DS, Durham SR, Kay AB. Co-expression of CD25 and CD3 in atopic allergy and asthma. Immunology 1992;75:659–663.

37. Robinson DS, Bentley AM, Hartnell AH, Kay AB, Durham SR. Activated memory T helper cells in bronchoalveolar lavage fluid from patients with atopic asthma: relation to asthma symptoms, lung function, and bronchial responsiveness. Thorax 1993;48:26–32.
38. Wilson JW, Djukanovic R, Howarth PH, Holgate ST. Lymphocyte activation in bronchoalveolar lavage and peripheral blood in atopic asthma. Am Rev Respir Dis 1992;145:958–960.
39. Walker C, Kaegi MK, Braun P, Blaser K. Activated T cells and eosinophilia in bronchoalveolar lavages from subjects with asthma correlated with disease severity. J Allergy Clin Immunol 1991;88:935–942.
40. Azzawai M, Johnson PW, Majumdar S, Kay AB, Jeffery PK. T lymphocytes and activated eosinophils in airway mucosa in fatal asthma and cystic fibrosis. Am Rev Respir Dis 1992;145:1477–1482.
41. Walker C, Virchow JC, Bruijnzeel PLB, Blaser K. T cell subsets and their soluble products regulate eosinophilia in allergic and non allergic asthma. J Immunol 1991;146:1829–1835.
42. Corrigan CJ, Hamid Q, North J, Barkans J, Moqbel R, Durham S, Kay AB. Peripheral blood CD4, but not CD8 T lymphocytes in patients with exacerbation of asthma transcribe and translate messenger RNA encoding cytokines which prolong eosinophil survival in the context of a Th2-type pattern: effect of glucocorticoid therapy. Am J Respir Cell Mol Biol 1995;12:567–578.
43. Gemou Engesaeth V, Kay AB, Bush A, Corrigan CJ. Activated peripheral blood CD4 and CD8 lymphocytes in childhood asthma: correlation with eosinopilia and disease severity. Paediatr Allergy Immunol 1994;5:170–177.
44. Alexander AB, Barkans J, Moqbel R, Barnes NC, Kay AB, Corrigan CJ. Serum interleukin 5 concentrations in atopic and non-atopic patients with glucocorticoid-dependent chronic severe asthma. Thorax 1994;49:1231–1233.
45. Collins PD, Marleau S, Griffiths-Johnson DA, Jose PJ, Williams TJ. Cooperation between interleukin 5 and the chemokine eotaxin to induce eosinophil accumulation in vivo. J Exp Med 1995;182:1169–1174.
46. Hamid Q, Azzawi M, Ying S, Moqbel R, Wardlaw AJ, Corrigan CJ, Bradley B, Durham SR, Collins JV, Jeffery PK, Quint DJ, Kay AB. Expression of mRNA for interleukin-5 in mucosal bronchial biopsies from asthma. J Clin Invest 1991;87:1541–1546.
47. Robinson DS, Hamid Q, Ying S, Tsicopoulos A, Barkans J, Bentley AM, Corrigan CJ, Durham SR, Kay AB. Predominant Th2-like bronchoalveolar T lymphocyte population in atopic asthma. N Engl J Med 1992;326:298–304.
48. Robinson DS, Ying S, Bentley AM, Meng Q, North J, Durham SR, Kay AB, Hamid Q. Relationships among numbers of bronchoalveolar lavage cells expressing messenger ribonucleic acid for cytokines, asthma symptoms, and airway methacholine responsiveness in atopic asthma. J Allergy Clin Immunol 1993;92:397–403.
49. Humbert M, Durham SR, Ying S, Kimmitt P, Barkans J, Assoufi B, Pfister R, Menz G, Robinson DS, Kay AB, Corrigan CJ. Bronchial mucosal interleukin-4

(IL-4) and IL-5 expression is a feature of both atopic and non-atopic asthma. Am J Respir Crit Care Med 1996;154:1497–1504.
50. Ying S, Humbert M, Barkans J, Corrigan CJ, Pfister R, Menz G, Larche M, Robinson DS, Durham SR, Kay AB. Expression of IL-4 and IL-5 mRNA and protein product by CD4+ and CD8+ T cells, eosinophils, and mast cells in bronchial biopsies obtained from atopic and non-atopic (intrinsic) asthmatics. J Immunol 1997;158:3539–3544.
51. Walker C, Bode E, Boer L, Hansel TT, Blaser K, Virchow J-C Jr. Allergic and nonallergic asthmatics have distinct patterns of T cell activation and cytokine production in peripheral blood and bronchoalveolar lavage. Am Rev Respir Dis 1992;146:109–115.
52. Sanderson CJ. Interleukin 5, eosinophils and disease. Blood 1992;79:3101–3109.
53. Bradding P, Roberts JA, Britten KM, Montefort S, Djukanovic R, Mueller R, Heusser CH, Howarth PH, Holgate ST. Interleukin-4, -5, and -6 and tumor necrosis factor-alpha in normal and asthmatic airways: evidence for the human mast cell as a source of these cytokines. Am J Respir Cell Mol Biol 1994;10:471–480.
54. Desreumaux P, Janin A, Colombel JF, Prin L, Plumas J, Emilie D, Torpier G, Capron A, Capron M. Interleukin 5 messenger RNA expression by eosinophils in the intestinal mucosa of patients with coeliac disease. J Exp Med 1992;175:293–296.
55. Ying S, Durham SR, Corrigan CJ, Hamid Q, Kay AB. Phenotype of cells expressing mRNA for TH2-type (interleukin-4 and interleukin-5) and TH1-type (interleukin-2 and interferon-γ) cytokines in bronchoalveolar lavage and bronchial biopsies from atopic asthmatics and normal control subjects. Am J Respir Cell Mol Biol 1995;12:477–487.
56. Gordon JR, Galli SJ. Release of both performed and newly synthesised tumour necrosis factor alpha (TNFα)/cachectin by mouse mast cells stimulated via the FCεRI. A mechanism for the sustained action of mast cell-derived TNFα during IgE-depemdent biological responses. J Exp Med 1991;174:103–107.
57. Moqbel R, Levi-Schaffer F, Kay AB. Cytokine generation by eosinophils. J Allergy Clin Immunol 1994;94:1183–1188.
58. Kupfer A, Mosmann TR, Kupfer H. Polarized expression of cytokines in cell conjugates of helper T cells and splenic B cells. Proc Natl Acad Sci USA 1991;88:775–779.
59. Salgame P, Abrams JS, Clayberger C, Goldstein H, Convit J, Modlin RL, Bloom BR. Differing lymphkine profiles of functional subsets of human CD4 and CD8 T cell clones. Science 1991;254:279–282.
60. Mosmann TR, Sad S. The expanding universe of T-cell subsets: Th1, Th2 and more. Immunol Today 1996;17:139–146.
61. Coyle AJ, Erard F, Bertrand C, Walti S, Pircher H, Le Gros G. Virus-specific CD8+ cells can switch to interleukin 5 production and induce airway eosinophilia. J Exp Med 1995;181:1229–1233.
62. Till S, Li B, Durham SR, Humbert M, Assoufi B, Huston D, Dickason R, Jeannin P, Kay AB, Corrigan CJ. Secretion of the eosinophil-active cytokines interleukin

5, granulocyte macrophage colony stimulating factor and interleukin 3 by bronchoalveolar lavage CD4+ and CD8+ T cell lines in atopic asthmatics. Eur J Immunol 1995;25:2727–2731.

63. Durham SR. Late asthmatic responses. Respir Med 1990;84:263–268.
64. Cartier A, Thomson NC, Frith PA, Roberts R, Hargreave FE. Allergen-induced increase in bronchial responsiveness to histamine: relationship to the late asthmatic response and change in airway calibre. J Allergy Clin Immunol 1982;70:170–177.
65. MacIntyre D, Boyd G. Site of airflow obstruction in immediate and late reactions to bronchial challenge with Dermataphagoides pteronyssinus. Clin Allergy 1983;13:213–218.
66. Bentley AM, Meng Q, Robinson DS, Hamid Q, Kay AB, Durham SR. Increases in activated T lymphcytes, eosinophils, and cytokine messenger RNA expression or IL-5 and GM-CSF in bronchial biopsies after allergen inhalation challenge in atopic asthmatics. Am J Respir Cell Mol Biol 1993;8:35–42.
67. Robinson DS, Hamid Q, Bentley AM, Ying S, Kay AB, Durham SR. $CD4^+$ T cell activation, eosinophil recruitment and interleukin 4 (IL-4), IL-5, and GM-CSF messenger RNA expression in bronchoalveolar lavage after allergen inhalation challenge of atopic asthmatics. J Allergy Clin Immunol 1993;92:313–324.
68. Broide DH, Direstein GS. Endobronchial allergen challenge in asthma: demonstration of cellular source of granulocyte macrophage colony-stimulating factor by in situ hybridization. J Clin Invest 1991;88:1048–1053.
69. Sedgwick JB, Calhoun WJ, Gleich GJ, Kita H, Abrams JS, Schwartz LB, Volovitz B, BenYaakov M, Busse W. Immediate and late airway response of allergic rhinitis patients to segmental antigen challenge. Am Rev Respir Dis 1991;144:1274–1281.
70. Virchow JC Jr, Walker C, Hafner D, Kortsik C, Werner P, Matthys H, Kroegel C. T cells and cytokines in bronchoalveolar lavage fluid after segmental allergen provocation in atopic asthma. Am J Respir Crit Care med 1995;151:960–968.
71. Bentley AM, Maestrelli P, Saetta M, Fabbri LM, Robinson DS, Bradley BL, Jeffery PK, Durham SR, Kay AB. Activated T-lymphocytes and eosinophils in the bronchial mucosa in isocyanate-induced asthma. J Allergy Clin Immunol 1992;89:821–829.
72. Bentley AM, Menz G, Storz CHR, Robinson DS, Bradley BL, Jeffery PK, Durham SR, Kay AB. Identification of T lymphocytes, macrophages and activated eosinophils in the bronchial mucosa in intrinsic asthma. Am Rev Respir Dis 1992;146:500–506.
73. Djukanovic R, Wilson JW, Britten KM, Wilson SJ, Walls AF, Roche WR, Howarth PH, Holgate ST. Effect of an inhaled corticosteroid on airway inflammation and symptoms in asthma. Am Rev Respir Dis 1992;145:669–674.
74. Wilson JW, Djukanovic R, Howarth PH, Holgate ST. Inhaled beclomethasone dipropionate downregulates airway lymphocyte activation in atopic asthma. Am J Respir Crit Care Med 1994;149:86–90.
75. Simon HU, Grotzer M, Nikolaizik WH, Blaser K, Schoni MH. High altitude climate therapy reduces peripheralblood T lymphocyte activation, eosinophilia, and bronchial obstruction in children with house-dust mite allergic asthma. Pediatric Pulmonology 1994;17:304–311.

76. Adelroth E, Rosenhall L, Johansson SA, Linden M, Venge P. Inflammatory cells and eosinophilic activity in asthmatics investigated by bronchoalveolar lavage. The effects of antiasthmatic treatment with budesonide or terbutaline. Am Rev Respir Dis 1990;142:91–99.
77. Trigg CJ, Manolitsas ND, Wang J, Calderon MA, McAulay A, Jordan SE, Herdman MJ, Jhalli N, Duddle JM, Hamilton SA, et al. Placebo-controlled immunopathologic study of four months of inhaled corticosteroids in asthma. Am J Respir Crit Care Med 1994;150:17–22.
78. Robinson DS, Hamid Q, Ying S, Bentley AM, Assoufi B, North J, Meng Q, Durham SR, Kay AB. Prednisolone treatment in asthma is associated with modulation of bronchoalveolar lavage cell interleukin-4, interleukin-5, and interferon-gamma cytokine gene expression. Am Rev Respir Dis 1993;148:401–406.
79. Leung DY, Martin RJ, Szefler SJ, Sher ER, Ying S, Kay AB, Hamid Q. Dysregulation of interleukin 4, interleukin 5, and interferon gamma gene expression in steroid-resistant asthma. J Exp Med 1995;181:33–44.
80. Krajewski AS, Wyllie AH. Inhibition of human T lymphocyte colony formation by methylprednisolone. Clin Exp Immunol 1981;46:206-213.
81. Carmichael J, Paterson IC, Diaz P, Crompton GK, Kay AB, Grant IWB. Corticosteroid resistance in chronic asthma. Br Med J 1981;282:1419-1422.
82. Poznansky MC, Gordon ACH, Douglas JG, Krajewski AS, Wylie AH, Grant IWB. Resistance to methylprednisolone in cultures of blood mononuclear cells from glucocorticoid-resistant asthmatic patients. Clin Sci 1984;67:639-645.
83. Poznansky MC, Gordon ACH, Grant IWB, Wylie AH.A cellular abnormality in glucocorticoid resistant asthma. Clin Exp Immunol1985;61:135-142.
84. Sher E, Leung DYM, Surs W, Kam JC, Zieg G, Kamada AK, Szefler SJ. Steroid-resistant asthma. Cellular mechanisms contributing to inadequate response to glucocorticoid therapy. J Clin Invest1994;93:33-39.
85. Kam J, Szefler SJ, Surs W, Sher E, Leung DYM. The combined effects of IL-2 and IL-4 alter the binding affinity of the glucocorticoid receptor. J Immunol 1993;151:3460-3466.
86. Adcock IM, Lane SJ, Brown CR, Lee TH, Barnes PJ. Abnormal glucocorticoid receptor-activator protein 1 interaction in steroid resistant asthma. J Exp Med 1995;182:1951-1958.
87. Schreiber SL, Crabtree GR. The mechanism of action of cyclosporin A and FK 506. Immunol Today 1992;13:136-141.
88. Alexander AG, Barnes NC, Kay AB. Trial of cyclosporin A in corticosteroid-dependent chronic severe asthma. Lancet 1992;339:324-328.
89. Lock SH, Kay AB, Barnes NC. Double-blind, placebo-controlled study of cyclosporin A as a corticosteroid-sparing agent in corticosteroid-dependent asthma. Am J Respir Crit Care Med 1996;153:509-514.
90. Sihra BS, Durham SR, Walker S, Kon OM, Barnes NC, Kay AB. Inhibition of the allergen-induced late asthmatic response by cyclosporin A. Thorax 1997;52: 447–452.
91. Tavernier J, Devos R, Cornelis S, Tuypens T, van der Heyden J, Fiers W,

Plaetinck G. A human high affinity interleukin 5 receptor (IL-5R) is composed of an IL-5 specific α chain and a β chain shared with the receptor for GM-CSF. Cell 1991;66:1175–1184.
92. Kitamura T, Sato N, Arai K, Miyajima A. Expression cloning of the human IL-3 receptor cDNA reveals a shared β subunit for the human IL-3 and GM-CSF receptors. Cell 1991;66:1165–1174.
93. Lopez AF, Elliott MJ, Woodcock J, Vadas MA. GM-CSF, IL-3 and IL-5: cross-competition on human haemopoietic cells. Immunol Today 1992;13:495–500.
94. Yamada T, Sun Q, Bungre J, Zeibecoglou K, Lopez A, Kay AB, Robinson DS. IL-3, IL-5, GM-CSF receptor α subunit and common β expression on peripheral blood leukocytes in asthma. J Allergy Clin Immunol 1998; in press.
95. Tavernier J, Tuypens T, Plaetinck G, Verhee A, Fiers W, Devos R. Molecular basis of the membrane-anchored and two soluble isoforms of the human interleukin 5 receptor α subunit. Proc Natl Acad Sci 1992;89:7041–7045.
96. Yasruel Z, Humbert M, Kotsimbos ATC, Ploysongsang Y, Minshall E, Durham SR, Pfister R, Menz G, Tavernier J, Kay AB, Hamid Q. Expresion of the membrane-bound and soluble interleukin-5 α receptor mRNA in the bronchial mucosa of atopic and non-atopic asthmatics. Am J Respir Crit Care Med 1997;155:1413–1418.
97. Sur S, Crotty TB, Kephart GM, Hyman BA, Colby TV, Reed CE, Hunt LW, Gleich GJ. Sudden-onset fatal asthma. A distinct entity with few eosinophils and relatively more neutrophils in the airway submucosa? Am Rev Respir Dis 1993;148:713–719.
98. Chand N, Harrison JE, Rooney S, Pillar J, Jkubicki R, Nolan K, Diamantis W, Sofia D. Anti-IL-5 monoclonal antibody inhibits allergic late phase bronchial eosinophila in guinea pigs: a therapeutic approach. Eur J Pharmacol 1992;211:121–123.
99. Foster PS, Hogan SP, Ramsay AJ, Matthaei KI, Young IG. IL-5 deficiency abolishes eosinophilia, airways hyperreactivity, and lung damage in a mouse asthma model. J Exp Med 1995;183:195–201.
100. Mauser PJ, Pitman AM, Fernandez X, et al. Effects of an antibody to interleukin-5 in a monkey model of asthma. Am J Respir Crit Care Med;152:467–472.

# 4

# Bone Marrow in Allergic Disease: The Role of Interleukin-5 as an Eosinophilopoietic Factor

**ROMA SEHMI and JUDAH A. DENBURG**

McMaster University
Hamilton, Ontario, Canada

## I. Introduction

Asthma is a complex disorder characterized by reversible airflow obstruction, airway hyperresponsiveness, and infiltration of the airways by activated inflammatory cells. Increasing evidence suggests that the clinical severity of asthma parallels the degree of eosinophilic inflammation and, as such, highlights a role for eosinophils in the pathology of asthma (1–4). However, the mechanisms underlying the development and persistence of tissue eosinophilia in allergic inflammation remain unresolved.

In this chapter we will discuss the evidence supporting the hypothesis that activation of specific hemopoietic pathways in the bone marrow may contribute to the allergic diathesis through increased production and traffic of bone marrow-derived lineage-committed inflammatory progenitor cells, such as those for eosinophils. In particular, we will discuss the evidence for a role of interleukin-5 (IL-5) in controlling hemopoiesis in the bone marrow during allergic inflammation. We will also raise the issue of the potential importance of IL-5 receptor (IL-5R) expression on progenitor cells as a site for therapeutic intervention by existing and potential antiallergic/antiasthma drugs.

## II. Interleukin-5: Background

Interleukin-5 is produced by T lymphocytes, eosinophils, and mast cells as a glycoprotein (40–45 kDa) with a unique disulphide-linked, antiparallel homodimeric structure (5). It is the most highly conserved member of a group of phylogenetically related cytokines, including also IL-3, IL-4, and granulocyte/macrophage colony-stimulating factor (GM-CSF), the genes which are closely linked on human chromosome 5 (6–8) and on chromosome 11 in the mouse (9).

Historically, two lines of evidence converged when it was demonstrated that two distinct biological activities were both properties of this molecule. On the one hand, Metcalf et al. demonstrated that supernatants from activated spleen cells induced eosinophil colony formation from mouse and human bone marrow (10,11). This line of investigation eventually culminated in the identification of eosinophil differentiation factor (EDF) (12,13). On the other hand, a number of activities were described to have effects on B cells in vitro, including T-cell replacing factor (TRF) (14). B-cell growth factor II (BCGFII) (15), and B-cell differentiation factor μ (BCDFμ) (16). BCGFII, shown to be identical to TFR (17), was later copurified with EDF through a series of protein separation techniques (18) and led to its designation as IL-5.

Of the cytokines which can support eosinophilopoiesis (IL-3, IL-5, and GM-CSF), IL-5 is unique in its ability to specifically promote the terminal differentiation and maturation of eosinophil/basophil lineage-committed progenitors in liquid and semisolid cultures (19,20). In addition, IL-5 prolongs eosinophil survival by delaying apoptotic death (21,22), primes and stimulates eosinophil chemotactic activity (23), increases eosinophil adhesion to endothelial cells (24), and enhances eosinophil effector function (21,25). In mice that overexpress the IL-5 transgene, IL-5 has been shown to be the predominant regulator of eosinophilia (26). However, the absence of any eosinophil-mediated tissue damage suggests that additional factors such as eotaxin may be required to activate these cells. A pivotal role for IL-5 in chronic allergic inflammation has been confirmed by the capacity of neutralizing anti-IL-5 mAb to inhibit antigen- or virus-induced airway hyperresponsiveness and eosinophil infiltration in the airways of mice, guinea pigs, and primates (27–33). Similar findings have also been observed in IL-5 deficient mice (34). More recent studies with intravenously administered IL-5 in guinea pigs (35) and in mice (28,36) highlighted an additional role for IL-5 in the transmigration of mature eosinophils from the bone marrow. The effect of IL-5 on bone marrow-derived progenitor cell differentiation during allergic inflammation has not been investigated to date; such investigations may provide valuable information into factors that contribute to the propagation of the eosinophilic element in chronic allergic inflammatory responses.

## III. IL-5 Receptor: Structure and Function

The human IL-5 receptor (IL-5R) has been identified in vitro on mature eosinophils and basophils in man, and in addition on B-lymphocytes in mice, but not on neutrophils or monocytes in either species (37). Molecular cloning of human cytokine receptors has revealed that IL-3R, IL-5R, and GM-CSFR are uniquely composed of heterodimeric structures consisting of a distinct α subunit that binds the cognate cytokine with low affinity and a common, shared β subunit; the latter, although failing to bind the ligand itself, forms high-affinity cytokine binding sites in association with the α subunit and activates specific signal transduction pathways (38,39). Deletion mutation experiments of IL-5R have now revealed that, like the β subunit, the proline-rich membrane proximal cytoplasmic domain of the α subunit is essential for signal transduction, in particular for mediating growth signals through IL-5R (40,41). In a recent study with transgenic mice that overexpress IL-5Rα, IL-5 was shown to stimulate multilineage growth activity, indicating that the lineage-restricted response of progenitor cells to IL-5 is likely due to the restricted expression of the α chain of IL-5R on progenitor cells (42).

The IL-5Rα subunit exists either as a membrane-bound or soluble isoform, depending on alternative splicing of the IL-5Rα subunit mRNA (39,43,44). The soluble isoform of the α subunit, which lacks the transmembrane and cytoplasmic domains, is secreted into the body fluids where it combines with IL-5 with the same affinity as the membranous isoform and antagonizes the action of IL-5 on its target cells (43,45). It has previously been reported that as much as 90% of the manufactured IL-5Rα subunit may be in the soluble (inactivating) isoform and as little as 10% may be in the membrane-anchored (activating) isoform, thereby potentially allowing the soluble isoform to function as a natural antagonist for IL-5 (39,43,44). In endobronchial biopsies from asthmatic subjects, it has recently been demonstrated that the level of mRNA expression for the membrane-bound isoform of IL-5Rα (mIL-5Rα) inversely correlated with $FEV_1$, whereas the expression of mRNA for the soluble isoform of IL-5Rα (sIL-5Rα) directly correlated with $FEV_1$ (46). These findings give rise to the view that generation of the two isoforms of IL-5Rα are, at least in part, inversely related and that the upregulation of mIL-5Rα mRNA transcripts may influence the eosinophil response and accompanying changes in airflow limitation in chronic asthma. The subject of IL-5R structure and function is reviewed in detail elsewhere in this volume.

## IV. Quantification of Progenitors

Over the last decade, work in our laboratory has focused on measuring hemopoietic progenitor cells associated with various allergic/asthmatic states. These studies require the use of assays to measure the quantity of lineage-committed progenitors, such as colony-forming assays, which are useful for measuring the sensitivity of samples to respond in vitro to added hemopoietic cytokines. Quantification of cells expressing various cell surface markers by flow cytometry also provides a means of identifying the absolute numbers of progenitors at various differentiative stages during hemopoiesis.

### A. Colony Assays

Progenitors for various lineages have, until recently, been identified and operationally defined primarily by colony-forming assays performed in semi-solid media, such as agar or methylcellulose. Clonogenic assays, developed independently by Pluznik and Sachs (47) and Bradley and Metcalf (48), are based on the culture of cell populations containing lineage-specific hemopoietic progenitors in the presence of hemopoietic support media, which can permit commitment to a given differentiation pathway. The lineage-specific colonies for a given number of cultured cells (quantified after a standard period of time) are, by definition, colony-forming units (CFU), each representing the progeny of a single progenitor cell under proper plating conditions. Based on a combination of distinct morphological characterisitics and immunohistochemical staining, the various CFU may be identified as erythroid-, megakaryocyte-, granulocyte/macrophage-, eosiniophil/basophil-, or lymphocyte-CFU (BFU-E, Meg-CFU, GM-CFU, Eo/B-CFU, pre-B- and pre-T-CFU) (Fig. 1). Thus the assay may be used to evaluate either the progenitor cell content of a cell sample (under conditions of standardized hemopoietic support media) or the hemopoietic properties of a new and uncharacterized growth factor. This assay method has played a crucial role in the characterization of all the hemopoietic cytokines shown in Figure 1. Its drawbacks are the length of time required to grow colonies (1 week or more), poor reproducibility due to the lack of standardization between institutions, and the assumption that colony growth under artificial in vitro conditions truly reflects the number of lineage-specific progenitors in vivo.

### B. Surface Markers

As outlined above, the inherent drawbacks of colony-forming assays make quantification of progenitor cells based on specific markers an attractive alternative. The advent of flow cytometric analyses facilitated the use of antibodies directed against cell-surface antigens as a rapid and highly reproducible means of marker analysis and cell sorting of progenitors both in human and animal systems. The markers of greatest interest include CD34 antigen, which is a monomeric, transmembrane, O-sialylated glycophosphoprotein (105–120 kDa) whose expression within the hemopoietic system is restricted to developmentally early lymphohemopoietic stem and progenitor cells (49–51) (Fig. 2). CD34 is therefore widely

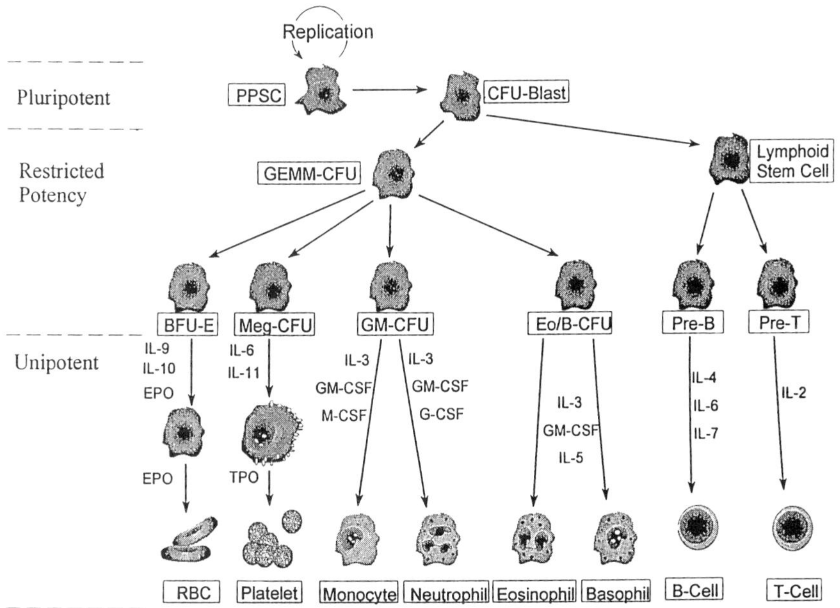


**Figure 1** Bone marrow hemopoietic pathways. Pluripotential stem cells (PPSC) under the influence of local cytokines give rise to blood cells of all lineages. It is possible that cytokines generated at sites of allergic inflammation or within the bone marrow microenvironment may stimulate specific hemopoiesis in an endocrine or paracrine fashion.

used as a tag for the enumeration, isolation, and manipulation of these cells. Despite this extensive use, the normal function of CD34 within hemopoiesis has remained enigmatic. In both man and mouse, CD34 is also expressed outside the hemopoietic system on vascular endothelium (52,53), high endothelial venules (54), and some fibroblasts (55), where it is thought to provide an adhesive binding site recognized by L-selectin on circulating lymphocytes (54). In a recent study, human CD34 ectopically expressed on murine hemopoietic cells was shown to increase adherence to bone marrow stromal cells, implicating a role for CD34 in the regulation and compartmentalization of stem cells (56).

Single-cell cloning experiments have revealed that $CD34^+$ cells coexpress varying levels of distinct surface markers at specific differentiative stages in the hemopoietic pathway (57). The earliest progenitor cells bear $CD34^{high}$, Thy-1/CDw90 (58), and A83/CDw109 (59) antigens, and later acquire *c-kit* (the protooncogene cell product which binds SCF) (60), $CD38^{low}$ (61), and $HLA\text{-}DR^{low}$ (62). Myeloid-lineage committed progenitors are characterized as $CD34^{low}$ $CD33^{high}$ cells (63), while B-lineage and T-lineage precursors bear $CD34^{low}$ $CD19^{high}$ cells and $CD34^{low}CD7^{high}$, respectively (64,65) (see Fig. 3).

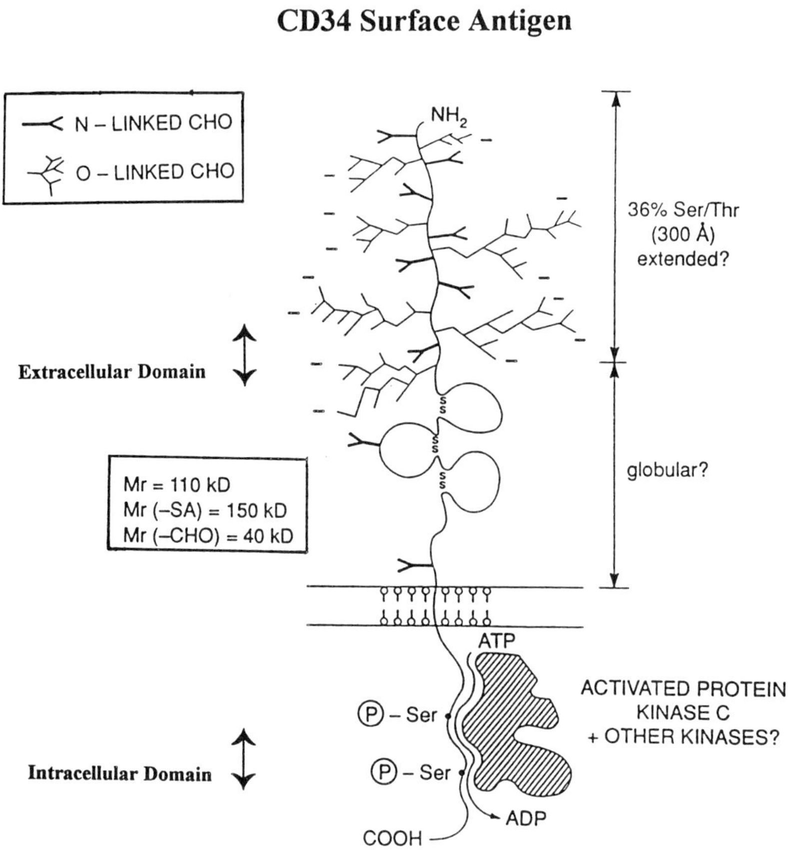


**Figure 2** Schematic representation of the structural characteristics of the human CD34 antigen. The full-length cDNA of human CD34 predicts a type 1 integral membrane protein of 40 kDa with a maximum of nine *N*-glycosylation sites and several *O*-linked glycosylation sites, producing an extended structure of the *N*-terminal domain of CD34 antigen. Between the *N*-terminal domain and the proximal extracellular domain is a cysteine-rich segment that exhibits a globular conformation. The cytoplasmic domain of 73 amino acids contains several potential phosphorylation sites for a variety of protein kinases (51). [Reproduced with permission from Sutherland et al., 1993 (51) and Stem Cells, all rights reserved].

Although the action of cytokines on early hemopoietic progenitors has been extensively investigated using liquid and semisolid cultures, little is known about the kinetics of expression of these receptors and their regulatory mechanisms on these cells. Recent studies of human bone marrow and peripheral blood cells have shown that high levels of the α subunit of IL-3 receptor (IL-3R) are ex-

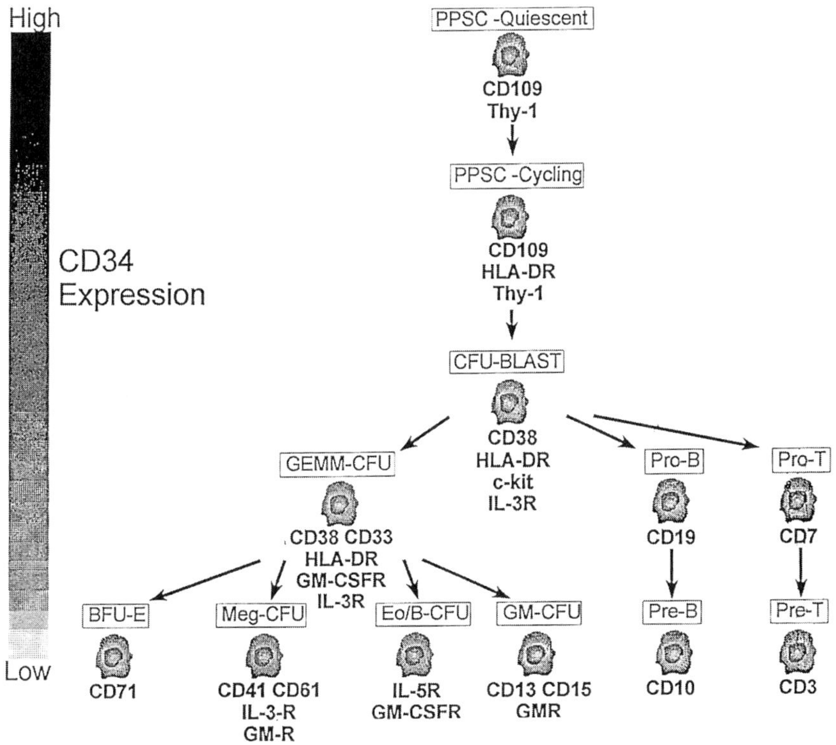


**Figure 3** Surface receptor expression on progenitor cells at various stages in the hemopoietic differentiation pathway. Cell sorting based on surface marker expression allows quantification of progenitor cell numbers.

pressed on primitive $CD34^+$ progenitors, and that this is attenuated as the cells become myeloid-lineage committed ($CD34^+CD33^+$) (66). Conversely, expression of the $\alpha$ subunit of GM-CSF receptor GM-CSFR), undetectable on $CD34^+CD33^-$ cells, is upregulated on $CD34^+CD33^{low/high}$ cells. Several early acting cytokines, including GM-CSF, IL-1, and IFN$\gamma$, upregulate the expression of IL-3R$\alpha$ on $CD34^+$ cells in vitro. Augmented expression of IL-5R$\alpha$ mRNA has been detected on a subline of the AML14 cell line that spontaneously differentiates to eosinophil myelocytes (67). Treatment with all-*trans* retinoic acid (ATRA), which causes a switch in the differentiative program of these cells toward neutrophils, causes a downregulation of IL-5R$\alpha$ mRNA, suggesting a lineage-specific association of IL-5R expression and the development of eosinophils (67).

Studies of progenitor cell surface markers in allergic disease have shown a close correlation between $CD34^+$ cell numbers and total colony-forming units

(Eo/B-CFU and GM-CFU) in cultures of progenitor cells with IL-5 and GM-CSF (68). These data indicate that enumeration of $CD34^+$ cells by flow cytometry is predictive of the colony-forming capacity of a biological sample and may be a useful alternative tool to clonogenic assays for enumerating progenitor cells. Furthermore, detailed analysis of surface marker expression on progenitor cells during allergic inflammatory responses may help to provide greater insight into the earliest phenotypic markers of eosinophil/basophil progenitors and the role of these cells in allergic inflammation.

### C. Identification of Human Eosinophil/Basophil Progenitor Cells

From data we have obtained, both in cultures of the human myeloid leukemic cell line (HL60) and in methylcellulose culture systems, it appears that the immunophenotype of an intermediate-stage eosinophil/basophil progenitor cell is $CD34^-CD35^+$ (69). However, clarification of the precise phenotype of either eosiniophil or basophil progenitors awaits further definition. Recent work on cultured eosinophils detected a hybrid Eo/B (70) previously recognized in several earlier studies of peripheral blood colonies and cord blood liquid cultures (19,71).

From studies on more primitive progenitors, present evidence suggests that both GM-CSF and IL-3 can support commitment of pluripotential $CD34^+CD33^-$ progenitors to the eosinophil lineage, with IL-5 responsible for terminal differentiation of less primitive myeloid lineage-committed progenitor cells (i.e., $CD34^-CD33^+$ cells) derived from $CD34^+CD33^-$ precursors (72). We have, however, now demonstrated for the first time the expression of IL-5R$\alpha$ directly on $CD34^+$ cells from cord blood cells and human bone marrow, indicating the existence of specific binding sites for IL-5 on more primitive progenitor cells than previously thought (73). This is supported by results from in situ hybridization studies demonstrating the colocalization of mRNA for membrane-bound IL-5R$\alpha$ to cord blood-derived progenitors immunostained with anti-CD34 antibody (see Fig. 4). It is therefore likely that the $CD34^+$ IL-5R$\alpha^+$ phenotype may be representative of the earliest eosinophil/basophil lineage-committed progenitors, although further cell sorting and cloning experiments are required to confirm these findings (Fig. 5).

## V. Evidence of Increased Progenitor Activity in Allergic Inflammation

Over the last decade our group has investigated the hypothesis that activation of specific hemopoietic pathways in the bone marrow may contribute to the allergic diathesis through increased production and traffic of lineage-committed inflammatory progenitor cells, which in turn would then contribute to the dis-

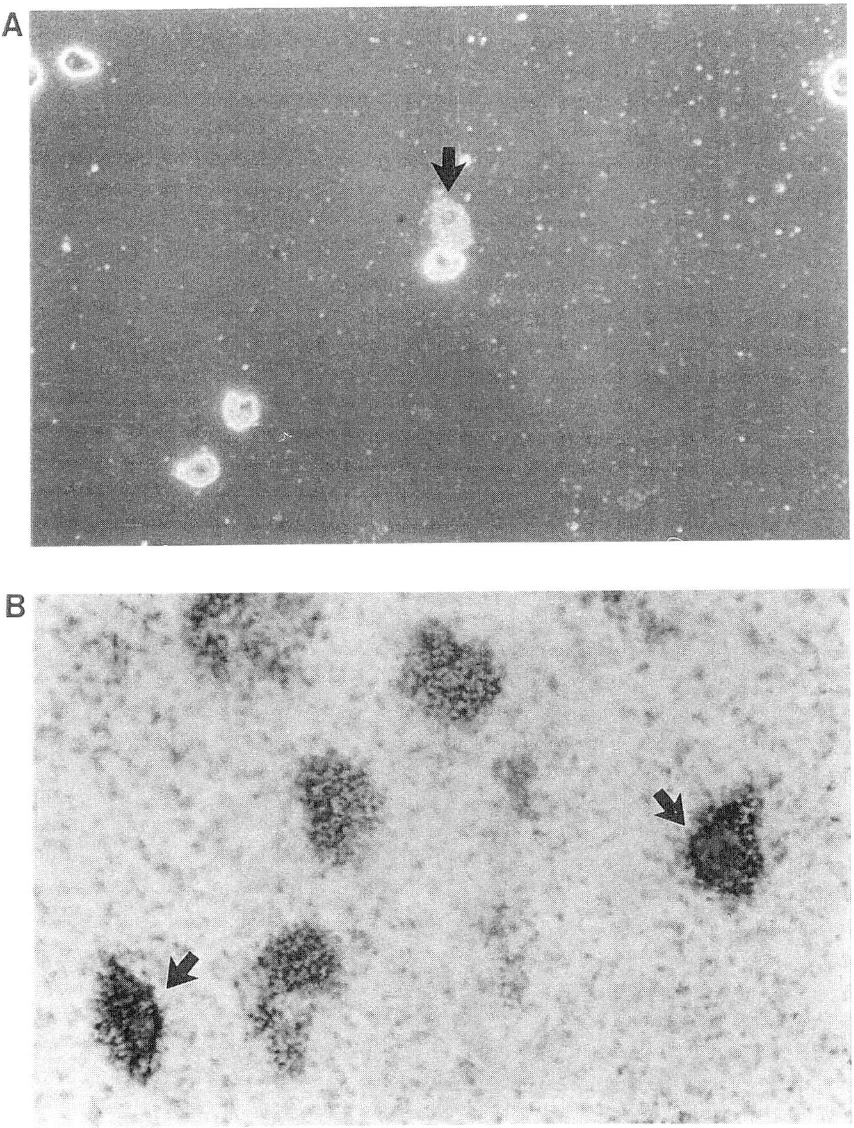


**Figure 4** Detection of mRNA for membrane-bound form of IL-5R$\alpha$ in human cord blood-derived CD34$^+$ cells.(**A,B**) CD34-enriched cell preparations were hybridized with $^{35}$S-labeled membrane-bound IL-5R$\alpha$ antisense riboprobe and simultaneously immunostained with a mouse anti-human CD34 (QBEND10). (**A**) Messenger RNA for membrane-bound IL-5R$\alpha$ was detected by autoradiography and visualized by dark-field illumination (arrow); (**B**) subcellular localization of membrane-bound IL-5R$\alpha$ mRNA in CD34$^+$ cells immunostained simultaneously with mouse anti-human CD34 and APAAP and viewed by bright-field illumination (arrow).

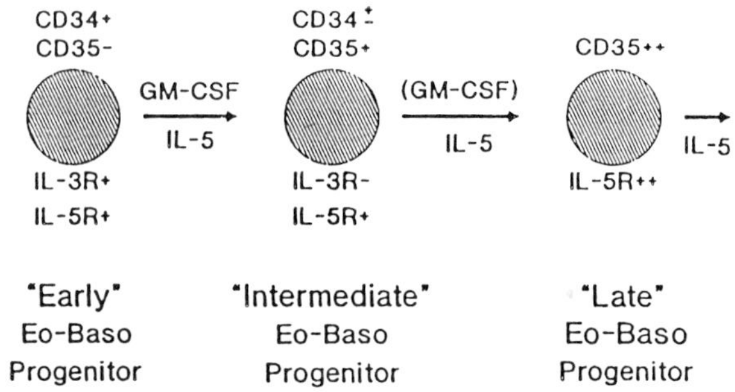


**Figure 5** Specific phenotypic changes on eosinophil/basophil lineage-committed progenitor cells. Based on our recent findings we postulate that IL-5R coexpressed on $CD34^+$ cells is representative of the earliest phenotypic change in lineage commitment to eosinophil/basophils. Studies on HL60 cells, which do not express CD34, demonstrate an up-regulation of CD35 expression when these cells are induced to differentiate toward eosinophil/basophil lineage. CD35 may be expressed on intermediate to late eosinophil/basophil progenitors.

ease process through the increased production of effector inflammatory cells, such as eosinophils (Fig. 6). Based on studies in human patients and animal models, a considerable body of evidence has been gathered to support the view that activation of specific hemopoietic pathways within the bone marrow does occur during allergic inflammation, and that this may contribute to disease activity or severity. This evidence, presented in the following sections, is summarized in Table 1.

### A. Increased Circulating Progenitors in Asthma/Allergy

The first observation of an association between allergic disease and increased numbers of inflammatory cell progenitors was made using colony assays of peripheral blood from atopic and nonatopic individuals. Atopics demonstrated greater numbers of Eo/B-CFU than controls (74,75). Furthermore, larger numbers of Eo/B-CFU were observed in atopic subjects when active disease was compared with quiescent atopic disease, suggesting a link between disease severity and progenitor numbers (75,76). We have now shown that increased numbers of IL-5-responsive eosinophil progenitors can be detected in the circulation of atopic compared with nonatopic subjects (68). In addition, using flow cytometric analyses, we have demonstrated significantly greater numbers of $CD34^+$ hemopoietic progenitor cells in the blood of atopics compared with normal control subjects (68,77). Interestingly, within the group of asymptomatic atopics, the highest levels of $CD34^+$ cell numbers were detected in subjects who were skin prick test positive for house dust mite and mold allergens.

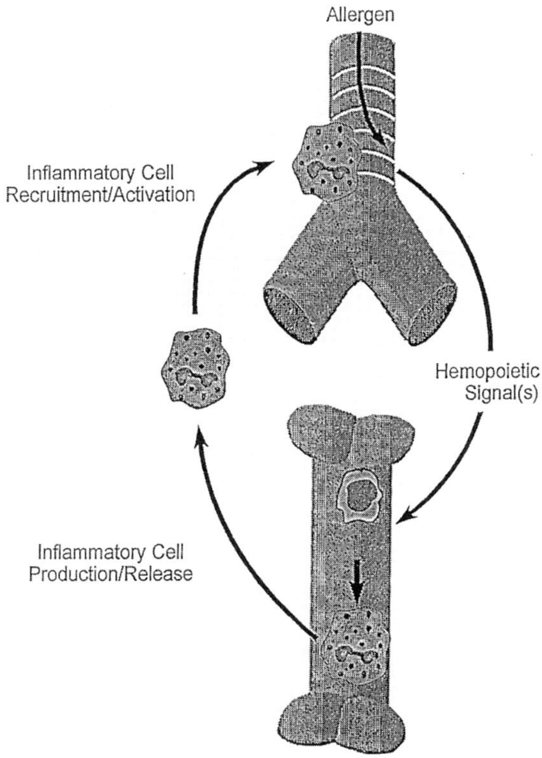


**Figure 6** Schematic representation of our working hypothesis that allergen exposure in atopic subjects may result in the production of a signal or signals which activate specific hemopoietic pathways within the microenvironment of the bone marrow. This results in increased production and traffic of lineage-committed inflammatory cell progenitors to the site of allergen challenge, where in situ differentiation of lineage committed progenitor cells in the presence of locally elaborated cytokines could provide an ongoing source of inflammatory effector cells.

This suggests that continual exposure to low levels of these allergens may have contributed to mild subclinical inflammation resulting in the elevation of blood progenitor numbers.

The link between disease severity and progenitor numbers was further investigated by observing the effect of allergen challenge both in vitro and in vivo on progenitor cell numbers in peripheral blood. Greater numbers of Eo/B-CFU were grown from the blood of atopics in the presence of antigen-stimulated lymphomononuclear cell conditioned medium, indicating the generation of a hemopoietic signal following in vitro allergen challenge. Evidence that

**Table 1** Summary of Findings Indicating Increased Hemopoietic Activity Associated with Allergic Inflammation or Asthma

| Model | Evidence |
|---|---|
| Atopics: compared to normal controls | ↑ circulating Eo/B-CFU (74,75)<br>↑ circulating IL-5 responsive Eo/B-CFU (68)<br>↑ circulating CD34$^+$ cells (68,77)<br>↑ bone marrow CD34$^+$ cells (68) |
| Atopics: during allergen season | ↑ fluctuating Eo/B-CFU (76,78)<br>circulating Eo/B-CFU inversely correlate with tissue eosinophils and metachromatic cells (75) |
| Asthmatics: during exacerbation | ↑ circulating Eo/B-CFU (79) |
| Asthmatics: during allergen challenge | ↑ circulating Eo/B-CFU (80)<br>↑ circulating CD34$^+$ cells (81)<br>↑ bone marrow Eo/B-CFU and GM-CFU (85)<br>↑ bone marrow CD34$^+$ cells expressing IL5Rα-subunit (73,86) |
| Dogs: following allergen challenge | ↑ bone marrow GM-CFU (82)<br>↑ serum hemopoietic activity (88,89)<br>↑ trafficking of bone marrow derived proliferating cells (84) |
| Mice: following allergen challenge | ↑ circulating and bone marrow eosinophils (28,36) |

comparable mechanisms were active in vivo was shown in allergic rhinitics who demonstrated fluctuating numbers of Eo/B-CFU during seasonal allergen exposure (75,78). The magnitude of increases in circulating progenitors was inversely correlated with systemic and nasal metachromatic cell infiltration and eosinophilia observed during natural exposure to allergen. These findings were followed by observations of selective and relevant fluctuations in Eo/B-CFU but not GM-CFU, numbers during exacerbations induced by withdrawal of inhaled corticosteroids as well as upon steroid-controlled resolution of the exacerbation (79). In atopic asthmatics following allergen inhalation challenge, a significant increase in blood Eo/B-CFU but not GM-CFU was observed 24 hr postallergen (80). These changes were only detected in subjects who developed late asthmatic responses. The link between disease severity and progenitor cell numbers was again evident since the increase in Eo/B-CFU was significantly negatively correlated with the degree of airway hyperresponsiveness measured at that time. Moreover, the relationship of progenitor fluctuations to preturbations of the airway mucosal surface (inhaled allergen or steroid) highlighted the notion that soluble factors derived from the inflamed airway may play a pivotal role in these responses (see below).

Recent data using surface marker analysis have shown that a significant increase in circulating $CD34^+$ cell numbers is detected in asthmatic subjects 24 hr postallergen challenge (81). In agreement with the colony-forming assays, these increases in $CD34^+$ cells were only detected in asthmatics who developed a late bronchoconstrictor response, not in isolated early responders.

### B. Increased Bone Marrow Progenitors in Asthma/Allergy

We assumed that the observed changes in circulating progenitors associated with allergic disease and asthma, outlined above, were reflective of specific hemopoietic events taking place in the bone marrow. This assumption is supported by the studies described below involving colony assays and surface marker measurements from bone marrow aspirates.

The first direct evidence for the involvement of the bone marrow-derived progenitor cells in allergen-driven airway responses was demonstrated in studies in a canine model of airway hyperresponsiveness. This model is similar to human disease in that the inhaled allergen (*Ascaris suum*) is associated with immediate bronchoconstriction and delayed airway hyperresponsiveness. However, unlike some human asthmatics, dogs do not develop late bronchoconstrictor responses and the postallergen inflammatory response is predominantly neutrophilic (82). Studies using this model have clearly shown that bone marrow-derived GM-CFU are significantly increased 24 hr postallergen inhalation challenge and that only small changes are observed following diluent challenge (82). Due to the lack, until recently (83), of available dog antibodies to progenitor cell surface antigens, such as CD34, it has not been possible to confirm these studies using surface marker assays. However, using bromo-deoxyuridine (BRDU), a thymidine analog taken up by the DNA of dividing cells and therefore a marker for proliferating cells, preliminary evidence from our group has provided evidence for the trafficking of progenitor cells, originating in the bone marrow, into the lungs via the peripheral circulation in response to allergen inhalation in dogs (84).

In accordance with the findings in animal models, we demonstrated that atopy itself or allergen challenge in human atopic asthmatics is also associated with higher numbers of bone marrow progenitors. Initially comparisons were made of surface marker levels between atopic and normal controls. Analysis of bone marrow samples from patients undergoing thoracotomy for cardiac surgery demonstrated significantly greater numbers of $CD34^+$ progenitor cells in atopics compared with nonatopic patients (68). Following these observations we studied human bone marrow progenitors from a group of mild atopic asthmatics in response to allergen challenge, in whom bone marrow aspirates were taken both pre- and 24 hr postallergen inhalation challenge (a time point associated with increases in circulating and airway eosinophils). As with the dogs, allergen inhalation in individuals who developed late asthmatic responses, airway hyperresponsiveness, and airway eosinophilia was associated with significant increases in Eo/B-CFU and GM-CFU in response to IL-5 and GM-CSF, respectively, as determined by colony-forming assays (85). In addition, no increases in either Eo-CFU or GM-CFU production in response to IL-3 was detected following allergen challenge in both groups of subjects. Interestingly, compared with isolated early responder asthmatics, who did not develop allergen-induced airway hyperresponsiveness or airway eosinophilia, late responder asthmatics showed significantly greater numbers of Eo/B-CFU in the presence of suboptimal concentrations of IL-5, suggesting a preferential increase in an IL-5 responsive progenitor element when eosinophilic inflammation is induced in the airways. These findings are consistent with our previous observations in which atopics gave significantly greater numbers of Eo/B-CFU in cultures with IL-5 compared with nonatopics (68). This view is further supported by our recent findings using surface marker analysis by flow cytometry in which the level of expression of CD34 and its coexpression with receptors for IL-5 and IL-3 were investigated in bone marrow aspirates taken pre- and postallergen challenge. Our results showed that a significant increase in the proportion of bone marrow $CD34^+$ progenitor cells expressing the $\alpha$ subunit for the IL-5 receptor was detected 24 hr postallergen in late responder asthmatics (73,86). Similar allergen-induced effects were not observed in isolated early responder asthmatics. Thus the data suggest that following allergen challenge in dual responder asthmatics, a fixed pool of bone marrow $CD34^+$ progenitors undergoes a distinct phenotypic change, resulting in increases in IL-5R$\alpha$ surface expression. These changes are associated with the development of delayed airway hyperresponsiveness to methacholine and sputum eosinophilia, suggesting that an IL-5 responsive subset of eosinophil/basophil progenitors is upregulated during atopy, and may play a role in the development of allergic airways inflammation.

Although the data presented herein do not prove a direct association between activation of the bone marrow and development of airway pathology as a result of increased inflammatory cell production, they are consistent with the concept that a feedback mechanism exists between tissues involved in allergic inflammation and distal sites, such as the bone marrow.

### C. Signaling Between Lung and Bone Marrow: A Possible Role for IL-5?

Based on the studies outlined above, it is clear that human allergic airway disease is associated with increased progenitor levels, both in the circulation and in the bone marrow. We have proposed that allergen exposure may result in the systemic release of tissue-derived signals which may provide communication between the allergic response and the bone marrow-peripheral blood axis, and result in activation of specific hemopoietic pathways within the microenvironment of the bone marrow, causing increased production and traffic of lineage-committed inflammatory cell progenitors to the site of allergen challenge (Fig. 6).

Evidence of the generation of a serum hemopoietic factor during airway allergen challenge, which can prime the bone marrow for increased production of granulocyte progenitor cells, was initially demonstrated in the same canine model of airway hyperresponsiveness referred to earlier. In these studies it was shown that serum taken from sensitized dogs, as early as 20 min, and also at 2 hr and 24 hr postallergen, stimulated increased production of GM-CFU from naive (preallergen) bone marrow in vitro (87). More recently it has been shown that serum taken 24 hr postallergen from an airway responder dog produced significant increases in progenitor (GM-CFU) growth in bone marrow aspirates taken from dogs that did not develop allergen-induced airway hyperresponsiveness (nonresponders) (88,89). In contrast, postallergen serum taken from the nonresponder dogs did affect progenitor cell growth in bone marrow aspirates taken from either the responder or nonresponder dogs. These findings suggest that allergen-induced increases in bone marrow progenitor formation depend on the generation of serum hemopoietic activity. The identity of this serum factor still remains to be elucidated.

Evidence for the generation of an antigen-specific T-cell-derived hemopoietic activity in humans was demonstrated when increased numbers of Eo/B-CFU were grown from the peripheral blood of atopic individuals in the presence of antigen-stimulated lymphomononuclear cell conditioned medium (74). In addition, in the model of allergic inflammation we have proposed, cytokines released by inflamed airway tissue structural cells can determine the pattern of accumulation of inflammatory effector cells. We have evidence that IL-3, IL-6, IL-8, G-CSF, M-CSF, GM-CSF, TNF-$\alpha$, TGF-$\beta$, and SCF are all expressed or produced in increased amounts by the epithelial cells and fibroblasts of chronically inflamed airways in patients with nasal polyposis, allergic rhinitis, asthma, and pulmonary fibrosis (90–94). Additionally, recent reports of selective IL-5 elaboration at sites of allergic inflammatory reactions, detected both at the mRNA (4,95,96) and protein levels (97), support the view that local tissue generation of cytokines in atopic disease (by T cells or other elements) may provide the appropriate microenvironmental trigger required to stimulate in situ differentiation of eosinophil/basophil lineage-committed progenitors. Furthermore, evidence of the local generation of IL-5 within the bone marrow, colocalized to T cells and $CD34^+$ cells, following allergen challenge in sensitized *balb/c* mice supports the view that this cytokine may play a pivotal role in expanding the eosinophilic element of allergic inflammatory responses at the level of the bone marrow (98).

In both guinea pig (35) and murine models (28,36), IL-5 has been shown to orchestrate the egress of eosinophils from bone marrow to blood. These findings suggest that the observed up-regulation of IL-5Rα expression on bone marrow CD34$^+$ cells following allergen challenge in dual-responder asthmatics may not only represent increased production of eosinophil lineage-committed progenitors, but also an increased transmigrational potential of these progenitors from the bone marrow to the circulation in response to IL-5 produced during an allergic inflammatory response (73). In agreement with this, Gibson et al. showed that significant increases in blood Eo/B-CFU were observed both during an acute asthma exacerbation and 24 hr post-Ag challenge in dual-responder asthmatics, while the numbers of blood GM-CFU remained unchanged (80).

In studies of nematode infection in IL-5 transgenic mice, Strath et al. showed that the level of blood eosinophilia may be controlled not only by the amount of IL-5 produced but by the frequency of eosinophil progenitors in the bone marrow during a chronic inflammatory response (99). In this regard, further investigation of the nature of the signals that modulate the expression of IL-5R on CD34$^+$ progenitor cells may provide insight into the control of eosinophil differentiation from pluripotential stem cells, and potentially may provide a novel therapeutic target for controlling the development of the eosinophilic component of the allergic inflammatory response in asthmatic airways.

## VI. Regulation of IL-5R Expression: A Potential Therapeutic Target in Asthma/Allergy

From in vitro studies, little is currently known regarding the effect of single cytokines or combinations of cytokines on the production of different mRNA splice variants of IL-5Rα subunits on normal progenitor cells. Studies with mature eosinophils have reported that preincubation with GM-CSF, but not IL-3, enhances expression of IL-5R (100). Preincubation of peripheral blood CD34$^+$ cells with GM-CSF and IL-3 enhances their subsequent ability to differentiate into eosinophils in response to IL-5 (101). While this finding implies up-regulation of IL-5R expression, this has not been formally demonstrated, at least not for progenitor cells.

The central question as to what controls both the transcriptional regulation of IL-5Rα subunits and the alternative splicing of the initial IL-5Rα subunit mRNA transcript remains to be determined. The effects of pharmacological agents such as ATRA and corticosteroids on IL-5R expression on progenitor cells is also unclear. ATRA inhibits eosinophil/basophil differentiation from pluripotential progenitor cells, while favoring neutrophil maturation (67,102).

Whether this occurs through receptor modulation on progenitors remains unresolved. ATRA was reported to reduce IL-5Rα mRNA expression in a myeloid leukemic cell line, AML14 (67), but it had no effect on IL-5Rα mRNA in the erythroleukemic cell line, TF1.4 (103). Down-regulation of the IL-5Rα subunit at the mRNA level in myeloid leukemic cell lines has also been shown to be due to factors that either promote eosinophil apoptosis, such as transforming growth factor $\beta_1$ (104). The in vivo inhibitory effect of corticosteroid on increases in peripheral blood Eo/B-CFU during an asthma exacerbation has been noted (79), but its effect at the level of bone marrow progenitors in down-modulating increased production of progenitor cells or their expression of IL-5R during allergic inflammation in man remains to be investigated.

Clearly, investigation of agents that can modulate the expression of IL-5R on $CD34^+$ progenitor cells may provide insight into the control of eosinophil differentiation and may provide novel therapeutic targets for controlling the development of eosinophilic responses in allergic inflammatory conditions, such as asthma (103,105).

## VII. Summary

In conclusion, there is clear evidence that allergic airway inflammation is accompanied by increased circulating and bone marrow inflammatory cell progenitors, and that this effect is mediated by hemopoietic signals, present in circulation following allergen exposure. Ongoing research in this area is directed at identifying the relevant hemopoietic signals and determining the importance of regulation of distinct phenotypic changes, leading to IL-5 responsiveness, in the progenitor cell population in both acute and chronic allergic-type inflammation. A more complete understanding of these fundamental concepts may provide the basis for the development of novel therapeutic interventions in allergy and asthma.

## References

1. Bousquet J, Chanez P, Lacoste YJ, Barnéon G, Chavanian N, Enander I, et al. Eosinophilic inflammation in asthma. N Eng J Med 1990;323:1033–1039.
2. Beasley R, Roche WR, Roberts JA, Holgate ST. Cellular events in the bronchi in mild asthma and after bronchial provocation. Am Rev Respir Dis 1989;139:806–817.
3. Azzawi M, Bradley B, Jeffery PK, Frew AJ, Wardlaw AJ, Knowles G, et al. Identification of activated T-lymphocytes and eosinophils in bronchial biopsies in stable atopic asthma. Am Rev Respir Dis 1909;142:1407–1413.
4. Hamid Q, Azzawi M, Ying S, Moqbel R, Wardlaw AJ, Corrigan CJ, et al. Ex-

pression of mRNA for interleukin-5 in mucosal bronchial biopsies from asthma. J Clin Invest 1991;87:1541–1546.
5. Milburn MV, Hassell AM, Lambert MH, Jordan SR, Proudfoot AE, Graber P, et al. A novel dimeric configuration revealed by the crystal structure of 2.4 Å resolution of human interleukin-5. Nature 1993;363:172–176.
6. Sutherland GR, Baker E, Callen DF, Campbell HD, Young IG, Sanderson CJ, et al. Interleukin-5 is at 5q31 and is detected in the 5q-syndrome. Blood 1988;71:1150–1152.
7. Van Leeuwen BH, Martinson ME, Webb GC, Young IG. Molecular organization of the cytokine gene cluster, involving the human IL-3, IL-4, IL-5 and GM-CSF genes of human chromosome 5. Blood 1989;73:1142–1148.
8. Chandrasekharappa SC, Rebelsky MS, Firak TA, Le-Beau MM, Westbrook CA. A long-range restriction map of the interleukin-4 and interleukin-5 linkage group on chromosome 5. Genomics 1990;6:94–99.
9. Lee JS, Campbell HD, Kozak CA, Young IG. The IL-4 and IL-5 genes are closely linked and are part of a cytokine gene cluster on mouse chromosome 11. Somat Cell Mol Genet 1989;15:143–152.
10. Metcalf D, Parker JW, Chester HM, Kincade PW. Formation of eosinophilic-like granulocyte colonies by mouse bone marrow cells. J Cell Physiol 1974;84:275–290.
11. Metcalf D, Cutler RL, Nicola NA. Clonal analysis of the response of HL60 human myeloid leukemia cells to biological regulators. Blood 1983;61:999–1005.
12. Warren DJ, Sanderson CJ. Production of a T cell hybrid producing a lymphokine stimulating eosinophil differentiation. Immunology 1985;54:615–623.
13. Sanderson CJ, Warren DJ, Strath M. Identification of a lymphokine that stimulates eosinophilic differentiation *in vitro*. Its relationship to interleukin 3 and functional properties of eosinophils produced in cultures. J Exp Med 1985;162:60–74.
14. Takatsu K, Tominaga A, Harada N, Mita S, Matsumoto M, Takahashi T, et al. T cell-replacing factor (TRF)/interleukin-5 (IL-5): molecular and functional properties. Immunol Rev 1988;102:107–135.
15. Swain SL, McKenzie DT, Dutton RW, Tonkonogy SL, English M. The role of IL-4 and IL-5: characterization of a distinct helper T-cell subset that makes IL-4 and IL-5 (Th2) and requires priming before induction of lymphokine secretion. Immunol Rev 1988;102:77–105.
16. Vitetta ES, Brooks K, Chen Y-W, Isakson P, Jones S, Layton J, et al. T cell-derived lymphokines that induce IgM and IgG secretion in activated murine B cells. Immunol Rev 1984;78:137–157.
17. Harada N, Kikuchi Y, Tominaga A, Takaki S, Takatsu K. BCGFII activity on activated B cells of a purified murine T cell replacing factor (TRF) from a T cell hybridoma (B151K12). J Immunol 1985;134:3944–3951.
18. Sanderson CJ, O'Garra A, Warren DJ, Klaus GGB. Eosinophil differentiation factor also has B cell growth activity. Proposed name interleukin 4. Proc Natl Acad Sci USA 1986;83:437–440.
19. Denburg JA, Telizyn S, Belda A, Messner H, Lim B, Jamal N, et al. Hetero-

geneity of human peripheral blood eosinophil-type colonies: evidence of a common basophil-eosinophil progenitor. Blood 1985;66:312–318.
20. Clutterbuck EJ, Herst EMA, Sanderson CJ. Human interleukin-5 (IL-5) regulates the production of eosinophils in human bone marrow cultures: comparisons and interaction with IL-1, IL-3, IL-6 and GM-CSF. Blood 1989;73:1504–1512.
21. Yamaguchi Y, Suda T, Eguchi M, Miura Y, Harada N, Tominaga A, et al. Purified interleukin-5 supports the terminal differentiation and proliferation of murine eosinophilic precursors. J Exp Med 1988;167:43–56.
22. Yamaguchi Y, Suda T, Ohta S, Tominaga K, Miura Y, Kasahara T. Analysis of the survival of mature eosinophils: interleukin-5 prevents apoptosis in mature human eosinophils. Blood 1992;78:2542–2547.
23. Sehmi R, Wardlaw AJ, Cromwell O, Kurihara K, Waltmann P, Kay AB. Interleukin-5 selectively enhances the chemotactic responsiveness of eosinophils obtained from normal but not eosinophilic subjects. Blood 1992;79:2952–2959.
24. Walsh GM, Hartnell A, Wardlaw AJ, Kurihara K, Sanderson CJ, Kay AB. IL-5 enhances the *in vitro* adhesion of human eosinophils, but not neutrophils, in a leucocyte integrin (CD11/CD18)-dependent manner. Immunology 1990;71:258–265.
25. Lopez AF, Sanderson CJ, Gamble JR, Campbell HD, Young IG, Vadas MA. Recombinant interleukin-5 is a selective activator of human eosinophil function. J Exp Med 1988;167:219–224.
26. Dent LA, Strath M, Mellor AL, Sanderson CJ. Eosinophilia in mice expressing interleukin-5. J Exp Med 1990;172:1425–1431.
27. Nagai H, Yamaguchi N, Inagaki N, Tsuruoka N, Hitoshi Y, Takatsu K. Effect of anti-IL-5 monoclonal antibody on allergic bronchial eosinophilia and airway hyperresponsiveness in mice. Life Sci 1993;53:PL243–PL247.
28. Kung T, Stelts DM, Zurcher JA, Adams III GK, Egan RW, Kreutner W, et al. Involvement of IL-5 in a murine model of allergic pulmonary inflammation: prophylactic and therapeutic effect of an IL-5 antibody. Am J Respir Cell Mol Biol 1995;13:360–365.
29. Chand RL, Seymour BW, Hudak S, Jackson J, Rennick D. Anti-IL-5 monoclonal antibody inhibits allergic late phase bronchial eosinophilia in guinea pigs: a therapeutic approach. Eur J Pharmacol 1992;211:121–123.
30. Gulbenkian AR, Egan RW, Fernandez X, Jones H, Kreutner W, Kung T, et al. Interleukin-5 modulates eosinophil accumulation in guinea pig lung. Am Rev Respir Dis 1992;146:263–265.
31. Van Oosterhout AJM, Van Ark I, Folkerts G, Van der Linde HL, Savelkoul HFJ, Verheyen KCP, et al. Antibody to interleukin-5 inhibits virus-induced airways hyperresponsiveness to histamine in guinea pigs. Am J Respir Crit Care Med 1995;151:177–183.
32. Mauser PJ, Pitman AM, Fernandez X, Foran SK, Adams GK III, Kreutner W, et al. Effects of antibody to interleukin-5 in a monkey model of asthma. Am J Respir Crit Care Med 1995;152:467–472.
33. Egan RW, Athwahl D, Chou C, Emtage S, Jehn C, Kung TT, et al. Inhibition of

pulmonary eosinophilia and hyperreactivity by antibodies to interleukin-5. Int Arch Allergy Immunol 1995;107:321–322.
34. Foster PS, Hogan SP, Ramsay AJ, Matthaei KI, Young IG. Interleukin 5 deficiency abolishes eosinophilia, airway hyperreactivity, and lung damage in a mouse asthma model. J Exp Med 1996;183:195–201.
35. Collins PD, Marleau S, Griffith-Johnson DA, Jose PJ, Williams TJ. Cooperation between interleukin-5 and chemokine eotaxin to induce eosinophil accumulation, in vivo. J Exp Med 1995;182:1169–1174.
36. Mould AW, Matthaei KI, Young IA, Foster PS. Relationship between interleukin-5 and eotaxin in regulating blood and tissue eosinophilia in mice. J Clin Invest 1997;99:1064–1071.
37. Lopez AF, Vadas MA, Woodcock J, Milton SE, Lewis A, Elliott MJ, et al. Selective interaction of the human eosinophil interleukin-5 receptor with interleukin-3 and granulocyte-macrophage colony stimulating factor. J Biol Chem 1991;266:24741–24747.
38. Murata Y, Takaki S, Migita M, Kikuchi Y, Tominaga A, Takatsu K. Molecular cloning and expression of the human interleukin-5 receptor. J Exp Med 1992;175:341–351.
39. Tavernier J, Devos R, Cornelis S, Tuypens T, Van der Heyden J, Fiers W, et al. A human high affinity interleukin-5 receptor (IL-5R) is composed of an IL-5 specific α-chain and a β-chain shared with a receptor for GM-CSF. Cell 1991;66:1175–1184.
40. Takaki S, Murata Y, Kitamura T, Miyajima A, Tominaga A, Takatsu K. Reconstitution of the functional receptors for murine and human interleukin-5. J Exp Med 1993;177:1523–1529.
41. Takagi M, Kanazawa H, Shiiba M, Takatsu K. A critical cytoplasmic domain of the interleukin-5 (IL-5) receptor α chain and its function in IL-5-mediated growth signal transduction. Mol Cell Biol 1994;14:7404–7413.
42. Takagi M, Takahiko H, Ichihara M, Takatsu K, Miyajima A. Multi-colony stimulating activity of interleukin 5 (IL-5) on hematopoietic progenitors from transgenic mice that express IL-5 receptor alpha subunit constitutively. J Exp Med 1995;181:889–899.
43. Koike M, Takatsu K. IL-5 and its receptor: which role do they play in the immune response. Int Arch Allergy Immunol 1994;104:1–9.
44. Devos R, Guisez Y, Cornelis S, Verhee A, Van der Heyden J, Manneberg M, et al. Recombinant soluble human interleukin-5 (hIL-5) receptor molecules: cross-linking and stoichiometry of binding to IL-5. J Biol Chem 1993;268:6581–6587.
45. Tavernier J, Tuypens T, Plaetnick G, Verhee A, Fiers W, Devos R. Molecular basis of membrane-anchored and two soluble isoforms of the human interleukin-5 receptor alpha-subunit. Proc Natl Acad Sci USA 1992;89:7041–7045.
46. Yasruel Z, Humbert M, Kotsimbos TC, Polysonsang Y, Minshall E, Durham SR, et al. Membrane-bound and soluble αIL-5 receptor mRNA in the bronchial mucosa of atopic and nonatopic asthmatics. Am J Respir Cell Mol Biol 1997;155:1413–1418.
47. Pluznik DH, Saks SL. The cloning of normal “mast” cells in tissue culture. J Cell Comp Physiol 1965;66:319–324.

48. Bradley TR, Metcalf D. The growth of mouse bone-marrow cells *in vitro*. Aus J Exp Biol Biol Sci 1966;44:287–289.
49. Civin C, Strauss LC, Brovall C, Fackler MJ, Schwartz JF, Shaper JH. Antigenic analysis of hematopoietic progenitor cell surface antigen defined by a monoclonal antibody raised against KG-la cells. J Immunol 1984;133:157–165.
50. Katz F, Tindle RW, Sutherland DR, Greaves MD. Identification of a membrane glycoprotein associated with hemopoietic progenitor cells. Leuk Res 1985;9:191–198.
51. Sutherland DR, Keating A. The CD34 antigen: structure, biology and potential clinical applications. J Hemother 1992;1:115–129.
52. Fina L, Molgaard HV, Robertson D, Bradley NJ, Monaghan P, Delia D, et al. Expression of the CD34 gene in vascular endothelial cells. Blood 1990;75:2417–2426.
53. Baumhueter S, Dybdal N, Kyle C, Lasky LA. Global vascular expression of murine CD34, a sialomucin-like endothelial ligand of L-selectin. Blood 1994;84:2554–2565.
54. Baumhueter S, Singer MS, Henzel W, Hemmerich S, Renz M, Rosen SD, et al. Binding of L-selectin to the vascular sialomucin CD34. Science 1993;262:436–438.
55. Greaves MF, Brown J, Molgaard HV, Spurr NK, Robertson D, Delia D, et al. CD34: a hemopoietic progenitor cell-associated molecule. Leukemia 1992;6:31–36.
56. Healy L, May G, Gale K, Grosveld F, Greaves MF, Enver T. The stem cell antigen CD34 functions as a regulator of hemopoetic cell adhesion. Proc Natl Acad Sci USA 1995;92:12240–12244.
57. Civin C, Trischman T, Fackler MJ, Bernstein I, Buhring H, Campos L, et al. Leukocyte typing. In: Knapp W, ed. Leukocyte Typing IV. Oxford: Oxford University Press, 1989:818–825.
58. Baum CM, Weismann IL, Tsukamoto A, Buckle A-M, Peault B. Isolation of a candidate human hematopoietic stem cell population. Proc Natl Acad Sci USA 1992;89:2804–2808.
59. Murray LJ, Bruno E, Yeo EL, Tsukamoto A, Hoffman R, Sutherland DR. CDw109 antibody 8A3 identifies a minor subset of $CD34^+$ foetal bone marrow cells that includes multilineage and megakaryocyte progenitor cells as well as hemopoietic stem cells [abstract]. Blood 1994;84:327.
60. Stobl H, Takimoto M, Majdic O, Hocker P, Knaff W. Antigenic analyses of human hematopoietic progenitor cells expressing the growth factor receptor *c-kit*. Br J Haematol 1992;82:287–294.
61. Hao Q-L, Shah AJ, Thiemann FT, Smogorzewska EM, Crooks GM. A functional comparison of $CD34^+CD38^-$ cells in cord blood and bone marrow. Blood 1995;86:3745–3753.
62. Scaland S, Duvert V, Caux C, Pandrau D, Favre C, Valle A, et al. Distribution of surface-membrane molecules in bone marrow and cord blood $CD34^+$ hemopoietic cells. Exp Hematol 1992;20:24–33.
63. Pierelli L, Teopili L, Menichella G, Rumi C, Paolini A, Lovino S, et al. Further investigations on the expression of HLA-DR, CD33 and CD13 surface antigens

on purified bone marrow and peripheral blood CD34$^+$ hemopoietic progenitor cells. Br J Haematol 1993;84:24–30.
64. Ryan D, Kossover S, Mitchell S, Frantz C, Hennessy L, Cohen H. Sub-populations of common acute lymphoblastic leukemia antigen-positive lymphoid cells in normal bone marrow identified by hemopoietic differentiation antigens. Blood 1986; 68:417–425.
65. Mossalayi MD, Dalloul AH, Bertho JM, Lecron JC, Goube de Laforest P, Debre P. *In vitro* differentiation and proliferation of purified human thymic and bone marrow CD7$^-$ CD2$^-$ T cell precursors. Exp Hematol 1990;18:326–331.
66. Hurata H, Arai T, Yokota T, Arai K. Differential expression of granulocyte-macrophage colony stimulating factor and IL-3 receptor subunits on human CD34$^+$ cells and leukemic cell lines. J Allergy Clin Immunol 1995;96:1083–1099.
67. Paul CC, Mahrer S, Tolbert M, Elbert BL, Wong I, Ackerman SJ, et al. Changing the differentiation program of hematopoietic cells: retinoic acid-induced shift of eosinophil-committed cells to neutrophils. Blood 1995;86:3737–3744.
68. Sehmi R, Howie K, Sutherland DR, Schragge W, O'Byrne PM, Denburg JA. Increased levels of CD34$^+$ hemopoietic progenitor cells in atopic subjects. Am J Respir Cell Mol Biol 1996;15:645–654.
69. Wong DA, Valent P, Bettleheim P, Switzer J, Denburg JA. Immunophenotypic analysis of HL60 cells during basophilic differentiation. Int Arch Allergy Immunol 1996;110:252–260.
70. Boyce JA, Friend D, Matsumoto R, Austen KF, Owen WF. Differentiation *in vitro* of hybrid eosinophil/basophil granulocytes: autocrine function of an eosinophil developmental intermediate. J Exp Med 1995;182:49–57.
71. Tanno Y, Bienenstock J, Richardson M, Lee TDG, Befus AD, Denburg JA. Reciprocal regulation of human basophil and eosinophil differentiation by seperate T-cell-derived factors. Exp Hematol 1987;15:24–33.
72. Ema H, Suda T, Nagayoshi K, Miura Y, Civin CI, Nakauchi H. Target cells for granulocyte-macrophage colony-stimulating factor, interleukin-3, and interleukin-5 in the differentiation pathways of neutrophils and eosinophils. Blood 1990;76:1956–1961.
73. Sehmi R, Wood LJ, Watson RM, Foley R, O'Byrne PM, Denburg JA. Increases in the proportion of bone marrow CD34$^+$ cells expressing the alpha-subunit of IL-5 receptors following allergen challenge in dual responder asthmatics [abstract]. J Allergy Clin Immunol 1997;99:S272.
74. Denburg JA, Telizyn S, Belda A, Dolovich J, Bienenstock J. Increased numbers of circulating basophil progenitors in atopic patients. J Allergy Clin Immunol 1985;76:466–472.
75. Otsuka H, Dolovich J, Befus AD, Bienenstock J, Denburg JA. Peripheral blood basophils, basophil progenitors and nasal metachromatic cells in allergic rhinitis. Am Rev Respir Dis 1986;136:710–717.
76. Otsuka H, Dolovich J, Befus AD, Telizyn S, Bienenstiock J, Denburg JA. Basophilic cell progenitors, nasal metachromatic cells and peripheral blood basophils in ragweed allergic patients. J Allergy Clin Immunol 1986;78:365–371.
77. Sehmi R, Howie K, Denburg J. Elevated levels of CD34$^+$ hemopoietic progenitor cells in atopic subjects [abstract]. J Allergy Clin Immunol 1995;1:A382.

78. Linden M, Svensson C, Andersson M, Greiff L, Andersson E, Denburg JA, et al. Increased numbers of circulating leukocyte progenitors in patients with allergic rhinitis during natural allergen exposure [abstract]. Am J Repir Crit Care Med 1994;149:A602.
79. Gibson PG, Dolovich J, Girgis-Gabardo A, Morris MM, Anderson M, Hargreave FE, et al. The inflammatory response in asthma exacerbation: changes in circulating eosinophils, basophils and their progenitors. Clin Exp Allergy 1990;20:661–668.
80. Gibson PG, Manning PJ, O'Byrne PM, Grigis-Gabardo A, Dolovich J, Denburg JA, et al. Allergen induced asthmatic responses. Relationship between increased airway responsiveness and increases in circulating eosinophils, basophils and their progenitors. Am Rev Respir Dis 1991;143:331–335.
81. Sehmi R, Wood LJ, Watson RM, Inman MD, O'Byrne PM, Denburg JA. Increases in circulating CD34$^+$ hemopoietic progenitors in allergen induced late asthmatic responses [abstract]. J Allergy Clin Immunol 1996;97:A277.
82. Woolley MJ, Denburg JA, Ellis R, Dahlback M, O'Byrne PM. Allergen induced changes in bone marrow progenitors and airways responsiveness in dogs and the effect of inhaled budesonide on these parameters. Am J Respir Cell Mol Biol 1994;11:600–606.
83. McSweeney PA, Rouleau KA, Strob R, Bolles L, Wallace PM, Bauchamp M, et al. Canine CD34: cloning of the cDNA and evaluation of an antiserum to recombinant protein. Blood 1996;6:1992–2003.
84. Wood LJ, Inman MD, Ellis R, Wattie J, Denburg JA, O'Byrne PM. Allergen-induced trafficking of inflammatory cells in dogs [abstract]. Am J Repir Crit Care Med 1997;155:A879.
85. Wood LJ, Inman MD, Watson RM, Foley R, Denburg JA, O'Byrne PM. Inhaled allergen-induced changes in bone marrow eosinophil/basophil progenitors in mild asthmatic subjects [abstract]. J Allergy Clin Immunol 1997;99(S364):A1485.
86. Sehmi R, Wood LJ, Watson RM, Foley R, Hamid Q, O'Byrne PM, et al. Allergen-induced increases in IL-5 receptor $\alpha$-subunit expression on bone marrow derived CD34$^+$ cells from asthmatic subjects: a novel marker of progenitor cells commitment towards eosinophilic differentiation. Journal of Clinical Investigation 1997; 100:2466–2475.
87. Inman MD, Denburg JA, Ellis R, Dahlback M, O'Byrne PM. Allergen-induced increase in bone marrow progenitors in airway hyperresponsive dogs: regulation by a serum hemopoietic factor. Am J Respir Cell Mol Biol 1996;15:305–311.
88. Inman MD, Ellis R, Wattie J, Dahlback M, Denburg JA, O'Byrne PM. Increased bone marrow progenitor growth after allergen challenge in dogs is dependent on a serum factor, not bone marrow responsiveness [abstract]. Am J Repir Crit Care Med 1997;155:879.
89. Inman MD, Denburg JA, Ellis R, Dahlback M, O'Byrne PM. Allergen-induced increase in bone marrow progenitors in airway hyperresponsive dogs: regulation by a serum hemopoietic factor. Am J Respir Cell Mol Biol 1997;15:339–347.
90. Denburg JA, Dolovich J, Ohtoshi T, Cox G, Gauldie J, Jordana M. The microenvironmental differentiation hypothesis of airway inflammation. Am J Rhinol 1990;4:29–32.

91. Ohnishi M, Ruhno J, Bienenstock J, Dolovich J, Denburg JA. Hemopoietic growth factor production by human nasal polyp epithelial scarpings: kinetics, cell source and relationship to clinical status. J Allergy Clin Immunol 1989;83:1091–1110.
92. Ohtoshi T, Tsuda T, Vancheri C, Abrams JS, Dolovich J, Denburg JA, et al. Human upper epithelial cell-derived granulocyte-macrophage colony-stimulating factor induces histamine containing cell differentiation of human progenitor cells. Int Arch Allergy Appl Immunol 1991;95:376–384.
93. Kim YK, Nakagawa N, Sulakvelidze I, Dolovich J, Denburg JA. Immunolocalization of stem cell factor in inflamed human nasal tissues [abstract]. J Allergy Clin Immunol 1996;97:A282.
94. Nakagawa N, Howie K, Switzer J, Marshall JS, Denburg JA. Human nasal polyp fibroblasts produce stem cell factor (SCF) [abstract]. J Allergy Clin Immunol 1995;95:A292.
95. Robinson DS, Hamid Q, Ying S, Tsicopoulos A, Barkans J, Bentley AM, et al. Predominant Th2-like bronchoalveolar T-lymphocyte population in atopic asthma. N Eng J Med 1992;326:298–304.
96. Robinson DS, Hamid Q, Bentley AM, Ying S, Kay AB, Durham SR. Activation of $CD4^+$ T cells, increased TH2-type cytokine mRNA expression and eosinophil recruitment in bronchoalveolar lavage after allergen inhalation challenge in patients with atopic asthma. J Allergy Clin Immunol 1993;92:313–324.
97. Brodie DH, Lotz M, Cuomo AJ, Coburn DA, Federman EC, Wasserman SI. Cytokines in symptomatic asthma airways. J Allergy Clin Immunol 1992;89:958–967.
98. Minshall E, Schleimer R, Cameron R, Minicozzi M, Egan RW, Eidelman DH, et al. IL-5 and aIL-5R mRNA expression in the bone marrow of sensitized BALB/c mice following allergen challenge [abstract]. Am J Repir Crit Care Med 1997;155:A735.
99. Strath M, Dent LA, Sanderson CJ. Infection of IL-5 transgenic mice with *Mesocestoides corti* induces very high levels of IL-5 but depressed production of eosinophils. Exp Hematol 1992;20:229–234.
100. Chihara J, Plumas J, Gruart V, Tavernier J, Prin L, Capron A, et al. Characterization of a receptor for interleukin 5 on human eosinophils: variable expression and induction by granulocyte-macrophage colony stimulating factor. J Exp Med 1990;172:1347–1351.
101. Shalit M, Sekhsaria S, Malech HL. Modulation of growth and differentiation of eosinophils from human peripheral blood $CD34^+$ cells by IL-5 and other growth factors. Cell Immunol 1995;160:50–57.
102. Gratas C, Menot ML, Dresch C, Chomienne C. Retinoic acid supports granulocytic but not erythroid differentiation of myeloid progenitors in normal bone marrow. Leukemia 1993;7:1156–1162.
103. Zanders ED. Interleukin-5 receptor alpha chain mRNA is down-regulated by transforming growth factor beta 1. Eur Cytokine Netw 1994;5:35–42.
104. Jacobson SEW, Ruscetti FW, Roberts AB, Keller JR. TGF-β is a bidirectional

modulator of cytokine receptor expression on murine bone marrow cells. Differential effects of TGF-β1 and TGF-β3. J Immunol 1993;151:4534–4544.
105. Devos R, Plaetnick G, Cornelis S, Guisez Y, Van der Heyden J, Tavernier J. Interleukin-5 and its receptors: a drug target for eosinophilia associated with chronic allergic disease. J Leuk Biol 1995;57:813–819.

# 5

# Eosinophils, Interleukin-5, and Cutaneous Disease

**KRISTIN M. LEIFERMAN**

Mayo Medical School, Mayo Clinic and Mayo Foundation
Rochester, Minnesota

## I. Introduction

The skin is an epithelial tissue that is in constant contact with the external environment. In addition to its structural components, immunologically functioning cells including mast cells and antigen-presenting cells are residents of skin tissue. As an epithelial tissue, the skin has analogous structural and functional relationships to the lung. Eosinophil activity in the lung, particularly in the pathogenesis of asthma, is increasingly well defined (1). Eosinophils are conspicuous cells when present in cutaneous tissues and are prominent in many skin diseases. On histologic staining with hematoxylin and eosin, the eosinophil is readily identifiable because of the intense avidity its distinctive cytoplasmic granules have for the acidic dye, eosin. Moreover, the histologic detection of eosinophils in skin lesions often contributes to the disease diagnosis. A summary of eosinophil-associated skin diseases is shown in Table 1 (2,3). In addition, eosinophils may be part of a disease process through degranulation, disruption, and deposition of granule proteins; a list of diseases in which eosinophil granule protein deposition has been found is shown in Table 2 (2). In these diseases, the eosinophil may not be readily apparent after histologic staining because the cell is no longer intact, having lost its morphologic identity.

**Table 1** Eosinophils and Cutaneous Disease

| |
|---|
| Diseases with peripheral and/or tissue eosinophilia |
| Atopic diseases |
| Parasitic diseases |
| Bullous diseases |
| Drug reactions |
| Hypereosinophilic syndrome |
| Eosinophilia myalgia syndrome |
| Toxic oil syndrome |
| Eosinophilic fasciitis |
| Urticaria and angioedema |
| Mastocytosis |
| Cutaneous T-cell lymphoma |
| Eosinophilic panniculitis |
| Reactions to arthropod bites and stings |
| Diseases histologically characterized by tissue eosinophilia (3) |
| Kimura's diseases and angiolymphoid hyperplasia with eosinophilia |
| Wells' syndrome (eosinophilic cellulitis) |
| Eosinophilic pustulosis (Ofugi's disease and erythema toxicum neonatorum) |
| Granuloma faciale |
| Eosinophilic ulcer of the tongue |

*Source*: Ref. 2.

By electron microscopy, the distinctive cytoplasmic granules of eosinophils show electron-dense cores and less dense matrices (32), and their contents have been investigated as a way of understanding the functions of eosinophils. Four strongly cationic proteins comprise the bulk of the granule: major basic protein (MBP), eosinophil peroxidase (EPO), eosinophil-derived neurotoxin (EDN), and eosinophil cationic protein (ECP). MBP constitutes the crystalloid core of the eosinophil granule whereas EPO, EDN, and ECP are localized in the granule matrix. Each of these granule proteins has toxic activity toward cells, in part, because of their strong basicity. Properties of eosinophil granule proteins have been recently reviewed (33).

Using immunohistology to stain for eosinophil granule proteins in cutaneous tissues, eosinophil involvement may be characterized by different patterns of staining as summarized in Table 3. Specific diseases show each of these staining patterns. For example, lesions of angiolymphoid hyperplasia with eosinophilia typically show many intact eosinophils with focal areas of extracellular protein staining, proportional to the number of infiltrating eosinophils, and urticarial and edematous lesions. Certain types of eczematoid dermatitis lesions show very few intact eosinophils with disproportionately extensive deposition of extracellular granule proteins.

**Table 2** Eosinophil Granule Protein Disposition in Cutaneous Disease

| |
|---|
| Urticarial and edematous lesions |
|   Chronic urticaria (4,5) |
|   Solar urticaria (6) |
|   Delayed pressure urticaria (7) |
|   IgE-mediated late-phase reaction (8) |
|   Episodic angioedema with eosinophilia (9–12) |
|   GM-CSF reactions (13) |
|   IL-2 capillary leak syndrome (14) |
|   Eosinophilic cellulitis (15) |
| Eczematoid dermatitis |
|   Atopic dermatitis (16–18) |
|   Onchocercal dermatitis (16) |
|   Pachydermatous eosinophilic dermatitis (19) |
|   Prurigo nodularis (20) |
| Blistering disorders |
|   Herpes (pemphigoid) gestationis (21) |
|   Bullous pemphigoid (22) |
|   Bullous morphea (23) |
|   Incontinenti pigmenti (24) |
| Vasculitis |
|   Recurrent cutaneous necrotizing eosinophilic vasculitis (25) |
|   Eosinophilic vasculitis in connective tissue disease (26) |
|   Churg-Strauss syndrome (27) |
| Miscellaneous |
|   Eosinophilia myalgia syndrome (28) |
|   Toxic oil syndrome (29) |
|   Fibrotic syndromes (30) |
|   Angiolymphoid hyperplasia with eosinophilia (31) |

*Source*: Ref. 2.

The factors determining eosinophil infiltration and granule protein deposition in tissue have been under investigation in recent years and involve at least three interrelated signals: chemoattractants, adhesion molecules, and activating cytokines including IL-5. First, members of both the C-X-C and C-C chemokine

**Table 3** Immunohistologic Staining Patterns for Eosinophil Granule Proteins

| |
|---|
| Many intact eosinophils, minimal or no extracellular protein deposition |
| Many intact eosinophils, focal extracellular protein deposition |
| Many intact eosinophils, massive extracellular protein deposition |
| Few intact eosinophils, disproportionately extensive extracellular protein deposition |

gene superfamilies are chemotactic for eosinophils. Eotaxin and RANTES are both members of the C-C chemokine gene superfamily. In addition to chemotactic activity for eosinophils, they activate eosinophil function as measured by production of reactive oxygen species (34,35). Although both are comparable in chemotactic activity, eotaxin is stronger in inducing reactive oxygen species and is selective for eosinophil recruitment (35). Second, eosinophils must transmigrate blood vessels to infiltrate tissues, and three gene superfamilies contribute to the signaling needed for transmigration (36). Selectins are involved in the early, high-sheer-force stage of leukocyte adhesion to endothelium, and integrins are cell-surface proteins that recognize counterreceptor members of the immunoglobulin gene superfamily. Together, the integrin-immunoglobulin family interactions promote flattening and migration of cells onto and through the endothelium. Following migration through vessels, eosinophils are present in the extracellular matrix where integrins, expressed on the cell surfaces, recognize as receptor substances such as the fibrous proteins, fibronectin, laminin and collagen, and the glycosaminoglycans, hyaluronic acid and chondroitin sulfate, which may exert effects on eosinophil activities (37). Ongoing studies suggest that integrin expression is critical for the effective functions of eosinophils, including degranulation (38). Third, additional lines of investigation indicate that eosinophils are recruited to and activated in tissues by cytokine activity from a subset of T cells, Th2 cells, which produce IL-5 in addition to other cytokines (39). Mast cells (40) and eosinophils themselves may also elaborate regulatory cytokines (41). It is likely that combinations of these factors regulate eosinophil activities and lead to the patterns of eosinophil involvement found in disease.

Once present and activated in tissues, eosinophils exert a variety of phlogistic effects which are likely pathogenically important in disease (32). The eosinophil granule proteins, MBP, EPO, and ECP are potent toxins to various targets including helminths, protozoa, bacteria, and normal mammalian cells (32) and are cytostimulants for basophil and mast cell mediator release (32,42,43) and for neutrophil (44) and platelet (45) activation. MBP, EPO, ECP, and EDN all directly affect blood vessels to increase vascular permeability (46), and all four proteins induce wheal and flare reactions in human skin (9). Activated eosinophils not only release granule proteins but also generate lipid mediators such as leukotriene $C_4$($LTC_4$) and platelet activating factor (PAF), generate reactive oxygen species, participate in antibody-dependent cytotoxicity reactions, and potentially act as antigen presenting cells. The oxidative products of eosinophils including superoxide anions, hydroxyl radicals, and singlet oxygen (47,48) are, like the granule proteins, damaging to cells. The small molecular weight mediators produced by eosinophils, PAF and $LTC_4$ (49–51), increase vascular permeability. PAF has several additional activities including attraction and activation of leukocytes in areas of inflammation and $LTC_4$ stimulates smooth muscle.

Eosinophils are also capable of synthesizing and secreting important inflammatory and regulatory cytokines (41,52,53); these include IL-1$\alpha$, transforming growth factor (TGF)$\alpha$ and $\beta_1$, granulocyte monocyte colony-stimulating factor (GM-CSF), IL-3, IL-5, IL-6, IL-8, tumor necrosis factor (TNF)$\alpha$, and macrophage inhibitory protein (MIP)-1$\alpha$. The stimuli that trigger eosinophils to produce cytokines are only now being elucidated, but the chemotactic factors, C5 and N-formyl methionyl-leucyl-phenylalanine (FMLP), have been found to induce production of IL-8 and GM-CSF by eosinophils (54). Through expression of MHC class II molecules and IL-1$\alpha$ production, eosinophils may act as specialized antigen presenting cells (41). Eosinophils may be involved in tissue repair by promoting collagen synthesis through release of TGF$\alpha$ and $\beta_1$ (55). They may also promote fibrosis by their ability to stimulate fibroblast DNA synthesis and extracellular matrix protein production (56). Thus the functional diversity of the eosinophil has manifold implications.

Three diseases will be used to illustrate interactions of eosinophils in cutaneous disease pathology: atopic dermatitis, bullous pemphigoid, and recurrent cutaneous necrotizing eosinophilic vasculitis.

## II. Atopic Dermatitis

Although a relationship between eosinophil activity and asthma has been increasingly well defined over the past 25 years, eosinophil activity in atopic dermatitis has been described more recently. Peripheral blood eosinophilia was recognized in association with atopic dermatitis (57), but systematic studies of infiltrating cells in lesions of atopic dermatitis showed minimal eosinophil infiltration (58). Measurement of peripheral blood eosinophils and serum MBP levels in a group of subjects including 16 patients with atopic dermatitis in the early 1980s showed that normal control subjects all had normal numbers of eosinophils and low MBP levels in peripheral blood; in contrast, over half of the patients with atopic dermatitis had elevated MBP levels in the peripheral blood including some patients with normal peripheral blood eosinophil counts (59). These results indicated that eosinophil granule proteins could be "escaping" from eosinophils in the disease process. To determine whether eosinophils in skin lesions of atopic dermatitis may have degranulated accounting for the increased granule protein levels in the peripheral blood, immunohistologic staining for eosinophil granule MBP was performed (16). Nineteen biopsy specimens of affected atopic dermatitis skin showing chronic dermatitis and 1 of unaffected skin were obtained from 18 patients, satisfying diagnostic criteria for atopic dermatitis. Biopsy specimens were taken simultaneously from affected and unaffected skin of one patient, and two biopsy specimens from affected skin of another patient were obtained 2 years apart. The biopsy specimens were stained by indirect immunofluorescence for eosinophil granule MBP. All 20 skin biopsy specimens from these patients showed extracellular MBP staining with few intact infiltrating eosinophils (Fig. 1) (16). The specimen from unaffected skin showed minimal but definite extracellular MBP staining in the upper dermis; in contrast, a specimen of affected skin from the same patient showed marked upper extracellular dermal MBP staining (60). Both specimens from the patient in whom biopsies of affected skin were obtained 2 years apart showed marked extracellular dermal MBP staining.

A striking finding in the atopic dermatitis specimens was the extensive extracellular MBP staining with very few intact eosinophils. The identifiable eosinophils were located predominantly within perivascular foci of mononuclear cell infiltration. The extracellular MBP staining was prominent throughout the entire upper dermis (Fig. 1). The localization of MBP principally in the upper dermis and the minimal staining of uninvolved skin suggests that eosinophils deposit granule proteins directly in the skin in atopic dermatitis (16).

Subsequently 22 patients with atopic dermatitis were studied; in addition to the collection of skin biopsy specimens, blood and urine specimens were obtained from 19 and 14 of the patients, respectively (17). Blood eosinophil counts were calculated by multiplying total white blood cell counts by percentages of eosinophils, and body surface involvement was estimated by the "rule of nines." Indirect immunofluorescence was performed to detect three eosinophil granule proteins—MBP, EDN, and ECP—in skin biopsy specimens. MBP, EDN, and ECP levels were measured in serum and urine by immunoassay. Relationships among the various parameters were statistically analyzed comparing the various parameters including tissue deposits of MBP, EDN, and ECP, serum and urine levels of MBP, EDN, and ECP, serum IgE levels, calculated eosinophil counts, and percent body surface involvement with atopic dermatitis lesions (17).

Lesional skin specimens from 16 of the 22 patients showed prominent extracellular staining of at least one eosinophil granule protein. The extracellular deposition was markedly out of proportion to the few infiltrating cells (17). Four of 19 patients from whom blood differential counts were available exhibited peripheral blood eosinophilia greater than 760 cells/μl. Levels of MBP, EDN, and ECP were elevated in 15 of 19, 14 of 19, and 10 of 19 serum specimens, respectively; mean MBP, EDN, and ECP serum levels in the 19 atopic dermatitis patients were elevated compared to 50 nonatopic, normal control subjects (17). Urine levels of MBP, EDN, and ECP were elevated in 3 of 14, 7 of 14, and 0 of 14 specimens, respectively (17).

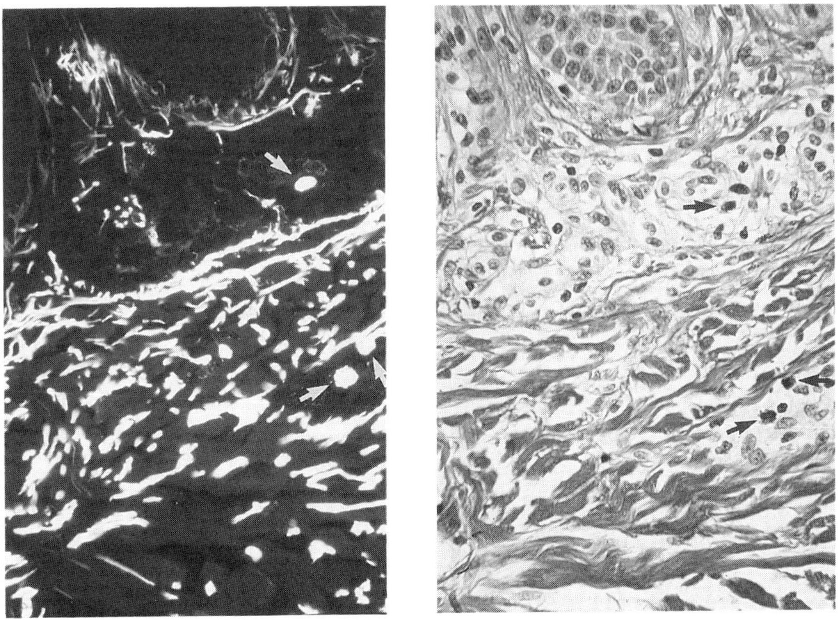

a b

**Figure 1** Immunohistology of atopic dermatitis skin lesion. (**a**) Photomicrograph of tissue section stained by indirect immunofluorescence for eosinophil granule major basic protein (MBP) showing very few intact eosinophils (brightly fluorescent ovals, arrows) and extensive extracellular deposition appearing as fibrils in the upper dermis (magnification 400×). A control serial section stained with rabbit IgG showed no specific fluorescence (not shown). (**b**) Photomicrograph of same tissue section as in (a) stained with hematoxylin and eosin. Eosinophils are identified by arrows. The extracellular MBP deposition is not visible with this stain (magnification 400×). Source: Ref. 16

Statistical comparisons showed eight significant positive correlations establishing a strong relationship between eosinophils and atopic dermatitis (17). Serum MBP and EDN levels were correlated ($r_s = 0.64$, $p < 0.007$) and serum EDN and ECP levels were correlated ($r_s = 0.63$, $p < 0.008$). Tissue MBP and EDN deposition was correlated ($r_s = 0.76$, $p < 0.0005$), as was tissue MBP and ECP deposition ($r_s = 0.67$, $p < 0.003$) and tissue EDN and ECP deposition ($r_s = 0.68$, $p < 0.002$). Urinary MBP levels correlated with serum EDN levels ($r_s = 0.60$, $p < 0.04$). Peripheral blood eosinophils correlated with MBP deposition in tissue ($r_s = 0.49$, $p < 0.04$). Finally and interestingly, disease activity as determined by body surface involvement was significantly correlated with serum MBP level ($r_s = 0.59$, $p < 0.02$) (17).

Various other reports have shown relationships between eosinophils and disease activity in patients with atopic dermatitis. Table 4 summarizes the findings. Peripheral blood eosinophilia roughly correlates with disease severity, and peripheral blood eosinophil counts decrease with therapeutic improvement (61–66). Studies have shown that increased numbers of hypodense eosinophils, that is, eosinophils which have lost density through activation, are present in the peripheral blood of patients with atopic dermatitis. Serum ECP levels have been found to be increased in atopic dermatitis patients in several studies and levels correlate with disease activity (62,64,67–75). Elevated ECP levels occur both in adults and in children (73–75), although children usually show lower ECP levels (67). Neither serum ECP levels nor serum MBP levels correlate with serum IgE levels in atopic dermatitis patients. The observed relationship between eosinophil granule proteins and disease activity provides strong support for the eosinophil's role in the disease.

Extracellular deposition of eosinophil granule proteins occurs in several in vivo models of hypersensitivity, including the IgE-mediated late-phase reaction (LPR) (8), which is induced by intradermal allergen injection in allergic subjects. The LPR is associated with release of eosinophil granule proteins into tissues and blister fluids bathing these tissues, with marked disruption of eosinophils and extracellular deposition of eosinophil granule proteins (8,76). Increased mRNA expression of several cytokines including IL-3, IL-4, IL-5, and GM-CSF is found in the cutaneous LPR (77) along with eosinophil survival-enhancing cytokines in LPR blister fluids (78). Likewise, in the nose, after antigen challenge, the LPR is accompanied by a dramatic increase in eosinophils and MBP and EDN levels in nasal lavage fluids along with eosinophil active cytokines in nasal secretions (79,80). Analyses of eosinophil granule proteins in the pulmonary LPR have shown that MBP, EDN, EPO, and ECP are elevated in bronchoalveolar lavage fluids, and IL-5 is the predominant eosinophil-active cytokine (81,82). Thus allergen challenge of sensitized patients causes eosinophil infiltration and granule protein release into the skin, nose, and lung.

**Table 4** Eosinophils in Atopic Dermatitis

| |
|---|
| Extensive deposition of eosinophil granule proteins in lesional tissue. |
| Increased peripheral blood eosinophils in severe disease which decrease with therapeutic improvement; hypodense eosinophils (activated phenotype) correlate best with disease activity. |
| Increased levels of eosinophil granule proteins in peripheral blood correlate with disease activity. |
| Eosinophil infiltration and extracellular granule protein deposition occur with patch test allergen provocation of lesions. |

*Source*: Ref. 18.

The late phase of the IgE-mediated reaction has been proposed as a model for chronic allergic inflammation, including that seen in atopic dermatitis (83,84). Histopathologic examinations of the cutaneous LPR have shown infiltration with mononuclear cells, neutrophils, basophils, and eosinophils along with edema and mast cell degranulation (85–87). Immunohistologic studies have shown extracellular deposition of eosinophil and neutrophil granule proteins beginning 1 hr after antigen challenge and persisting during the LPR to 56 hr or longer (8). Eosinophil infiltration occurs quickly after antigen challenge, with eosinophils marginating in blood vessels as early as 15 min after challenge (8). Both extracellular eosinophil and neutrophil granule protein deposition are prominent at the peak of the reaction, 6 to 8 hr after antigen challenge (8). In contrast to the LPR, neutrophil granule proteins are largely absent in established lesions of atopic dermatitis, and patients with atopic dermatitis do not have elevated elastase levels in the peripheral blood (17).

Allergen challenge models, in addition to the LPR, have been studied in an effort to simulate the pathogenic mechanisms in atopic dermatitis. These studies further establish links between eosinophils and the pathophysiology of the disease. Biopsies of patch test sites provoked by topical aeroallergen applications in atopic dermatitis patients showed that lymphocytes and eosinophils infiltrate the dermis 2 to 6 hr after allergen application. By 24 to 48 hr, eosinophils infiltrated the epidermis and had released ECP (88). Following house dust mite antigen provocation with epicutaneous patch testing, activated eosinophils were present in the dermis in contact with antigen-presenting cells in the skin of atopic dermatitis patients (89). Moreover, in these specimens, eosinophil granules were present outside of intact cells, and ECP was present in macrophage-like dermal cells (89). These studies demonstrate direct relationships between eosinophil activity and eczematous dermatitis development. Although certain immunohistologic comparisons between the IgE-mediated LPR and atopic dermatitis differ, the possibility remains that they are part of the same inflammatory process. In atopic dermatitis, exposure to allergen is likely to result from transdermal, ingestational, or inhalational exposures, rather than intradermal injection as used to induce the LPR. Disease expression may be modified based on antigen processing and presentation by immunocompetent cells in various skin compartments. Furthermore, the LPR studies have been performed in patients with allergic rhinitis. Antigen exposure in atopic dermatitis skin may induce a different inflammatory response than does intradermal antigen exposure in patients with respiratory allergies. Finally, in atopic dermatitis, repeated or continuous antigen exposure may affect inflammatory reactivity, enhancing eosinophil participation while diminishing neutrophil participation as has been observed in a primate model of antigen challenge in the lung (90).

Cutaneous biopsy specimens from LPRs at 24 hr showed mRNA expression for IL-3 in 8 of 14 patients, IL-4 in 10 of 14 patients, IL-5 in 11 of 14 patients, and GM-CSF in 13 of 14 patients (77). Only 5 of 14 patients showed mRNA expression for IL-2 and none of the 14 for IFN-γ. These findings demonstrate that cells infiltrating cutaneous LPRs have mRNA for IL-3, IL-4, IL-5, and GM-CSF, supporting the hypothesis that the LPR is associated with preferential activation of cells producing a Th2 cell cytokine profile. The studies further indicate that expression of these cytokines is associated with eosinophil induction and activation in the LPR.

Studies to determine cytokine expression have shown different patterns in patients with atopic dermatitis. One study comparing "atopic" dermatitis with "nonatopic" atopic dermatitis (i.e., atopic dermatitis with identifiable and without identifiable IgE relationships, respectively) showed that a Th2-type cytokine profile was observed in patients with "atopic" atopic dermatitis (91). These patients' peripheral blood lymphocytes spontaneously released IL-4 and IL-5, whereas "nonatopic" atopic dermatitis patients displayed high IL-5 but low IL-4 levels. Supernatants from lesional skin biopsies showed similar findings with increased IL-4 levels present in "atopic" atopic dermatitis skin biopsies and IL-5 levels increased in both "atopic" and "nonatopic" atopic dermatitis specimens (91). In another study comparing cytokine mRNA expression, both acute and chronic lesions had significantly greater numbers of cells with mRNA for IL-4 and IL-5 compared to uninvolved skin, but chronic atopic dermatitis lesions had significantly fewer IL-4 mRNA-expressing cells and significantly more IL-5 mRNA-expressing cells than acute lesions (92). The chronic lesions also showed more eosinophil infiltration than either the acute lesions or uninvolved skin (92). Considering the effects of IL-5 in promoting differentiation, adhesion, and enhanced survival of eosinophils, these studies emphasize the potential important involvement of eosinophils in chronic atopic dermatitis and may explain the persistent evidence for eosinophil activity in chronic allergic inflammation.

## III. Bullous Pemphigoid

Bullous pemphigoid is an immunobullous disease in which patients develop blistering of the skin in association with circulating antibodies that bind specifically to normal skin basement membrane zone components. The etiopathogenesis of the disease is not completely understood (93). The presence of antibody alone does not result in blister formation. Complement deposition and activation at the basement membrane zone, involving both the classic complement pathway as well as the alternative pathway, appear important. In animal models, leukocytes are required to induce basement membrane zone separation. In human disease, eosinophils prominently infiltrate lesions of bullous pemphigoid. Tense blisters, erosions, and crusts may all be seen in bullous pemphigoid along with erythematous macules, papules, and urticarial plaques (93).

To determine the involvement of eosinophils in the development of bullous pemphigoid lesions, skin biopsies from three patients were studied immunohistologically (22). The three patients showed clinical, histological, and immunohistological findings typical of bullous pemphigoid, and none of these patients had been treated before biopsy specimens were obtained. Histopathologic changes in hematoxylin and eosin-stained sections of mature lesions showed lymphohistiocytic infiltration, many eosinophils, and subepidermal blistering. Direct immunofluorescence of perilesional tissue in all three patients showed the characteristic pattern of linear IgG and C3 staining at the basement membrane zone. Indirect immunofluorescence of serum on monkey esophagus substrate showed an IgG anti-basement membrane zone titer of 1:2560 in one patient and was negative in the other two (22).

Biopsy specimens from three or four lesions in different stages of development from each patient were immunohistologically stained for three eosinophil granule proteins: MBP, ECP, and EDN. Skin specimens from areas appearing as erythema, wheal, blister, crusted, and healing lesions were obtained. In prebullous lesions, including areas of erythema and wheals, intact eosinophils were clustered in the papillary dermis and diffusely distributed in the mid-dermis; few eosinophils were observed in the epidermis. Extracellular eosinophil granule protein deposition was striking and out of proportion to the number of infiltrating eosinophils (22). In blistered lesions and crusted areas, extracellular eosinophil granule protein deposition was prominent and eosinophils were more numerous in the epidermis and clustered at the edges of the dermal-epidermal separation (Fig. 2); eosinophils were also present in blister cavities (22). In healing lesions, eosinophil infiltration was less than in the active lesions; however, extracellular eosinophil granule protein deposition persisted in the dermis. Uninvolved skin showed very slight MBP, ECP, and EDN staining with no infiltration of intact cells (22).

Electron microscopic examination of lesional tissues from two patients showed infiltration with lymphocytes, histiocytes, and eosinophils in the blistering lesions (22). Mainly intact eosinophils were found scattered in the papillary dermis in an erythematous lesion; some of the eosinophils were in close proximity or contacting the basement membrane zone. Degenerating eosinophils in a prebullous lesion were observed near hemidesmosomes in a disrupted area of the basement membrane zone. Prominent eosinophil disruption with free granules was found on both sides of the basement membrane zone in proximity to hemidesmosomes in areas of degenerating basement membrane zone in blistering lesions (22).

Eosinophil granule proteins were measured in serum, urine, and blister fluid. Eosinophil granule protein levels were increased in all of these fluids but were most strikingly increased in blister fluids. All three patients showed elevated MBP and EDN levels in the serum and urine. Two patients also showed

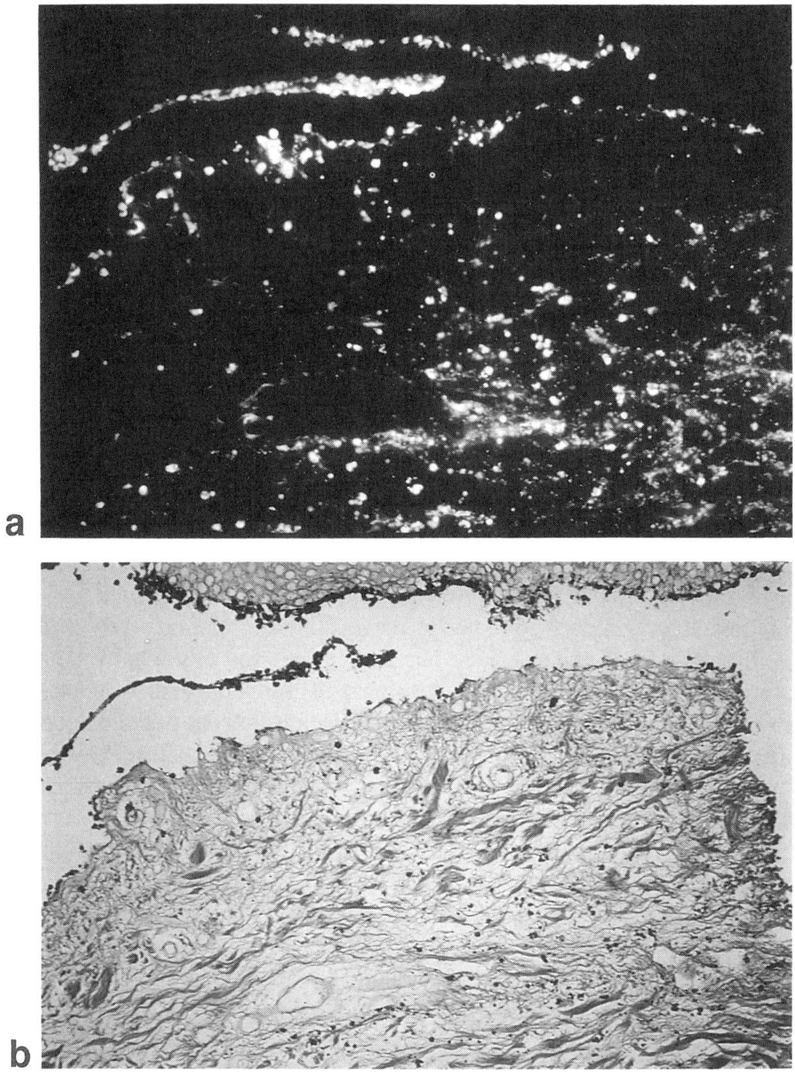


**Figure 2** Immunohistology of bullous pemphigoid lesion. (**a**) Photomicrograph of tissue section stained by indirect immunofluorescence for MBP showing extensive cellular and extracellular staining in and around a subepidermal blister and in the mid-dermis (magnification 160×). A control serial section stained with rabbit IgG showed no specific fluorescence (not shown). (**b**) Photomicrograph of the same field as in (a) counterstained with hematoxylin and eosin demonstrating a subepidermal blister and inflammatory cell infiltration. The extent of the MBP staining is not apparent with this stain (magnification 160×).

elevated ECP serum levels, and one showed an elevated ECP urine level. A second serum sample from one of the patients, obtained after treatment when blistering had resolved, showed normal eosinophil granule protein levels (22). In an eosinophil survival assay, blister fluid from all three bullous pemphigoid patients enhanced eosinophil survival. Eosinophil survival-enhancing activity in two of the blister fluids was blocked by antibodies to IL-5 and IL-3 and slightly by anti-GM-CSF. The quantity of blister fluid from the other patient was insufficient to perform blocking studies (22).

These findings demonstrate the prominence of eosinophil activity at all stages of lesional development in bullous pemphigoid. Previous studies showed that bullous pemphigoid blister fluids contained high levels of ECP and MBP (94–96). A recent study suggests that gelatinase, produced and deposited by eosinophils at the site of blister formation, contributes to dermal-epidermal separation in bullous pemphigoid (97). Moreover, using in vitro models of basement membrane zone, eosinophils have been found to elaborate a matrix metalloproteinase that degrades basement membrane zone components (98). Interestingly, the release and the activation of matrix metalloproteinase by eosinophils are dissociated. For example, PAF alone strongly enhances release of matrix metalloproteinase from eosinophils but does not enhance matrix metalloproteinase enzymatic activity in the eosinophil; IL-5 is required for both to occur. It appears that combinations of signals including activation by IL-5 may be necessary for eosinophils to elaborate enzymatically active factors for basement membrane zone degradation as may be occurring in bullous pemphigoid.

## IV. Recurrent Cutaneous Necrotizing Eosinophilic Vasculitis

A vasculitis with nearly exclusive eosinophil infiltration has been identified through histopathologic examination of skin biopsy specimens (25). Clinical characterization of three patients with this histopathologic presentation showed that all three patients presented with recurrent pruritic and purpuric papular skin lesions along with angioedema. Urticarial plaques and palpable purpura had also developed. Occasionally the patients noted annular erythematous, edematous lesions and vesicular lesions. The skin lesions showed prompt response to systemic glucocorticoid therapy, requiring alternate-day glucocorticoids to maintain disease control in two of the patients. Swelling and itching were prominent symptoms (25).

All three patients had marked peripheral blood eosinophilia. Urine and blood cultures, multiple stool examinations for ova and parasites, and serologic studies for underlying connective tissue diseases or infection were negative. Bone marrow biopsy specimens were examined from all patients; slight to moderate increases in eosinophil precursors without neoplastic changes were found (25).

Electrocardiograms, chest roentgenograms, and urinalyses were normal. An abdominal computed tomographic scan and echocardiogram in one patient were also negative. No deposition of immunoglobulins along vessel walls was found on direct immunofluorescence testing of frozen specimens. One patient showed a striking elevation of serum IgE level. Two of the patients had elevated erythrocyte sedimentation rates (25).

Hepatic vein occlusion developed in one patient and transient lymphadenopathy with hepatosplenomegaly and alopecia totalis developed in another. There was no evidence of cardiac, pulmonary, or other visceral organ involvement in any of the patients. None of the patients had asthma or allergic rhinitis. No other systemic symptoms including fever, weight loss, arthralgia, myalgia, or peripheral neuropathy developed during disease observation of 2 to 23 years (25).

Two or more skin biopsy specimens from each patient all showed necrotizing vasculitis of small dermal vessels with fibrinoid necrosis of vessel walls and exclusive eosinophil infiltration throughout the dermis with minimal or no leukocytoclasis. The epidermis was normal except for occasional intraepidermal vesicles with eosinophil infiltration. Indirect immunofluorescence for eosinophil granule MBP (Fig. 3) and EDN showed marked staining of MBP and EDN in affected small dermal vessels and in surrounding areas of the skin tissues (25). Electron microscopic examination of an early skin lesion from one patient showed adherence of abnormal eosinophils and free eosinophil granules to endothelial cells in walls of small vessels in association with damage to endothelial cells. The eosinophils showed loss of cytoplasmic granule core density, loss of cellular organelles, and chromatolysis of nuclei. Abnormalities of endothelial cells consisted of nuclear pyknosis, swelling and destruction of mitochondria, and destruction of cellular membranes. Degenerating eosinophils with scattered clusters of free granules were found between collagen bundles in addition to the vascular location (25).

Immunostaining for adhesion molecules showed vascular cell adhesion molecule (VCAM)-1 on endothelial cells of involved small vessels with very late activation antigen (VLA)-4 staining cells in the immediate area of the positive vessels. Intracellular adhesion molecule (ICAM)-1 expression was prominent and strongest in the affected vessels of the superficial dermis. E-selectin was not expressed on involved vessels. No VCAM-1 staining or VLA-4 positive cells were observed in uninvolved vessels (25).

Eosinophil survival assay using serum from one patient showed prolongation of eosinophil survival that was abolished by antibodies to IL-5. In contrast, antibodies to IL-3 and GM-CSF failed to inhibit the enhanced survival. Prolonged eosinophil survival was also observed with serum samples from another patient, but it was not possible to characterize the cytokines present and a serum sample from the third patient was not available (25).

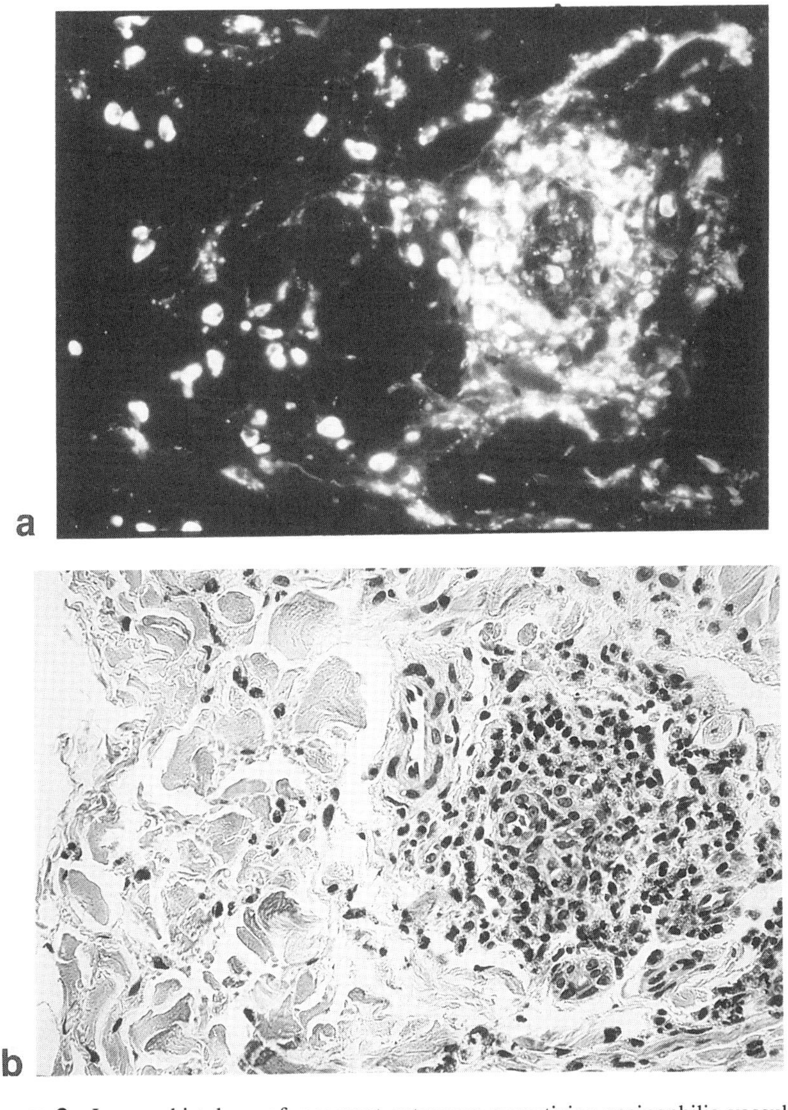

**Figure 3** Immunohistology of recurrent cutaneous necrotizing eosinophilic vasculitis lesion. (a) Photomicrograph of tissue section stained by indirect immunofluorescence for MBP showing striking cellular and extracellular staining in small vessel walls and surrounding dermis (magnification 400×). A control serial section stained with rabbit IgG showed no specific fluorescence (not shown). (b) Photomicrograph of same field as in (a) stained with hematoxylin and eosin demonstrating prominent vascular infiltration by eosinophils; the extensive extracellular protein deposition is not observable with this stain (magnification 400×).

These three patients presented with an interesting glucocorticoid-responsive pruritic, cutaneous eruption associated with angioedema that histologically showed eosinophil vascular inflammation and destruction. The selective recruitment of eosinophils via the expression of VCAM-1 and endothelial cells is likely important in this syndrome as well as in other diseases associated with eosinophil infiltration as eosinophils expressed the integrin VLA-4, which is a ligand for VCAM-1. In addition, IL-5 likely contributed to the peripheral blood eosinophilia as well as the activation of the cells in the tissue in this disorder (25).

Eosinophils have been associated with edema in a number of conditions, and eosinophils show several activities that may provoke edema formation as summarized in Table 5 (9,99). Eosinophil granule proteins have direct effects on blood vessels causing an increase in vascular permeability (46). Extracellular MBP has been localized around dermal blood vessels in edematous skin reactions including chronic urticaria and episodic angioedema (4,9). Moreover, eosinophils elaborate $LTC_4$ (50,51) and PAF (49) both of which promote vasopermeability. Also, eosinophil granule proteins induce histamine release from rat mast cells and human basophils which may further increase vasopermeability (42,43). Although MBP does not appear to induce histamine release from human mast cells (100), MBP induces histamine release from human basophils. An added wave of mediator release from basophils may be the explanation for the marked edema that is characteristic of the LPR.

In this syndrome of recurrent necrotizing eosinophilic vasculitis, periorbital and acral edema was prominent in the patients. Electron microscopic examinations showed degenerating eosinophils with free eosinophil granules in the dermis and immunofluorescent localization of eosinophil granule proteins showed prominent MBP deposition in and around cutaneous blood vessels (25). The presence of IL-5 in serum and the VCAM-1 expression on the endothelium of affected vessels likely contributed to the selective adherence and localization of activated eosinophils; subsequently, release of cytotoxic eosinophil granule proteins may have contributed to the edema and ultimately resulted in destruction of the endothelium in this unique syndrome.

**Table 5** Eosinophils and Edema

| |
|---|
| Eosinophil granule proteins induce wheal and flare reactions in human skin. |
| Eosinophils elaborate leukotriene $C_4$ and platelet activating factor which promote vasopermeability. |
| EPO with $H_2O_2$ and halide and MBP alone induce histamine release from mast cells and basophils. |
| Eosinophil granule proteins have direct effects on blood vessels. |
| Eosinophil granule proteins are deposited around blood vessels in edematous skin lesions. |

*Source*: Ref. 18

## V. Conclusion

Investigative observations of eosinophils in cutaneous diseases along with recent studies defining activities of eosinophils support a role for the eosinophil as a primary participant in the pathogenesis of several cutaneous disorders. Multiple signaling mechanisms appear to control eosinophil infiltration, activation, and degranulation at inflammatory sites. Considering its effects on eosinophils, IL-5 likely is an important factor in directing eosinophil activities in certain diseases. The eosinophil possesses proteins that are toxic to a variety of cells and induce activation of cells such as basophils with release of histamine and other vasoactive substances. Potent oxidants and toxic cationic proteins from eosinophils likely achieve high concentrations at points of granule deposition, thus mediating damage to tissues. Because eosinophils disrupt in tissue, they may not be recognized as an infiltrating cell in tissues. Nevertheless, granule protein deposition as well as other toxic activities may cause tissue damage in the absence of morphologically identifiable cells. Therefore, contributions of the eosinophil to the pathophysiology of cutaneous diseases may not be recognized by simple identification of tissue eosinophils. Recent studies, including those defining the effects of IL-5 on eosinophils and the presence of IL-5 in disease, are providing important information about recruitment and activation of eosinophils in cutaneous inflammation.

## Acknowledgment

This work was supported by grants from the National Institutes of Health (AR 36008, AI 34577, and AI 15231), the Mayo Foundation, and the Kieckhefer Foundation.

Portions of this chapter have been taken in part and used with permission from:

Leiferman KM. Cutaneous eosinophilic diseases. In: Fitzpatrick TB, Eisen AZ, Wolff K, Freeberg IM, Austen KF, Katz SI, Goldsmith LA, eds. Dermatology in General Medicine, Fifth Edition. New York: McGraw-Hill, in press.

Leiferman KM, Gleich GJ. The role of eosinophils in atopic dermatitis. In: Leung DYM, ed. Atopic Dermatitis: From Pathogenesis to Treatment. Austin, TX: R. G. Landes, 1996:145–183.

Ott NL, Gleich GJ, Peterson EA, Fujisawa T, Sur S, Leiferman KM. Assessment of eosinophil and neutrophil participation in atopic dermatitis: comparison with the IgE-mediated late phase reaction. J Allergy Clin Immunol 1994;94:120–128.

Borrego L, Maynard B, Peterson EA, George T, Iglesias L, Peters MS, Newman W, Gleich GJ, Leiferman KM. Deposition of eosinophil granule proteins precedes blister formation in bullous pemphigoid: comparison with neutrophil and mast cell granule proteins. Am J Pathol 1996;148:897–909.

Chen K-R, Pittelkow MR, Su WPD, Gleich GJ, Newman W, Leiferman KM. Recurrent cutaneous necrotizing eosinophilic vasculitis: a novel eosinophil mediated syndrome. Arch Dermatol 1994;130:1159–1166.

## References

1. Gleich GJ. The eosinophil and bronchial asthma: current understanding. J Allergy Clin Immunol 1990;85:422–436.
2. Leiferman KM. Cutaneous eosinophilic diseases. In: Fitzpatrick TB, Eisen AZ, Wolff K, Freeberg IM, Austen KF, Katz SI, Goldsmith LA, eds. Dermatology in General Medicine, Fifth Edition. New York: McGraw-Hill, in press.
3. Peters MS. The eosinophil. In: Callen JP, ed. Advances in Dermatology. Chicago: Yearbook, 1987:129.
4. Peters MS, Schroeter AL, Kephart GM, Gleich GJ. Localization of eosinophil granule major basic protein in chronic urticaria. J Invest Dermatol 1983;81:39–43.
5. Sodhi N, Peterson EA, Schroeter AL, Reed CE, Gleich GJ, Butterfield JH, Leiferman KM. Inflammatory cells in chronic urticaria [abstract]. J Allergy Clin Immunol 1990;85:204.
6. Leiferman KM, Norris PG, Murphy GM, Hawk JLM, Winkelmann RK. Evidence for eosinophil degranulation with deposition of granule major basic protein in solar urticaria. J Am Acad Dermatol 1989;21:75–80.
7. McEvoy MT, Peterson EA, Kobza-Black A, English JSC, Dover JS, Murphy GM, Bhogal B, Greaves MW, Winkelmann RK, Leiferman KM. Immunohistological comparison of granulated cell proteins in induced immediate dermographism and delayed pressure urticaria. Br J Dermatol 1995;133:853–860.
8. Leiferman KM, Fujisawa T, Gray BH, Gleich GJ. Extracellular deposition of eosinophil and neutrophil granule proteins in the IgE-mediated cutaneous late phase reaction. Lab Invest 1990;62:579–589.
9. Gleich GJ, Schroeter AL, Marcoux JP, Sachs MI, O'Connell EJ, Kohler PF. Episodic angioedema associated with eosinophilia. N Engl J Med 1984;310:1621–1626.
10. Katzen DR, Leiferman KM, Leung DYM. Hypereosinophilia and recurrent angioedema in a 2-1/2 year old girl. Am J Dis Child 1986;140:62–64.
11. Wolf C, Pehamberger H, Breyer S, Leiferman KM, Wolff K. Episodic angioedema with eosinophilia. J Am Acad Dermatol 1989;20:21–27.
12. Butterfield JH, Leiferman KM, Abrams J, Silver JE, Bower J, Gonchoroff N, Gleich GJ. Elevated serum levels of interleukin-5 in patients with the syndrome of episodic angioedema and eosinophilia. Blood 1992;79:688–692.
13. Mehregan DR, Fransway AF, Edmonson JH, Leiferman KM. Cutaneous reactions to granulocyte monocyte colony stimulating factor. Arch Dermatol 1992;128:1055–1059.

14. van Haelst-Pisani C, Kovach JS, Kita H, Leiferman KM, Gleich GJ, Silver JE, Dennin R, Abrams JS. Administration of interleukin-2 (IL-2) results in increased plasma concentrations of IL-5 and eosinophilia in patients with cancer. Blood 1991;78:1538–1544.
15. Peters MS, Schroeter AL, Gleich GJ. Immunofluorescence identification of eosinophil granule major basic protein in the flame figures of Wells' syndrome. Br J Dermatol 1983;109:141–148.
16. Leiferman KM, Ackerman SJ, Sampson HA, Haugen HS, Venencie PY, Gleich GJ. Dermal deposition of eosinophil-granule major basic protein in atopic dermatitis: comparison with onchocerciasis. N Engl J Med 1985; 313:282–285.
17. Ott NL, Gleich GJ, Peterson EA, Fujisawa T, Sur S, Leiferman KM. Assessment of eosinophil and neutrophil participation in atopic dermatitis: comparison with the IgE-mediated late phase reaction. J Allergy Clin Immunol 1994;94:120–128.
18. Leiferman KM, Gleich GJ. The role of eosinophils in atopic dermatitis. In: Leung DYM, ed. Atopic Dermatitis: From Pathogenesis to Treatment. Austin, TX: R. G. Landes, 1996:145–183.
19. Jacyk WK, Simson IW, Slater DN, Leiferman KM. Pachydermatous eosinophilic dermatitis. Br J Dermatol 1996;134:469–474.
20. Perez GL, Peters MS, Reda AM, Butterfield JH, Peterson EA, Leiferman KM. Mast cells, neutrophils and eosinophils in prurigo nodularis. Arch Dermatol 1193; 129:861–866.
21. Scheman AJ, Hordinsky MD, Groth DW, Vercellotti GM, Leiferman KM. Evidence for eosinophil degranulation in the pathogenesis of herpes gestationis. Arch Dermatol 1989;125:1079–1083.
22. Borrego L, Maynard B, Peterson EA, George T, Iglesias L, Peters MS, Newman W, Gleich GJ, Leiferman KM. Deposition of eosinophil granule proteins precedes blister formation in bullous pemphigoid: comparison with neutrophil and mast cell granule proteins. Am J Pathol 1996;148:897–909.
23. Daoud MS, Su WPD, Leiferman KM, Perniciaro C. Bullous morphea: clinical, pathologic and immunopathologic evaluation of thirteen cases. J Am Acad Dermatol 1994;30:937–943.
24. Thyresson NH, Goldberg NC, Tye MJ, Leiferman KM. Localization of eosinophil granule major basic protein in incontinentia pigmenti. Pediatr Dermatol 1991;8:102–106.
25. Chen K-R, Pittelkow MR, Su WPD, Gleich GJ, Newman W, Leiferman KM. Recurrent cutaneous necrotizing eosinophilic vasculitis: a novel eosinophil mediated syndrome. Arch Dermatol 1994;130:1159–1166.
26. Chen K-R, Su WPD, Pittelkow MR, Conn DL, George T, Leiferman KM. Eosinophilic vasculitis in connective tissue disease. J Am Acad Dermatol 1996;35:173–182.
27. Drage LA, Davis MDP, deCastro F, VanKeulen V, Gleich GJ, Leiferman KM. Eosinophil and neutrophil involvement in Churg-Strauss syndrome [abstract]. J Cutan Pathol 1997;24:95.
28. Martin RW, Duffy J, Engel AG, Lie JT, Bowles CA, Moyer TP, Gleich GJ. The

clinical spectrum of the eosinophilia-myalgia syndrome associated with L-tryptophan ingestion. Clinical features in 20 patients and aspects of pathophysiology. Ann Intern Med 1990;113:124–134.
29. Ten RM, Kephart GM, Posada M, Abaitua I, Soldevilla L, Kilbourne EM, Dunnette SL, Gleich GJ. Participation of eosinophils in the toxic oil syndrome. Clin Exp Immunol 1990;82:313–317.
30. Noguchi H, Kephart GM, Colby TV, Gleich GJ. Tissue eosinophilia and eosinophil degranulation in syndromes associated with fibrosis. Am J Pathol 1992;140:521–528.
31. Helander SD, Peters MS, Kuo TT, Su WPD. Kimura's disease and angiolymphoid hyperplasia with eosinophilia: new observations from immunohistochemical studies of lymphocyte markers, endothelial antigens and granulocyte proteins. J Cutan Pathol 1995;22:319–326.
32. Gleich GJ, Adolphson CR, Leiferman KM. Eosinophils. In: Gallin JI, Goldstein IM, Snyderman R, eds. Inflammation, Basic Principles and Clinical Correlates. New York: Raven Press, 1992:663–700.
33. Kita H, Gleich GJ. The eosinophil: structure and functions. In: Kaplan AP, ed. Allergy. Philadelphia: W. B. Saunders, 1997:148–178.
34. Kapp A, Zek-Kapp G, Czech W, Schopf E. The chemokine RANTES is more than a chemoattractant: characterization of its effect on human eosinophil oxidative metabolism and morphology in comparison with IL-5 and GM-CSF. J Invest Dermatol 1994;102:906–914.
35. Elsner J, Hochstetter R, Kimmig D, Kapp A. Human eotaxin represents a potent activator of the respiratory burst of human eosinophils. Eur J Immunol 1996;26:1919–1925.
36. Bochner BS, Schleimer RP. The role of adhesion molecules in human eosinophil and basophil recruitment. J Allergy Clin Immunol 1994;94:427–438.
37. Teti A. Regulation of cellular functions by extracellular matrix. J Am Soc Nephrol 1992;2(suppl 10):S83–S87.
38. Horie S, Kita H. CD11b/CD17 (Mac-1) is required for degranulation of human eosinophils induced by human recombinant granulocyte-macrophage colony-stimulating factor and platelet-activating factor. J Immunol 1994;152:5457–5467.
39. Mosmann TR, Coffman RL. TH1 and TH2 cells: different patterns of lymphokine secretion lead to different functional properties. Annu Rev Immunol 1989;7:145–173.
40. Bradding P, Feather IH, Wilson S, Bardin PG, Heusser CH, Holgate ST, Howarth PH. Immunolocalization of cytokines in the nasal mucosa of normal and perennial rhinitic subjects. The mast cell as a source of IL-4, IL-5, and IL-6 in human allergic mucosal inflammation. J Immunol 1993;151:3853–3865.
41. Moqbel R, Levi-Schaffer F, Kay AB. Cytokine generation by eosinophils. J Allergy Clin Immunol 1994;94:1183–1188.
42. O'Donnell MC, Ackerman ST, Gleich GJ, Thomas LL. Stimulation of basophil and mast cell histamine release by eosinophil major basic protein. J Exp Med 1983;157:1981–1991.
43. Zheutlin LM, Ackerman SJ, Gleich GJ, Thomas GJ, Thomas LL. Stimulation of

basophil and rat mast cell histamine release by eosinophil granule-derived cationic proteins. J Immunol 1984;133:2180–2185.
44. Moy JN, Gleich GJ, Thomas LL. Noncytotoxic activation of neutrophils by eosinophil granule major basic protein: effect on superoxide anion generation and lysosomal enzyme release. J Immunol 1990;145:2626–2632.
45. Rohrbach MS, Wheatley CL, Slifman NR, Gleich GJ. Activation of platelets by eosinophil granule proteins. J Exp Med 1990;172:1271–1274.
46. Minnicozzi M, Duran WN, Gleich GJ, Egan RW. Eosinophil granule proteins increase microvascular macromolecular transport in the hamster cheek pouch. J Immunol 1994;153:2664–2670.
47. Kanofsky JR, Hoogland H, Wever R, Weiss SJ. Singlet oxygen production by human eosinophils. J Biol Chem 1988;263:9692–9696.
48. Petreccia DC, Nauseef WM, Clark RA. Respiratory burst of normal human eosinophils. J Leukocyte Biol 1987;41:283–288.
49. Lee TC, Lenihan DJ, Malone B, Roddy LL, Wasserman SI. Increased biosynthesis of platelet-activating factor in activated human eosinophils. J Biol Chem 1984;259:5526–5530.
50. Weller PF, Lee CW, Foster DW, Corey EJ, Austen KF, Lewis RA. Generation and metabolism of 5-lipoxygenase pathway leukotrienes by human eosinophils: predominant production of leukotriene C4. Proc Natl Acad Sci USA 1983;80:7626–7630.
51. Shaw RJ, Walsh GM, Cromwell O, Moqbel R, Spry CJF, Kay AB. Activated human eosinophils generate SRS-A leukotrienes following physiological (IgG-dependent) stimulation. Nature 1985;316:150–152.
52. Hansel TT, Braun RK, DeVries IJ, Boer C, Boer L, Rih S, Walker C. Eosinophils and cytokines. Agents Actions 1993;43(suppl):197–208.
53. Moqbel R. Eosinophils, cytokines, and allergic inflammation [review]. Ann NY Acad Sci 1994;725:223–233.
54. Miyamasu M, Hirai K, Takahashi Y, Lida M, Yamaguchi M, Koshino T, Takaishi T, Morita Y, Ohta K, Kasahara T, Ito K. Chemotactic agonists induce cytokine generation in eosinophils. J Immunol 1995;154:1339–1349.
55. Elovic A, Wong DT, Weller PF, Matossian K, Galli SJ. Expression of transforming growth factors-alpha and beta 1 messenger RNA and product by eosinophils in nasal polyps. J Allergy Clin Immunol 1994;93:864–869.
56. Birkland TP, Cheavens MD, Pincus SH. Human eosinophils stimulate DNA synthesis and matrix production in dermal fibroblasts. Arch Dermatol Res 1994;286:312–318.
57. Rajka G. Atopic dermatitis. Major Prob Dermatol 1975;3:42.
58. Mihm MC, Soter NA, Dvorak HF, Austen KF. The structure of normal skin and the morphology of atopic eczema. J Invest Dermatol 1976;67:305–312.
59. Wassom DL, Loegering DA, Solley GO, Moore SB, Schooley RJ, Fauci AS, Gleich GJ. Elevated serum levels of the eosinophil granule major basic protein in patients with eosinophilia. J Clin Invest 1981;67:651–661.
60. Leiferman KM. Current perspective on the role of eosinophils in dermatologic diseases. J Am Acad Dermatol 1991;24:1101–1112.

61. Sanda T, Yasue T, Oohashi M, Yasue A. Effectiveness of house dust-mite allergen avoidance through clean room therapy in patients with atopic dermatitis. J Allergy Clin Immunol 1992;89:653–657.
62. Kagi MK, Joller-Jemelka H, Wuthrich B. Correlation of eosinophils, eosinophil cationic protein and soluble interleukin-2 receptor with the clinical activity of atopic dermatitis. Dermatology 1992;185:88–92.
63. Mukai H, Noguchi T, Kamimura K, Nishioka K, Nishiyama S. Significance of elevated serum LDH (lactate dehydrogenase) activity in atopic dermatitis. J Dermatol 1990;17:477–481.
64. Suagai T, Shoji A, Nagareda T. Changes of ECP values, number of eosinophils and EG2 eosinophils in the peripheral blood following oral ketotifen in patients with atopic dermatitis. Skin Res 1992;34:368–386.
65. Uehara M, Izukura R, Sawai T. Blood eosinophilia in atopic dermatitis. Clin Exp Dermatol 1990;15:264–266.
66. Businco L, Meglio P, Ferrara M. The role of food allergy and eosinophils in atopic dermatitis. Pediatr Allergy Immunol 1993;4:33–37.
67. Knapp A. The role of eosinophils in the pathogenesis of atopic dermatitis—eosinophil granule proteins as markers of disease activity. Allergy 1993;48:1–5.
68. Paganelli R, Fanales-Belasio E, Carmini D, Scala E, Meglio P, Businco L, Aiuti F. Serum eosinophil cationic protein in patients with atopic dermatitis. Int Arch Allergy Appl Immunol 1991;96:175–178.
69. Czech W, Krutmann J, Schopf E, Kapp A. Serum eosinophil cationic protein (ECP) is a sensitive measure for disease activity in atopic dermatitis. Br J Dermatol 1992;126:351–355.
70. Juhlin L, Venge P. Eosinophilic cationic protein (ECP) in skin disorders. Acta Dermatol Venereol (Stockh) 1991;71:495–501.
71. Krutmann J, Czech W, Diepgen T, Niedner R, Kapp A, Schopf E. High-dose UVA1 therapy in the treatment of patients with atopic dermatitis. J Am Acad Dermatol 1992;26:225–230.
72. Sugai T, Sakiyama Y, Matsumoto S. Eosinophil cationic protein in peripheral blood of pediatric patients with allergic diseases. Clin Exp Allergy 1992;22:275–281.
73. Tsuda S, Kato K, Miyasato M, Sasai Y. Eosinophil involvement in atopic dermatitis as reflected by elevated serum levels of eosinophil cationic protein. J Dermatol 1992;19:208–213.
74. Kapp A, Czech W, Krutmann J, Schoepf E. Eosinophil cationic protein in sera of patients with atopic dermatitis. J Am Acad Dermatol 1991;24:555–558.
75. Jakob T, Hermann K, Ring J. Eosinophil cationic protein in atopic eczema. Arch Dermatol Res 1991;283:5–6.
76. Zweiman B, Atkins PC, von Allmen C, Gleich GJ. Release of eosinophil granule proteins during IgE-mediated allergic skin reactions. J Allergy Clin Immunol 1991;87:984–992.
77. Kay AB, Ying S, Varney V, Gaga M, Durham SR, Moqbel R, Wardlaw AJ, Hamid Q. Messenger RNA expression of cytokine gene cluster, interleukin 3 (IL-3), IL-4, IL-5, and granulocyte/macrophage colony-stimulating factor, in allergen-induced late-phase cutaneous reactions in atopic subjects. J Exp Med 1991;173:775–778.

78. Charlesworth EN, Nish WA, Charlesworth MG, Valtier S, George T, Leiferman KM. Standard high dose immunotherapy decreases the production of IL-3, IL-5 and GM-CSF during the cutaneous late-phase response (LPR) to antigen. J Allergy Clin Immunol 1993;91:252.
79. Bascom R, Pipkorn U, Proud D, Dunnette S, Gleich GJ, Lichtenstein LM, Naclerio RM. Major basic protein and eosinophil-derived neurotoxin concentrations in nasal-lavage fluid after antigen challenge: effect of systemic corticosteroids and relationship to eosinophil influx. J Allergy Clin Immunol 1989;84:338–346.
80. Sim TC, Grant JA, Hilsmeier KA, Fukuda Y, Alam R. Proinflammatory cytokines in nasal secretions of allergic subjects after antigen challenge. Am J Respir Crit Care Med 1994;149:339–344.
81. Sedgwick JB, Calhoun WJ, Gleich GJ, Kita H, Abrams JS, Schwartz LB, Volovitz B, Ben-Yaakov M, Busse WW. Immediate and late airway response of allergic rhinitis patients to segmental antigen challenge. Characterization of eosinophil and mast cell mediators. Am Rev Respir Dis 1991;144:1274–1281.
82. Ohnishi T, Kita H, Weiler D, Sur S, Sedgwick JB, Calhoun WJ, Busse WW, Abrams JS, Gleich GJ. IL-5 is the predominant eosinophil-active cytokine in the antigen-induced pulmonary late-phase reaction. Am Rev Respir Dis 1993;147:901–907.
83. Gleich GJ. The late phase of the immunoglobulin-E mediated reaction: a link between anaphylaxis and common allergic disease? J Allergy Clin Immunol 1982;70:160–169.
84. Sampson HA. Late-phase response to food in atopic dermatitis. Hosp Pract (Off) 1987;22:111–128.
85. Charlesworth EN, Hood AF, Soter NA, Kagey-Sobotka A, Norman PS, Lichtenstein LM. Cutaneous late-phase response to allergen: mediator release and inflammatory cell infiltration. J Clin Invest 1989;83:1519–1526.
86. Dolovich J, Hargreave FE, Chalmers R, Shier KJ, Gauldie J, Bienenstock J. Late cutaneous allergic responses in isolated IgE-dependent reactions. J Allergy Clin Immunol 1973;52:38–46.
87. Solley GO, Gleich GJ, Jordon RE, Schroeter AL. The late phase of the immediate wheal and flare skin reaction: its dependence upon IgE antibodies. J Clin Invest 1976;58:408–420.
88. Bruijnzeel PL, Kuijper PH, Kapp A, Warringa RA, Betz S, Bruijnzeel-Koomen CA. The involvement of eosinophils in the patch test reaction to aeroallergens in atopic dermatitis: its relevance for the pathogenesis of atopic dermatitis. Clin Exp Allergy 1993;23:97–109.
89. Maeda K, Yamamoto K, Tanaka Y, Anan S, Yoshida H. The relationship between eosinophils, OKT6-positive cells and house dust mite (HDM) antigens in naturally occurring lesions of atopic lesions. J Dermatol Sci 1992;3:151–156.
90. Gundel RH, Gerritsen ME, Gleich GJ, Wegner CD. Repeated antigen inhalation results in a prolonged airway eosinophilia and airway hyperresponsiveness in primates. J Appl Physiol 1990;68:779–786.
91. Kagi MK, Wuthrich B, Montano E, Barandun J, Blaser K, Walker C. Differential cytokine profiles in peripheral blood lymphocyte supernatants and skin biop-

sies from patients with different forms of atopic dermatitis, psoriasis and normal individuals. Int Arch Allergy Immunol 1994;103:332.

92. Hamid Q, Boguniewicz M, Leung DYM. Differential in situ cytokine gene expression in acute versus chronic atopic dermatitis. J Clin Invest 1994;94:870–876.
93. Korman N. Bullous pemphigoid. J Am Acad Dermatol 1987;16:907–924.
94. Czech W, Schaller J, Schopf E, Kapp A. Granulocyte activation in bullous diseases: release of granular proteins in bullous pemphigoid and pemphigus vulgaris. J Am Acad Dermatol 1993;29:210–215.
95. Tsuda S, Miyasato M, Iryo K, Nakama T, Kato K, Sasai Y. Eosinophil phenotypes in bullous pemphigoid. J Dermatol 1992;19:270–279.
96. Wintroub BU, Dvorak AM, Mihm MC, Gleich GJ. Bullous pemphigoid: cytotoxic eosinophil degranulation and release of eosinophil major basic protein [abstract]. J Invest Dermatol 1981;76:310.
97. Stahle-Backdahl M, Inoue M, Giudice GJ, Parks WC. 92-kD gelatinase is produced by eosinophils at the site of blister formation in bullous pemphigoid and cleaves the extracellular domain of recombinant 180-kD bullous pemphigoid autoantigen. J Clin Invest 1994;93:2022–2030.
98. Okada S, Kita H, George TJ, Gleich GJ, Leiferman KM. Migration of eosinophils through basement membrane components in vitro: role of metalloproteinase-9. Am J Resp Cell Mol Biol, 1997; 17:519–528.
99. Leiferman KM, Peters MS, Gleich GJ. The eosinophil and cutaneous edema. J Am Acad Dermatol 1986;15:513–517.
100. Okayama Y, el-Lati SG, Leiferman KM, Church MK. Eosinophil granule proteins inhibit substance P-induced histamine release from human skin mast cells. J Allergy Clin Immunol 1994;93:900–909.

# 6

# Perinatal and Early Childhood Cytokine Responses to Environmental Allergens

**CLAUDIA MACAUBAS, SUSAN L. PRESCOTT, TROY SMALLACOMBE, AKIHIRO YABUHARA, THIERRY VENAILLE, BARBARA HOLT, PETER D. SLY, and PATRICK HOLT**

TVW Telethon Institute for Child Health Research
West Perth, Western Australia

## I. Introduction

Allergic diseases such as asthma are associated with Th2-polarized T-cell immunity. This observation seems to fit with what we know about the main role of the most typical Th2 cytokines. IL-4 is a key factor for IgE production (1) and IL-5 is critical for eosinophil production (2). More direct evidence concerning Th2 cytokines and asthma comes from studies showing expression of IL-4 and IL-5 mRNA in bronchoalveolar lavage of asthmatic patients and circulating T lymphocytes (3–5). To understand how these different patterns of T-cell immunity develop over a lifetime is a central point in the study of the etiology of allergic diseases, as this knowledge may lead to improvements in therapy. Several lines of evidence suggest that the immune response that results in an allergic condition in adult life initiates in infancy (6). For example, production of IgE antibodies is initiated in early life, being transient for nonatopics but persisting in atopic children (7).

In fact, the initial priming of T-cell responses may have already occurred "in utero" (6). These responses are subsequently reshaped during postnatal allergen exposure, probably via immune deviation (8). The result is the eventual development of stable allergen-specific T-cell memory polarized toward Th1 (in nonatopics) or Th2 (in atopics). The underlying Th1/Th2 switching process is influenced by genetic (9) and environmental factors (10) that are poorly understood. In particular, there is growing evidence that the immunological environment at the fetal/maternal interface is naturally skewed toward a Th2 profile (11,12), and the bias appears to be preserved for varying periods into infancy, which may account for the presence of the high-risk "window" for allergic sensitization in early postnatal life (13).

## II. Allergen-Specific Cytokine Responses at Birth

Our ongoing studies with cord blood mononuclear cells (CBMC) from full-term newborns demonstrated that lymphoproliferative responses to both inhalant and food classes of allergens are present at birth, with over 80% of individuals proliferating to at least one allergen tested (14,15). Responses to Der pI, the major allergen from the house dust mite, are very common, with about 70% of the cord blood showing positive responses. Ovalbumin and β-lactoglobulin induce proliferative responses in approximately 40% of babies. This responsiveness was not related to allergic family history (FH), as a similar proportion of FH-positive and FH-negative risk babies responded to each of these allergens. In contrast to these responses to allergen, responses to tetanus toxoid are rare (3% of all babies) and of low magnitude.

These results agree with a range of reports (6) that detected proliferative responses of cord blood mononuclear cells to several allergens. We next analyzed the production of allergen-specific cytokine response by neonatal lymphocytes, from which very little information is available. Because of limits in the sensitivity of the available assays for detection of cytokine protein, we analyzed the production of cytokine-specific mRNA by semiquantitative reverse transcriptase-polymerase chain reaction (RT-PCR).

We observed that at birth a high proportion of babies in both FH-positive and FH-negative groups showed an increase in IL-4- and IL-5-specific mRNA production by CBMC in response to allergen stimulation. At the population level, the only response that achieved statistical significance was production of IL-5 mRNA induced by OVA in the FH-positive group (Fig. 1; 14,15). The IFN-γ mRNA responses to the allergens were lower in frequency and magnitude, and at the population level were not significantly different from control. In addition, IFN-γ responses could only be detected by using 47 cycle numbers in the PCR, suggesting a very low frequency of cells producing this cytokine.

As mentioned earlier, the low levels of cytokine protein produced in these responses were an obstacle for detection by ELISA. However, it was possible to measure allergen-specific IL-10 protein production in supernants of 24 hr from 85% of CBMC cultures. Significant increases in production of specific IL-10

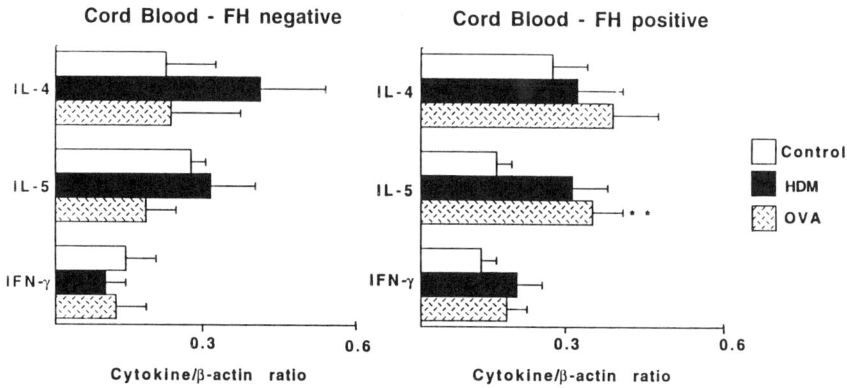


**Figure 1** Allergen-specific cytokine mRNA production by cord blood classified by family history of atopy. Cytokine mRNA is expressed as a ratio to β-actin. Data showed as mean ± SEM (** $p < 0.01$). (From Refs. 14 and 15).

protein in response to HDM and OVA were detected for both FH-positive and FH-negative groups (Fig. 2; 14,15).

The production of food- and aeroallergen-specific cytokine mRNA by CBMC supports earlier findings that the neonatal immune system is commonly

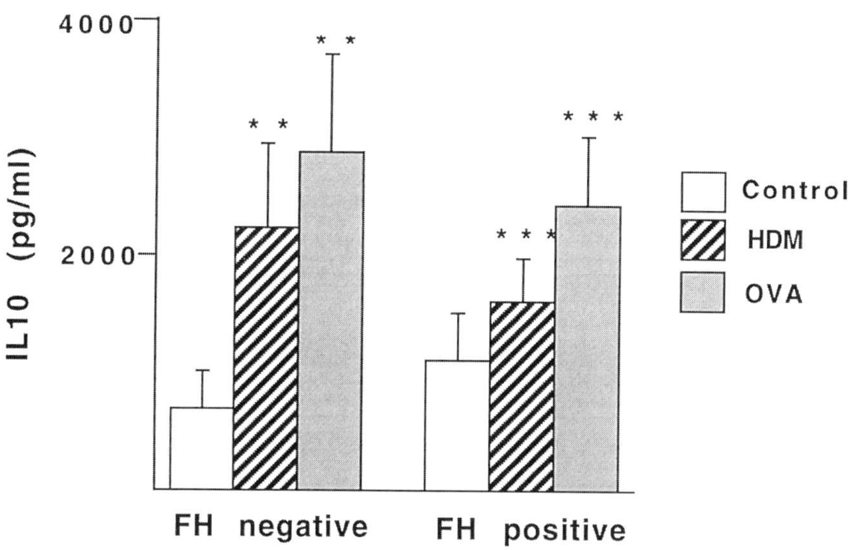


**Figure 2** Allergen-specific production of IL-10 protein by cord blood classified by family history of atopy. Data represent mean ± SEM (* $p < 0.05$; ** $p < 0.01$; *** $p < 0.001$). (From Refs. 14 and 15).

primed "in utero" to both types of antigen (6). It is also consistent with evidence suggesting that a successful pregnancy environment is biased toward production of Th2 cytokines like IL-10 (16), while Th1 cytokines appear associated with fetal loss (17).

Interestingly, the IL-5 responses in children with positive FH of atopy suggest that the polarization process may already have been initiated at birth for individuals at high risk of developing atopy. Further evidence comes from previous observation (6) confirmed in our sample of a decreased IFN-γ production by cord blood cells of newborns at high risk of atopy following policlonal stimulation.

## III. Allergen-Specific Cytokine Responses in Infancy and Early Childhood

Cross-sectional analysis of a group of infants about 2 years of age (mean age 17.9 months) showed major differences when the population was analyzed based on family history of allergy. The FH-positive group showed a mixed cytokine response to HDM and OVA, characterized by IL-4, IL-5, and IFN-γ mRNA production. In contrast, the FH-negative group displayed only a low-level Th2 response involving IL-5-specific mRNA to OVA allergen (Fig. 3; 18). In this study peripheral mononuclear cells were analyzed, and clonal studies are necessary to define the profile of cells producing cytokines.

Extending the analysis to an older age group, we tested a group of 5-year-old children. At this age, more objective markers of atopy can be used, and we selected the children based on their skin prick test reactivity (SPT) to HDM.

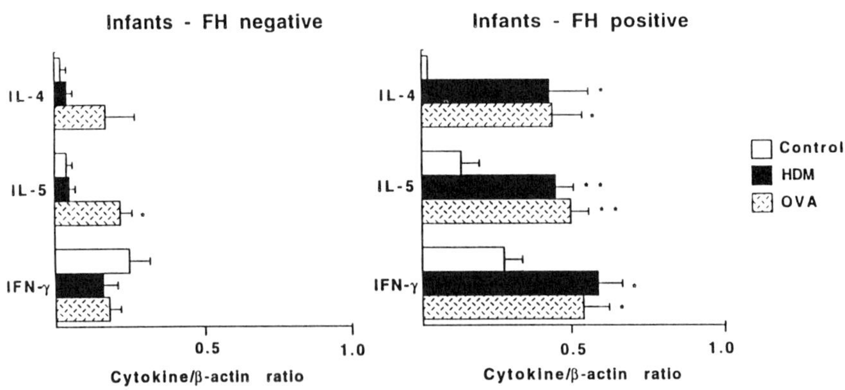


**Figure 3** Allergen-specific cytokine mRNA production by infants (mean age 17.9 months) classified by family history of atopy. Cytokine mRNA is expressed as a ratio to β-actin. Data is shown as mean ± SEM (* $p < 0.05$; ** $p < 0.01$). (From Ref. 18).

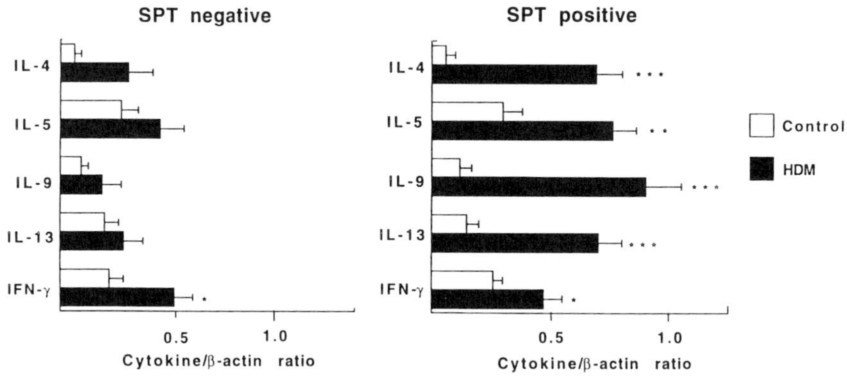


**Figure 4** HDM-specific cytokine mRNA production by 5-year-olds classified by skin prick test to HDM. Cytokine mRNA is expressed as a ratio to β-actin. Data is shown as mean ± SEM (* $p < 0.05$; ** $p < 0.01$; *** $p < 0.001$). (From Ref. 18).

Analysis of mRNA production by peripheral mononuclear cells in this age group showed a strong and consistent Th2 pattern in the atopic group, characterized by increased production of specific IL-4, IL-5, IL-9, and IL-13 mRNA responses to HDM, concomitant with increased production of IFN-γ mRNA (Fig. 4; 18). In contrast, the nonatopic group demonstrates IFN-γ responses to HDM lacking any significant contribution from Th2 cytokines. Occasional responses to OVA were observed, but these were not significant on a population basis in either group except production of IL-13 mRNA for atopic children (Fig. 5; 18).

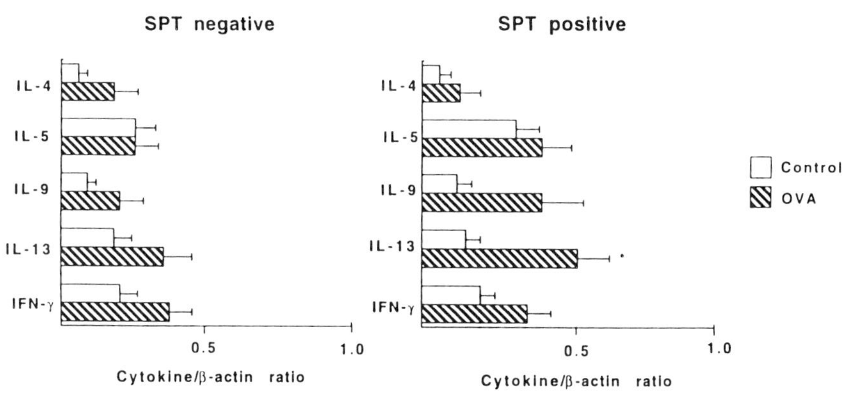


**Figure 5** OVA-specific cytokine mRNA production by 5-year-olds classified by skin prick test to HDM. Cytokine mRNA is expressed as a ratio to β-actin. Data is shown as mean ± SEM (* $p < 0.05$; ** $p < 0.01$; *** $p < 0.0001$). (From Ref. 18).

Two points emerge from these studies: First, that on a population basis, a Th2 pattern equivalent to adults is established for atopic children within the first 2 to 5 years of life. Nonatopic children, in contrast, express a Th1-like profile, with IFN-γ expression and notable absence of Th2 responses. Longitudinal studies are needed to address in greater detail the cytokine profile at the individual subject level. Given this time frame, however, we can start addressing more specific questions about how the T-cell response in atopic individuals is skewed toward a potentially pathologic Th2 or sometimes Th0 type of response.

The second point refers to the different course of respective responses to food and inhalant allergens, since previous studies have suggested that there is an almost reciprocal relation between responses to these allergens with age: food responses tend to appear early and decline during infancy, while inhalant allergies come later in life, persisting in atopic individuals (7,19). What are the mechanisms for this tolerance? Is response to food allergens characterized by deletion or anergy, in contrast to immune deviation which seems to predominant for inhalant allergens?

## IV. Conclusions

The accumulating evidence points to the initiation of immune response to allergens very early in life. We demonstrate that proliferative and allergen-specific cytokine responses can be detected at birth, suggesting that priming occurred in utero. This early response is elicited by both inhalant (HDM) and food allergens (OVA). The cytokine profile appears polarized toward Th2-type cytokines, significantly IL-5 mRNA and IL-10 protein, while the production of IFN-γ to specific allergen seems impaired at this early age.

At about 2 years of age Th0-like responses to both HDM and OVA allergens are detected and seem to correlate better with family history of atopy than with symptomology. At 5 years of age, a strong Th2 cytokine pattern to HDM is observed in atopic children, along with a weak IFN-γ response. In marked contrast, the response of the nonatopic group to HDM is dominated by IFN-γ. For both groups at this age, cytokine-specific responses to OVA were markedly decreased, possible reflecting distinct tolerance mechanisms.

The association between Th2 cytokines like IL-5 and allergic diseases reflects a dynamic process that may have been initiated long before "the first breath was ever taken" (20).

## References

1. Del Prete G, Maggi E, Parronchi P, Chretien I, Tiri A, Macchia D, Ricci M, Banchereau J, De Vries J, Romagnani S. IL-4 is an essential factor for the IgE

synthesis induced in vitro by human T cell clones and their supernatants. J Immunol 1988;140:4193–4198.

2. Clutterbuck EJ, Hirst EM, Sanderson CJ. Human interleukin-5 (IL-5) regulates the production of eosinophils in human bone marrow cultures: comparison and interaction with IL-1, IL-3, IL-6, and GMCSF. Blood 1989;73:1504–1512.
3. Robinson DS, Hamid Q, Ying S, Tsicopoulos A, Barkans J, Bentley AM, Corrigan C, Durham SR, Kay AB. Predominant TH2-like bronchoalveolar T-lymphocyte population in atopic asthma. N Eng J Med 1992;326:298–304.
4. Corrigan CJ, Hamid Q, North J, Barkans J, Moqbel R, Durham S, Gemou-Engesaeth V, Kay AB. Peripheral blood CD4 but not CD8 T-lymphocytes in patients with exacerbation of asthma transcribe and translate messenger RNA encoding cytokines which prolong eosinophil survival in the context of a Th2-type pattern: effect of glucocorticoid. Am J Resp Cell Mol Biol 1995;12:567–578.
5. Lai CK, Ho AS, Chan CH, Tang J, Leung JC, Lai KN. Interleukin-5 messenger RNA expression in peripheral blood CD4+ cells in asthma. J Allergy Clin Immunol 1996;97:1320–1328.
6. Holt PG. Primary allergic sensitization to environmental antigens: perinatal T cell priming as a determinant of responder phenotype in adulthood. J Exp Med 1996;183:1613–1621.
7. Hattevig G, Kjellman B, Björkstén B. Appearance of IgE antibodies to ingested and inhaled allergens during the first 12 years of life in atopic and non-atopic children. Pediatr Allergy Immunol 1993;4:182–186.
8. Holt PG. Immunoprophylaxis of atopy: light at the end of the tunnel? Immunol Today 1994;15:484–489.
9. Daniels SE, Bhattacharrya S, James A, Leaves NI, Young A, Hill MR, Faux JA, Ryan GF, le Souef PN, Lathrop GM, Musk AW, Cookson WO. A genome-wide search for quantitative trait loci underlying asthma. Nature 1996;383:247–250.
10. Bjorksten, B. Risk factors in early childhood for the development of atopic diseases. Allergy 1994;49:400–407.
11. Lin H, Mosmann TR, Guilbert L, Tuntipopipat S, Wegmann TG. Synthesis of T helper 2-type cytokines at the maternal-fetal interface. J Immunol 1993;151:4562–7453.
12. Krishnan L, Guilbert LJ, Russell As, Wegmann TG, Mosmann TR, Belosevic M. Pregnancy impairs resistance of C57BL/6 mice to *Leishmania major* infection and causes decreased antigen-specific IFN-gamma response and increased production of T helper 2 cytokines. J Immunol 1996;156:644–652.
13. Holt PG, McMenamin C, Nelson D. Primary sensitisation to inhalant allergens during infancy. Pediatr Allergy Immunol 1990;1:3–13.
14. Prescott SL, Macaubas C, Yabuhara A, Venaille TJ, Holt BJ, Habre W, Loh R, Sly PD, Holt PG. Developing patterns of T cell memory to environmental allergens in the first two years of life. Int Arch Allergy Immunol 1997;113:75–79.
15. Prescott S, Macaubas C, Holt BJ, Smallacombe T, Loh R, Sly PD, Holt PG. Transplacental priming of the human immune system to environmental allergens: universal skewing of initial T-cell responses towards the Th2 cytokine profile. J Immunol, in press.
16. Chaouat G, Assal Meliani A, Martal J, Raghupathy R, Elliot J, Mosmann T,

Wegmann TG. IL-10 prevents naturally occurring fetal loss in the CBA × DBA/2 mating combination, and local defect in IL-10 production in this abortion-prone combination is corrected by in vivo injection of IFN-tau. J Immunol 1995;154:4261–4268.

17. Krishnan L, Guilbert LJ, Wegmann TG, Belosevic M, Mosmann TR. T helper 1 response against *Leishmania major* in pregnant C57BL/6 mice increases implantation failure and fetal resorptions. Correlation with increased IFN-gamma and TNF and reduced IL-10 production by placental cells. J Immunol 1996;156:653–662.
18. Yabuhara A, Macaubas C, Prescott SL, Venaille TJ, Holt BJ, Habre W, Sly PD, Holt PG. Th-2-polarised immunological memory to inhalant allergens in atopics is established during infancy and early childhood. Clin Exp Allergy, 1997; 27:1261–1269.
19. Holt PG, O'Keeffe P, Holt BJ, Upham JW, Baron-Hay MJ, Suphioglu C, Knox B, Stewart GA, Thomas WR, Sly PD. T-cell "priming" against environmental allergens in human neonates: sequential deletion of food antigen reactivity during infancy with concomitant expansion of responses to ubiquitous inhalant allergens. Pediatr Allergy Immunol 1995;6:85–90.
20. Brown MA, Halonen MJ, Martinez FD. Cutting the cord: Is birth already too late for primary prevention of allergy? Clin Exp Allergy 1997;27:4–6.

# 7

# The Role of Interleukin-5 in Allergic Airways Disease

**PAUL S. FOSTER, SIMON P. HOGAN, KLAUS I. MATTHAEI, and IAN G. YOUNG**

Australian National University
Canberra, Australia

## I. Introduction

It is now generally accepted that inflammatory cells play an important role in the clinical expression and pathogenesis of asthma (1–3). Investigation of respiratory secretions and biopsy samples from asthmatics has shown a correlation between the presence of activated inflammatory cells in the airways and changes in airway morphology and the existence of airway hyperreactivity (4–15). The inflammatory infiltrate consists of eosinophils, mast cells, monocytes, and neutrophils. The recruitment and activation of these cells appears to be controlled by T lymphocytes through the secretion of cytokine and chemotactic agents following antigenic stimulation. The precise roles that particular inflammatory cells and mediators play in the complex inflammatory cascade leading to morphological and functional changes in the airways in asthma remain to be defined.

A number of investigations have shown a correlation between the accumulation of activated $CD4^+$ T cells and eosinophils and disease severity (4–9,11–17). There is also increasing evidence of the role of T lymphocytes and eosinophils in asthma from the studies with animal models (18–21). Of the cytokines produced by allergen-specific T lymphocytes, IL-4 and IL-5 may be particularly important because of their potential to promote the recruitment and activation of airway mast cells and eosinophils (13,22). Increased levels of IL-4 and IL-5 are found in respiratory secretions from atopic asthmatics (13) and increases in the number of cells in the BALF expressing elevated mRNA levels for these cytokines has been shown to correlate with bronchial hyperresponsiveness (23,24).

IL-5 is a key regulator of the eosinophil lineage, promoting the growth, differentiation, and activation of eosinophils (25–28). IL-4 is believed to regulate commitment to the $CD4^+$ Th2 lineage and to regulate IgE isotype switching in B lymphocytes (29–34). IgE and allergen-specific immunoglobulins may be important in mast cell activation and eosinophil degranulation (34–37). Both IL-4 and IL-5 may also regulate eosinophil recruitment by activating adhesion systems at the vascular endothelium (38,39).

Recently mouse models that mimic late-phase asthmatic responses have been used as an investigative tool for exploring the pathophysiology of allergic airways disease. Systemic ovalbumin sensitization followed by aerosol challenge has been shown to induce pronounced airways disease, with enhanced bronchial hyperreactivity and pathological changes similar to those observed in severe asthma (40). The pathological changes include epithelial detachment, plugging of the airways, and a pronounced infiltration of inflammatory cells, particularly eosinophils and lymphocytes. The use of cytokine-deficient mice in conjunction with the aeroallergen model provides a new approach for investigating the role of cytokines in airway inflammation. Using this model we have studied mice deficient in IL-5 and IL-4 to determine the role played by these two cytokines in allergic airways disease.

## II. Role of IL-5 in Allergic Airways Disease

We have made a major study of the involvement of IL-5 in allergic airways inflammation and in the recruitment of eosinophils using IL-5-deficient mice. IL-5-deficient mice (41) make no detectable IL-5 protein or IL-5 mRNA. They are healthy and fertile and no indirect effects on other related cytokine levels have been detected (42). The mice are unable to mount the characteristic helminth-induced eosinophilia (41,43), but initial studies have shown no effects on conventional B cells or T-cell-dependent antibody responses (41). Although IL-5-deficient mice cannot elicit a pronounced eosinophilia in response to inflammatory stimulation following parasite infection or aeroallergen challenge they still produce basal levels of eosinophils that appear morphologically and functionally normal (42–44). However, IL-5 deficiency, presumably through the inability to mount an eosinophilia compromises host defense against several helminth parasites (42). More recent studies have suggested that IL-5-deficient mice have functional deficiencies in peritoneal B1 lymphocytes (45) and in IgA production (46). Therefore, although the major effect of IL-5 deficiency is on the eosinophil lineage, caution needs to be observed in interpreting all effects seen in IL-5-deficient mice in terms of eosinophils.

Dramatic effects were obtained when IL-5-deficient mice were examined in the ovalbumin aeroallergen model. In IL-5$^{-/-}$ mice, the airway hyperreactivity, pulmonary eosinophilia, and gross morphological changes normally resulting from aeroallergen challenge were absent (40). Accumulation of lymphocytes in the lungs still occurred, although not to the same extent as in IL-5$^{+/+}$ animals. However, ova-specific IgE levels were comparable in IL-5$^{-/-}$ and IL-5$^{+/+}$ aeroallergen-challenged mice. When IL-5 production was restored using a recombinant vaccinia virus expressing IL-5, eosinophilic inflammation, lung pathology, and airway hyperreactivity were fully reconstituted (40).

The role of T lymphocytes in this model was confirmed by adoptive transfer experiments. Allergic airways disease in IL-5$^{-/-}$ mice could be reconstituted by transfer of CD4$^+$ Th2-type cells from ovalbumin-sensitized and aerosol-challenged IL-5$^{+/+}$ mice to IL-5$^{-/-}$ mice which had been challenged but not presensitized with ovalbumin (47). Clearly the IL-5 produced by the transferred T lymphocytes from the IL-5$^{+/+}$ mouse is sufficient to generate airways disease in the IL-5$^{-/-}$ mice. Other experiments using vaccinia virus-derived IL-5 have indicated that although IL-5 is necessary it is not sufficient on its own to induce pronounced lung eosinophilia or airways disease and that other signals derived from activated T lymphocytes are also required (40). Overall these investigations implicate eosinophils as the primary inflammatory cell involved in the changes of pulmonary structure and function observed in the aeroallergen model.

## III. Role of IL-4 in Allergic Airways Disease

An analysis of the role of IL-4 in allergic inflammation of the airways was also carried out using IL-4-deficient mice (48). These mice are defective in IgE production and have impaired CD4$^+$ Th2 cell responses (33). Surprisingly, in view of the established role of IL-4 and IgE as regulators of allergic disease, no major role for IL-4 in airways inflammation was identified. When the IL-4-deficient mice were tested in the ovalbumin model of allergic airways disease, it was found that recruitment of eosinophils to the lungs was impaired but the characteristic lung damage and airway hyperreactivity was not attenuated (48). Airways disease in IL-4$^{-/-}$ mice could, however, be inhibited by pretreatment with anti-IL-5 mAb or anti-CD4$^+$ mAb, both of which abolished blood and airway eosinophilia. These findings provide further support for a central role of IL-5 and eosinophils in allergic airways disease and indicate that IL-4 and IgE do not play an obligatory role in this model.

The IL-$4^{-/-}$ mice therefore show a disease pathology analogous to intrinsic asthmatics where there is no correlation between disease and elevated IgE levels, although eosinophilia is still present. Furthermore, respiratory secretions in such individuals show increased levels of IL-5 (but not of IL-4) and the presence of activated $CD4^+$ T cells (3,49).

## IV. Discussion

In recent years animal models have been used to study the role of IL-4 and IL-5 in the induction of allergic airways disease, but the findings have been controversial. The ovalbumin sensitization/aerosol challenge model used in our experiments generated many of the features of lung pathology seen in severe asthma, including epithelial detachment, airway plugging, and a pronounced inflammatory infiltrate consisting mainly of eosinophils and lymphocytes. Airway hyperresponsiveness is also induced. Our results with cytokine-deficient mice, which are summarized above, have consistently indicated a central role of IL-5 and eosinophils in the development of allergic airways disease and no obligatory role for IL-4. The role of IL-5 is also supported by other animal studies and clinical investigations (4,15,18–21). However, there are other studies where a correlation between increased eosinophil numbers and the development of airway hyperreactivity was not found and which have indicated that IL-4 and IgE-dependent mechanisms may be important for both cytokine production by Th2 cells and for eosinophil-associated airway dysfunction (50). Although the ovalbumin aeroallergen model is in common use, it is important to note that the protocols used vary widely and this should not be overlooked when comparing the findings of different laboratories. For example, Brusselle et al. have also examined IL-$4^{-/-}$ mice using an ovalbumin aeroallergen model. Analogous to our results, they found that eosinophil accumulation was significantly reduced in IL-4-deficient mice but their protocol produced much milder pathology in the lung; inflammation was localized, pathological changes to the airways were not induced, and hyperreactivity was not established.

Results may also be somewhat dependent on the strain of mouse used. Such an explanation (51) has been put forward to try and reconcile the findings we have reported for a central role for IL-5 using C57BL/6 mice (40), with the conclusion that IL-4 is the key cytokine in allergic airways disease derived from experiments with BALB/c mice (50). Interestingly, in recent experiments in this laboratory with BALB/c mice, pretreatment with anti-IL-5 mAb (52) abolished airway eosinophilia and pathology and significantly reduced but did not completely abolish airway hyperresponsiveness. Thus, although there are strain differences in the mechanisms generating airway hyperresponsiveness, our results indicate that IL-5 and eosinophils are also playing a major role in the induction of allergic airways disease in BALB/c mice.

Despite some apparently contradictory findings in the literature, the consistency of our own findings lead us to conclude that there is an obligatory and specific role of IL-5 in regulating blood and airway eosinophilia and in the induction of lung damage and airway hyperresponsiveness, thereby defining IL-5 as a potential therapeutic target for the relief of airway dysfunction in asthma.

## References

1. Gleich GJ, Adolphson CR. The eosinophilic leukocyte: structure and function. Adv Immunol 1986;39:177–253.
2. Djukanovic R, Wilson JW, Britten KM, Wilson SJ, Walls AF, Roche WR, Howarth PH, Holgate ST. Quantitation of mast cells and eosinophils in the bronchial mucosa of symptomatic atopic asthmatics and healthy control subjects using immunohistochemistry [see comments]. Am Rev Respir Dis 1990;142:863–871.
3. Bochner BS, Undem BJ, Lichtenstein LM. Immunological aspects of allergic asthma. Annu Rev Immunol 1994;12:295–335.
4. De Monchy JG, Kauffman HF, Venge P, Koeter GH, Jansen HM, Sluiter JH, De Vries K. Bronchoalveolar eosinophilia during allergen-induced late asthmatic reactions. Am Rev Respir Dis 1985;131:373–376.
5. Fukuda T, Dunnette SL, Reed CE, Ackerman SJ, Peters MS, Gleich GJ. Increased numbers of hypodense eosinophils in the blood of patients with bronchial asthma. Am Rev Respir Dis 1985;132:981–985.
6. Gleich GJ, Flavahan NA, Fujisawa T, Vanhoutte PM. The eosinophil as a mediator of damage to respiratory epithelium: a model for bronchial hyperreactivity. J Allergy Clin Immunol 1988;81:776–781.
7. Wardlaw AJ, Dunnette S, Gleich GJ, Collins JV, Kay AB. Eosinophils and mast cells in bronchoalveolar lavage in subjects with mild asthma. Relationship to bronchial hyperreactivity. Am Rev Respir Dis 1988;137:62–69.
8. Beasley R, Roche WR, Roberts JA, Holgate ST. Cellular events in the bronchi in mild asthma and after bronchial provocation. Am Rev Respir Dis 1989;139:806–817.
9. Frick WE, Sedgwick JB, Busse WW. The appearance of hypodense eosinophils in antigen-dependent late phase asthma. Am Rev Respir Dis 1989;139:1401–1406.
10. Motojima S, Frigas E, Loegering DA, Gleich GJ. Toxicity of eosinophil cationic proteins for guinea pig tracheal epithelium in vitro. Am Rev Respir Dis 1989;139:801–805.
11. Bousquet J, Chanez P, Lacoste JY, Barneon G, Ghavanian N, Enander I, Venge P, Ahlstedt S, Simony-Lafontaine J, Godard P, Michel F-B. Eosinophilic inflammation in asthma [see comments]. N Engl J Med 1990;323:1033–1039.
12. Broide DH, Gleich GJ, Cuomo AJ, Coburn DA, Federman EC, Schwartz LB,

Wasserman SI. Evidence of ongoing mast cell and eosinophil degranulation in symptomatic asthma airway. J Allergy Clin Immunol 1991;88:637–648.
13. Walker C, Kaegi MK, Braun P, Blaser K. Activated T cells and eosinophilia in bronchoalveolar lavages from subjects with asthma correlated with disease severity. J Allergy Clin Immunol 1991;88:935–942.
14. Fukuda T, Numao T, Akutsu I, Makino S. Platelet-activating factor (PAF)-induced chemotaxis and PAF binding to human eosinophils. J Lipid Mediat 1992;5:145–149.
15. Ohashi Y, Motojima S, Fukuda T, Makino S. Airway hyperresponsiveness, increased intracellular spaces of bronchial epithelium, and increased infiltration of eosinophils and lymphocytes in bronchial mucosa in asthma [see comments]. Am Rev Respir Dis 1992;145:1469–1476.
16. Azzawi M, Bradley B, Jeffery PK, Frew AJ, Wardlaw AJ, Knowles G, Assoufi B, Collins JV, Durham S, Kay AB. Identification of activated T lymphocytes and eosinophils in bronchial biopsies in stable atopic asthma. Am Rev Respir Dis 1990;142:1407–1413.
17. Bentley AM, Menz G, Storz C, Robinson DS, Bradley B, Jeffery PK, Durham SR, Kay AB. Identification of T lymphocytes, macrophages, and activated eosinophils in the bronchial mucosa in intrinsic asthma. Relationship to symptoms and bronchial responsiveness. Am Rev Respir Dis 1992;146:500–506.
18. Chand N, Harrison JE, Rooney S, Pillar J, Jakubicki R, Nolan K, Diamantis W, Sofia RD. Anti-IL-5 monoclonal antibody inhibits allergic late phase bronchial eosinophilia in guinea pigs: a therapeutic approach. Eur J Pharmacol 1992;211:121–123.
19. Gavett SH, Chen X, Finkelman F, Wills Karp M. Depletion of murine $CD4^+$ T lymphocytes prevents antigen-induced airway hyperreactivity and pulmonary eosinophilia. Am J Respir Cell Mol Biol 1994;10:587–593.
20. Eum SY, Haile S, Lefort J, Huerre M, Vargaftig BB. Eosinophil recruitment into the respiratory epithelium following antigenic challenge in hyper-IgE mice is accompanied by interleukin-5-dependent bronchial hyperresponsiveness. Proc Natl Acad Sci USA 1995;92:12290–12294.
21. Haczku A, Chung KF, Sun J, Barnes PJ, Kay AB, Moqbel R. Airway hyperresponsiveness, elevation of serum-specific IgE and activation of T cells following allergen exposure in sensitized Brown-Norway rats. Immunology 1995;85:598–603.
22. Bradley BL, Azzawi M, Jacobson M, Assoufi B, Collins JV, Irani AM, Schwartz LB, Durham SR, Jeffery PK, Kay AB. Eosinophils, T-lymphocytes, mast cells, neutrophils, and macrophages in bronchial biopsy specimens from atopic subjects with asthma: comparison with biopsy specimens from atopic subjects without asthma and normal control subjects and relationship to bronchial hyperresponsiveness. J Allergy Clin Immunol 1991;88:661–674.
23. Robinson D, Hamid Q, Ying S, Bentley A, Assoufi B, Durham S, Kay AB. Prednisolone treatment in asthma is associated with modulation of bronchoalveolar lavage cell interleukin-4, interleukin-5, and interferon-gamma cytokine gene expression. Am Rev Respir Dis 1993;148:401–406.

24. Robinson DS, Ying S, Bentley AM, Meng Q, North J, Durham SR, Kay AB, Hamid Q. Relationships among numbers of bronchoalveolar lavage cells expressing messenger ribonucleic acid for cytokines, asthma symptoms, and airway methacholine responsiveness in atopic asthma. J Allergy Clin Immunol 1993;92:397–403.
25. Campbell HD, Tucker WQ, Hort Y, Martinson ME, Mayo G, Clutterbuck EJ, Sanderson CJ, Young IG. Molecular cloning, nucleotide sequence, and expression of the gene encoding human eosinophil differentiation factor (interleukin-5). Proc Natl Acad Sci USA 1987;84:6629–6633.
26. Lopez AF, Sanderson CJ, Gamble JR, Campbell HD, Young IG, Vadas MA. Recombinant human interleukin-5 is a selective activator of human eosinophil function. J Exp Med 1988;167:219–224.
27. Sanderson CJ, Campbell HD, Young IG. Molecular and cellular biology of eosinophil differentiation factor (interleukin-5) and its effects on human and mouse B cells. Immunol Rev 1988;102:29–50.
28. Yamaguchi Y, Hayashi Y, Sugama Y, Miura Y, Kasahara T, Kitamura S, Torisu M, Mita S, Tominaga A, Takatsu K. Highly purified murine interleukin-5 (IL-5) stimulates eosinophil function and prolongs in vitro survival. IL-5 as an eosinophil chemotactic factor. J Exp Med 1988;167:1737–1742.
29. Snapper CM, Paul WE. Interferon-gamma and B cell stimulatory factor-1 reciprocally regulate Ig isotype production. Science 1987;236:944–947.
30. Finkelman FD, Katona IM, Mosmann TR, Coffman RL. IFN-gamma regulates the isotypes of Ig secreted during in vivo humoral immune responses. J Immunol 1988;140:1022–1027.
31. Bergstedt Lindqvist S, Moon HB, Persson U, Moller G, Heusser C, Severinson E. Interleukin 4 instructs uncommitted B lymphocytes to switch to IgG1 and IgE. Eur J Immunol 1988;18:1073–1077.
32. Swain SL, Weinberg AD, English M, Huston G. IL-4 directs the development of Th2-like helper effectors. J Immunol 1990;145:3796–3806.
33. Kopf M, Le Gros G, Bachmann M, Lamers MC, Bluethmann H, Köhler G. Disruption of the murine IL-4 gene blocks $Th_2$ cytokine responses. Nature 1993;362:245–248.
34. Dubucquoi S, Desreumaux P, Janin A, Klein O, Goldman M, Tavernier J, Capron A, Capron M. Interleukin-5 synthesis by eosinophils: association with granules and immunoglobulin-dependent secretion. J Exp Med 1994;179:703–708.
35. Looney RJ, Ryan DH, Takahashi K, Fleit HB, Cohen JH, Abraham GN, Anderson CL. Identification of a second class of IgG Fc receptors on human neutrophils. A 40 kilodalton molecule also found on eosinophils. J Exp Med 1986;163:826–836.
36. Gounni AS, Lamkhioued B, Ochiai K, Tanaka Y, Delaporte E, Capron A, Kinet JP, Capron M. High-affinity IgE receptor on eosinophils is involved in defence against parasites. Nature 1994;367:183–186.
37. Kaneko M, Swanson MC, Gleich GJ, Kita H. Allergen-specific IgG1 and IgG3 through Fc gamma RII induce eosinophil degranulation. J Clin Invest 1995;95:2813–2821.

38. Walsh GM, Hartnell A, Wardlaw AJ, Kurihara K, Sanderson CJ, Kay AB. IL-5 enhances the in vitro adhesion of human eosinophils, but not neutrophils, in a leucocyte integrin (CD11/18)-dependent manner. Immunology 1990;71:258–265.
39. Schleimer RP, Sterbinsky SA, Kaiser J, Bickel CA, Klunk DA, Tomioka K, Newman W, Luscinskas FW, Gimbrone MA Jr, McIntyre BW, Bochner BS. IL-4 induces adherence of human eosinophils and basophils but not neutrophils to endothelium. Association with expression of VCAM-1. J Immunol 1992;148:1086–1092.
40. Foster PS, Hogan SP, Ramsay AJ, Matthaei KI, Young IG. Interleukin-5 deficiency abolishes eosinophilia, airways hyperreactivity, and lung damage in a mouse asthma model [see comments]. J Exp Med 1996;183:195–201.
41. Kopf M, Brombacher F, Hodgkin PD, Ramsay AJ, Milbourne EA, Dai WJ, Ovington KS, Behm CA, Kohler G, Young IG, Matthaei KI. IL-5-deficient mice have a developmental defect in CD5+ B-1 cells and lack eosinophilia but have normal antibody and cytotoxic T cell responses. Immunity 1996;4:15–24.
42. Matthaei KI, Foster PS, Young IG. The role of IL-5 in vivo: studies with IL-5 deficient mice. in New perspectives in eosinophils. Role in inflammation associated with allergy, asthma and parasitic disease (Cordeiro R, Moqbel R & Weller PF editors) Memorias Instituto Oswaldo Cruz 1997; 92:63–68.
43. Takamoto M, Ovington KS, Behm CA, Sugane K, Young IG, Matthaei KI. Eosinophilia, parasite burden and lung damage in *Toxocara canis* infections in C57BL/6 mice genetically deficient in IL-5. Immunology 1997;90:511–517.
44. Mould AW, Matthaei KI, Young IG, Foster PS. Relationship between interleukin-5 and eotaxin in regulating blood and tissue eosinophilia in mice. J Clin Invest 1997;99:1064–1071.
45. Bao S, Beagley KW, Murry AM, Caristo V, Matthaei KI, Young IG, Husband AJ. Intestinal IgA Plasma cells of theB-1 lineage are IL-5 dependent. Immunology, 1998, in press.
46. Whittle BL, Smith RM, Matthaei KI, Young IG, Verma NK. Interleukin-5 expressed by an attenuated strain of *Salmonella* serotype Dublin enhances specific mucosal IgA response *in vivo*. Journal of Medical Microbiology, 1997; 46(12):1029–1038.
47. Hogan SP, Koskinen A, Matthaei KI, Young IG, Foster PS. IL-5 producing $CD4^+$T-cells play a pivotal role in the induction of eosinophilia and allergic airways disease in mice. American Journal of Respiratory and Critical Care Medicine, 1998; 157(1): 210–218.
48. Hogan SP, Mould AM, Kikutani H, Ramsay AJ, Foster PS. Aeroallergen-induced eosinophilic inflammation, lung damage and airways hyperreactivity in mice can occur independently of IL-4 and allergen-specific immunoglobulins. J Clin Invest 1997;99:1329–1339.
49. Walker C, Bode E, Boer L, Hansel TT, Blaser K, Virchow JC Jr. Allergic and nonallergic asthmatics have distinct patterns of T-cell activation and cytokine production in peripheral blood and bronchoalveolar lavage. Am Rev Respir Dis 1992;146:109–115.

50. Corry DB, Folkesson HG, Warnock ML, Erle DJ, Matthay MA, Wiener Kronish JP, Locksley RM. Interleukin-4, but not interleukin-5 or eosinophils, is required in a murine model of acute airway hyperreactivity [see comments]. J Exp Med 1996;183:109–117.
51. Drazen JM, Arm JP, Austen KF. Sorting out the cytokines of asthma [comment]. J Exp Med 1996;183:1–5.
52. Hogan SP, Koskinen A, Foster PS. Interleukin-5 and eosinophils induce airways damage and bronchial hyperreactivity during allergic airways inflammation in BALB/c mice. Immunol Cell Biol, in press.

# 8

# Cytokine Control of the Development of a T-Helper 2 Response

**ANDREW N. J. McKENZIE**

MRC Laboratory of Molecular Biology
Cambridge, United Kingdom

## I. T-Helper Cell Differentiation Pathways

In general IL-5 production forms part of a tightly regulated immune response that is characterized by the coordinate expression of related cytokines such as IL-4 and IL-13. This chapter discusses the induction and expansion of responses in which IL-5 and its family members play leading roles.

The ability of cytokines to modulate immune responses has made them clinically important molecules, with a wide spectrum of potential applications. Cells of the immune system secrete a spectrum of immunoregulatory proteins called cytokines, including interferons (IFN), colony-stimulating factors (CSF), chemokines, and interleukins. During immune responses to foreign antigens, and normal hematopoiesis, the expression of these cytokines is strictly regulated. In many instances these cytokines are not restricted to a single function, but display multiple biological activities, leading to the formation of highly complex cytokine networks.

Early reports based on clinical observations indicated that an inverse relationship existed between humoral immune responses and delayed-type hypersensitivity reactions (1). More recently these phenomena have been shown to be controlled by T lymphocytes which secrete factors known to regulate antibody production, inflammation, and cell lineage commitment and differentiation. Indeed, the discovery and molecular cloning of an array of T-cell-derived cytokines enabled Mosmann et al. (2–5) to determine cytokine secretion profiles from a range of T-cell clones, allowing their subdivision into distinct populations. Over recent years the expression patterns of additional novel cytokines have been assessed, and where applicable they have been included into a model of polarized cytokine secretion by helper T-cell populations. At one end of the spectrum helper T cells, referred to as Th1 cells, secrete IL-2, interferon-$\gamma$ (IFN-$\gamma$), and lymphotoxin $\alpha$, and are important in the induction of delayed-type hypersensitivity reactions and the production of complement-fixing and opsonizing antibodies. Another T-cell population, termed Th2, is characterized by the production of IL-4, IL-5, IL-6, IL-9, IL-10, and IL-13. Th2 cells primarily regulate humoral immune responses (including the production of IgE) and promote the differentiation of mast cells and eosinophils. IL-3 and granulocyte macrophage colony-stimulating factor (GM-CSF) are produced by both subsets.

Although polarization of T-cell cytokine expression has been well described in the mouse system, it has taken longer to assess such differentiation in human systems. This inconsistency is probably due to the disparate conditions in which mouse and human T cells have been derived. Mice have generally been multiply challenged with antigens before isolation of T cells from spleen or lymph node, whereas human T cells have generally been isolated from the peripheral blood of healthy donors, before being stimulated in vitro with polyclonal activators. However, polarized Th1 and Th2 cell populations have now been recorded in studies using T cells from human donors with chronic disease (6,7).

While this general model has proved extremely useful in presenting a simple rationale for the development of T-cell-driven immune responses, it should be recognized that an ongoing immune response in vivo can also result in a broad range of cytokine secreting T-cell populations that cannot be conveniently characterized by cytokine secretion profile, since individual cells may express a unique subset of cytokines. Indeed, many researchers now refer to “Th2-like” or “Th1-like” responses to describe immune reactions that are skewed toward a particular cytokine spectrum. Such a definition allows the incorporation of other cytokine secreting cells such as $CD8^+$ T cells and hematopoietic cells such as mast cells, basophils, and eosinophils that may also modulate an immune response.

## II. Factors Affecting T-Cell Differentiation

It is of fundamental importance of to understand how apparent commitment of helper T cells to their divergent cytokine producing lineages occurs, and why certain stimuli such as those present in asthma, allergy, and parasitic helminth infections predispose to the production of IL-4, IL-5, and IL-13. It is widely accepted that IL-12 and IFN-$\gamma$ are prerequisite for the development of Th1 responses (8) and that IL-4 is a fundamental element in the development of Th2 responses (9,10). However, it is also true that factors other than IL-4 appear important in initiating this response. It also remains unclear how the initiation of helper T-cell differentiation occurs, although factors including the route of antigenic challenge, the type of antigen presenting cell (APC), the cytokine milieu at the site of challenge, and the dose of the antigen are all believed to influence the skewing of helper T-cell phenotypes.

### A. Dose of Antigen

A number of studies have implicated antigenic dose in determining the development of differentiated $CD4^+$ helper T cells into Th1 or Th2 subpopulations, but it has been difficult to circumvent the problems encountered with heterogeneity of the immune response. Using T-cell receptor transgenic mice it has been possible to show that, in the absence of variation of MHC genotype and the presence of a single TCR, naive $CD4^+$ T cells develop a Th2-like phenotype at low antigen doses and Th1-like characteristics at high doses (11). However, this study also emphasized the role played by the immediate cytokine environment in which the cells were cultured, with the presence of extremely low levels of IFN-$\gamma$ causing a dominant Th1 response even in the presence of low doses of antigen (11). It is argued that the low antigen doses characteristic of allergic responses to inhaled allergens may in part explain the preferential activation of a Th2-like response and the resultant IgE response and eosinophilia. However, the role of antigenic dose is far from proven, and it appears that complex antigens can mediate divergent effects from those of the peptide antigen used in the transgenic study. Indeed, Bretscher et al. (12) have shown that if "susceptible" BALB/c mice are injected with a small number of *Leishmania major* parasites they acquire resistance typical of a Th1 response, to subsequent challenge with larger, normally pathogenic doses.

### B. Route of Challenge

It is apparent that the route of antigen challenge can influence the progression of helper T-cell differentiation, due to the type of APC that are initially encountered and the cytokines they disgorge. The events responsible for the initial development of Th1 lineages in response to microbial pathogens are relatively clear. This is because cells including macrophages and dendritic cells produce IL-12 in response to microbial infection or the by-products of pathogens (13). This innate immune response is rapid, occurring within 24 hr of challenge and results in a cytokine microenvironment, complemented by the additional secretion of IFN-γ from NK cells that induces naive T cells to develop into Th1 populations. Thus subsequent effector functions are dominated by cell-mediated responses and complement fixing humoral responses.

The initial sources of IL-4 production are somewhat less clear, since unlike IL-12, IL-4 is not secreted by macrophages. A number of proposals have been made concerning the origins of the primary IL-4 production. $NK1^+$ T cells are known to rapidly secrete significant levels of IL-4 upon activation in vivo using antibodies to CD3, and thus were proposed as a unique source of early IL-4 (14). However, recent studies have shown that even in the absence of the $NK1^+$ T-cell population, Th2 responses to parasites or protein antigens are unimpaired (15,16). The only affected responses were those to the polyclonal stimulators, anti-CD3 and anti-IgD (17).

It has also been suggested that naive $CD4^+$ T cells themselves may supply the original source of IL-4. However, evidence supporting this claim has been difficult to obtain since the manipulation of the $CD4^+$ lineage will inevitably lead to a perturbation of the IL-4 response. Furthermore, the effects reported by a number of studies do not rule out the presence of other mediators of Th2 differentiation. If IL-4-deficient animals were irradiated and then reconstituted with a variety of combinations of $CD4^+$ or $CD4^-$ spleen cells from IL-4-deficient or wild-type mice, it was found that IL-4-producing wild-type $CD4^+$ T cells still appeared even in the absence of all other IL-4-producing cells (18). Thus either the donor $CD4^+$ cells are capable of producing their own primary IL-4 or another factor(s) elicits IL-4 production.

Indeed a Th2 differentiation pathway which appears to parallel that for Th1 cells has recently been described by Rincon et al. (19). Using $CD4^+$ T cells and APC from IL-6-deficient mice the authors show that the presence of IL-6 can stimulate IL-4-dependent development of a Th2 cell lineage. However, it is unclear when or how this IL-6 response is invoked in favor of an IL-12-dominated response.

Certain other tissues, including mucosal membranes and the peritoneal cavity, contain significant numbers of eosinophils and mast cells which are known to produce considerable levels of Th2-like cytokines including IL-4, IL-5, and IL-13 (20,21), thus these non-T cells are in a unique position to supply cytokines important in initiation of Th2-like development. Indeed a recent report by Sabin et al. (22) indicates that IL-5, released by mast cells in response to *Schistosoma mansoni* eggs, causes the recruitment of eosinophils, and that these eosinophils are responsible for perpetuating the response by releasing IL-4.

### C. Receptor Regulation

The regulation of receptor expression is a downstream effect that appears to be involved in stabilizing the phenotypes of Th cell subpopulations. It has been shown that IFN-γ inhibits the proliferation of Th2 cell populations but not Th1 subsets, due to the down-regulation of IFN-γRβ chain on Th1 cells (23). Furthermore, IL-12Rβ has been shown to be modulated on T cells in response to IL-4 or IFN-γ (24,25). IL-4 acts by inhibiting IL-12Rβ expression thereby leading to a loss in IL-12 signaling (26), while IFN-γ can act on immature Th2 cells to maintain IL-12Rβ expression and thereby sustain IL-12 responsiveness (24). Such expression patterns may thus allow for the control of certain Th2 cell responses where IL-4 expression has not yet reached a critical threshold.

### D. Costimulation

In concert with the secreted cytokines and their receptors, a host of cell surface molecules also participate in the maturation of immune reactions characterized by polarized T-cell responses. The costimulatory molecules B7-1 (CD80) and B7-2 (CD86), and their coreceptors CD28 and CTLA4, are clearly involved in the activation and development of T-cell responses, but exactly how they mediate their effects is not well characterized. Using antibodies to either B7-1 or B7-2 it has been possible to influence the outcome of immune reactions, though the results of such studies would suggest that the timing of treatment and the initial cytokine profiles encountered can cause apparently opposite outcomes (27). This may have much to do with the APC at the point of challenge and which particular B7 molecule is abundant. Recent studies using mice deficient in B7-1, B7-2, or both B7-1 and B7-2 have indicated that route of challenge can significantly affect humoral responses, with an absence of antigen-specific IgG1 and IgG2a following intravenous immunization of B7-2-deficient animals (28). It will be interesting to ascertain how the cytokine profiles vary in such situations.

It is apparent from the details discussed in the previous sections that there are multiple sources of stimuli that are able to modulate a Th cell response, depending on the type of antigen challenge encountered at specific locations. The following sections will describe how certain Th2 cytokine family members interact to produce the various facets of a Th2 response.

## III. Coordinated Cytokine Family Expression

There is now well-documented evidence that eosinophilia is primarily regulated by the production of IL-5, and IgE by the expression of IL-4 and by the re-

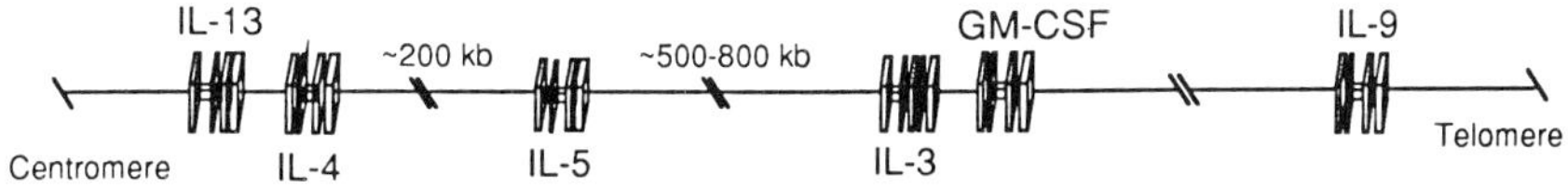


**Figure 1** Chromosomal organization of the IL-4 gene family.

cently described IL-13 (29–34). However, it is also evident that a number of other cytokines, including IL-3, GM-CSF, IL-9, and IL-10 influence the immediate inflammatory responses elicited during allergic reactions. It is noteworthy that the genes encoding inducers of hemopoiesis and immune regulation, including IL-3, IL-4, IL-5, IL-13, and GM-CSF, are located in a cluster on mouse chromosome 11 and in the syntenic region of human chromosome 5q31 (35,36) (see Fig. 1). With the exception of IL-3 (which has five exons), the genes within this cluster share a common intron-exon structure consisting of four exons and three introns (35). Chromosomal mapping studies have shown that the human IL-13 gene is upstream and probably within 20 kb of the IL-4 gene (37) and we have recently found that the mouse IL-13 gene is 10 kb upstream of the mouse IL-4 gene and arranged in tandem (A. McKenzie, unpublished data). Physical linkage has also been demonstrated between the IL-4 genes and IL-5 genes in humans and the mouse, with approximately 310 kb separating them in the former (38) and approximately 110 to 180 kb in the latter (39). The IL-3 and GM-CSF genes are extremely closely linked ($\sim$10 kb) and map in the region of 600 to 1000 kb from IL-5 (40). The structural relationship and juxtaposition of the IL-3, IL-4, IL-5, IL-13, and GM-CSF genes suggest that they have evolved through gene duplication events. Although these cytokines may show coordinate expression patterns, it is evident that they are also individually regulated.

### A. IL-4 and IL-13

Two cytokines that are often produced coordinately with IL-5 are IL-4 and IL-13. IL-13 is a recently described cytokine (30–32) that is produced principally by activated T cells, and although expression is primarily associated with the Th2 lineage, human Th1 and Th0 cell clones may also make IL-13 (34). Using in vitro culture systems, the biological activities of IL-4 and IL-13 have been found to overlap.

#### *B-Cell Responses*

IL-13 is a potent inducer of CD23 on purified human B cells, and also increases expression of MHC class II, sIgM, CD71, and CD72 (33,41). However, expression of CD19, CD20, CD25, CD40, MHC class I, B7, ICAM-1, LFA-1, and LFA-3 are not changed significantly (33).

Until the discovery of IL-13, IL-4 was the only cytokine known to induce IgE switching in human or mouse B cells. Considerable levels of IgE are synthesized by purified human B cells costimulated by IL-13 or IL-4 and ligation of CD40 (33,42,43), though only IL-4 has been reported to have this function in the mouse (34,44). However, IL-4-deficient mice infected with *Plasmodium chabaudi* malaria produce IgE (45), as do mice infected with murine acquired immunodeficiency syndrome (46), indicating that IL-4-independent switching to IgE does occur in the mouse, and this may be attributable to IL-13. Recent evidence suggests that mast cells and basophils, which can make IL-4, can also ligate CD40 on B cells and induce IgE secretion (47). IL-13 can also be produced by activated mast cells (20), thus it will be important to determine the possible role of IL-13 in mast cell-induced IgE secretion.

### *Monocyte and Macrophage Responses*

IL-4 and IL-13 have been shown to modulate monocyte function in a number of experimental systems. They are capable of synergizing with stem cell factor (SCF) and granulocyte colony-stimulating factor (G-CSF) to enhance the proliferation of $Lin^{-}Sca\text{-}1^{+}$ bone marrow progenitor cells, but are unable to influence the SCF-induced proliferation of the more mature $Lin^{-}Sca\text{-}1^{-}$ progenitor cells. While SCF, in combination with G-CSF, causes $Lin^{-}Sca\text{-}1^{+}$ cells to differentiate into granulocytes, the addition of IL-13 results in the almost exclusive generation of macrophages (48). Thus, IL-13 and IL-4 also influence early myelopoiesis.

In common with IL-4 and IL-10, IL-13 inhibits the production by human LPS-activated monocytes of a number of proinflammatory cytokines, including IL-1α, IL-1β, IL-6, IL-8, G-CSF, and tumor necrosis factor α (TNF-α) (49), and the transcription of IFN-α and the α (p35) and β (p40) chains of IL-12 (49). In addition, IL-4, IL-13, and IL-10 enhance the production of IL-1 receptor antagonist (IL-1ra) by monocytes (49,50) and both IL-13 and IL-4 have recently been shown to increase the production of the IL-1 "decoy" receptor in human polymorphonuclear cells (51), suggesting that IL-13 and IL-4 may mediate the reversal of inflammatory reactions. Indeed, IL-13 and IL-4 can both act to inhibit nitric oxide (NO) production and this can impair intracellular parasite killing by activated macrophages (52,53). In contrast, IL-13 has been reported to induce the expression of vascular cell adhesion molecule-1 (VCAM-1) on endothelial and mesothelial cells (54), suggesting that IL-13 may be capable of mediating the recruitment of eosinophils and basophils, which express the VLA-4 counterreceptor for VCAM-1, to endothelial cells. It should be emphasized that although IL-4 and IL-13 are potent suppressors of inflammatory responses, they do not simply "turn off" macrophages, but are able to up-regulate molecules important in antigen presentation.

The ability of both IL-4 and IL-13 to modulate monocyte function has also proven effective in inhibiting HIV replication in cultured human peripheral blood monocytes, and although the virus is not eradicated there is significant reduction of viral protein, reverse transcriptase levels, and cytopathic effects in monocytes treated before or after viral infection (55). Exactly how IL-13 and IL-4 repress HIV replication, or what role this might play in the course of an infection, remains unclear.

*T-Cell Responses*

In vitro assays have failed to show a concordance of IL-13 and IL-4 responses on T cells. As mentioned earlier IL-4 has been shown to facilitate the induction of Th2 cell development in vitro and in vivo (9,10), however, it is also apparent that IL-4-independent mechanisms of Th2 cell differentiation occur. This has been demonstrated in IL-4-deficient mice which still have residual levels of Th2 cells (10,56) and under certain stimulations can still produce IgE (45,46), leading to the proposal that Th precursor or Th0 T cells may be IL-4-independent while chronically stimulated Th cells are IL-4 dependent (10). Moreover, low doses of antigen induce Th2 cell development even in the presence of saturating concentrations of anti-IL-4 monoclonal antibody (11). Furthermore, studies involving the administration of the immunosuppressant cyclosporin A have shown that despite inhibiting IL-4 production, Th2 biasing is observed (57). Significantly, IL-13 production is enhanced by cyclosporin A treatment, possibly implicating this cytokine in Th2 polarization (57). Our own experiments using IL-13-deficient mice suggest that IL-13 plays a direct role in the development of Th2 cell responses in vivo (McKenzie, unpublished data). Although the molecular mechanism by which this occurs is unclear it is possible that IL-13 either mediates its effects directly on the developing T cells or by suppressing IL-12 (or a similar factor) from antigen presenting cells.

It is intriguing that IL-4 and IL-13 appear to share so many functions, and the relatedness of the responses have been explained, at least in part, by studies showing that both of these cytokines can cross-compete for IL-4 receptor α (IL-4Rα) (58–61). However, the exact constitution of the receptor complexes engaging the individual cytokines is poorly understood, although recent molecular cloning has identified that IL-13 can bind to at least two distinct receptor chains (IL-13Rα1 and IL-13Rα2) to which IL-4 does not bind (61–65). These receptor subunits, which are structurally related to IL-5Rα, do not appear to be coordinately regulated, and their mRNA was detected in a broad range of tissues. Further investigation is required to elucidate how the spatial and temporal expression of these receptors is linked with the expression patterns of IL-13 and IL-4. The situation is complicated further by the interaction of IL-4 with IL-2Rγc(γc) chain (66,67), a complex that has not been shown for IL-13 (68,69). It is noteworthy that coexpression of IL-13Rα1 with γc actually causes a reduction in the number of IL-13 binding sites on COS cells, possibly due to the interaction of γc with IL-4Rα on these cells (62). Thus, while a number of receptor associated intracellular signaling pathways are common to IL-13 and IL-4, such as Janus kinase 1 (JAK-1) and signal transducer and activator of transcription 6 (STAT-6) (69), others may be more specific.

Given the receptor interaction that occurs between IL-4 and IL-13, it is tempting to speculate that differential expression of IL-13/IL-4 receptor components may influence cell lineage development such as that seen for T cells. The presence of IL-13 receptors on freshly isolated primary human T cells has been proven functionally by the ability of IL-13 to inhibit $CD4^+$ and $CD8^+$ T-cell chemotaxis (70) and by the detection of IL-13Rα1 mRNA expression in purified peripheral T cells (64). Evidence from the human system suggests that IL-13 is produced by a population of naive T cells which do not make IL-4 (57), hence IL-13 may be uniquely placed in the differentiation pathway of Th2 cells. Thus IL-13 may initially bind to its receptor on T cells, being outcompeted subsequently by IL-4 which may recruit IL-2Rγc into its receptor complex, displacing IL-13 and evoking a proliferative response. Recent data would also suggest that cell surface expression of the IL-13 receptor is then down-regulated or its signaling functions restricted in a manner similar to that described for the IFN-γ receptor on Th1 cells (23), since expression of IL-13Rα1 mRNA has been found to be down-regulated upon stimulation of purified peripheral T cells with anti-CD3 or phorbol ester (64), and IL-13 only induces STAT activation in fresh peripheral blood leucocytes (PBL), but not in preactivated PBL, while IL-4 is able to stimulate STAT activation in both fresh and preactivated cells (69).

Thus although IL-13 and IL-4 share at least a subset of intracellular signaling pathways, including the localization of STAT-6 to the nucleus, their mechanism of activation may differ (69). Recent studies using mice in which the *Stat6* gene has been disrupted have identified a severe Th2 block (71,72), and since both IL-13 and IL-4 have been shown to signal through STAT-6 the resultant phenotype may be due to the combined effect of interrupting the downstream signaling pathways of both cytokines (73). The presence of active STAT-6 sites in the IL-4 promoter (74) and IL-4Rα promoter (75) indicates that IL-13-induced STAT-6 could play a role in modulating IL-4 and IL-4Rα expression, which subsequently drives T-cell expansion.

It is evident that complex interrelated roles exist for IL-13 and IL-4 in the development of immune reactions, and though apparently redundant, the elaborate nature of their receptor components implies that much remains to be discovered concerning their individual status.

In summary it is evident that the concept of polarized helper T-cell subsets has improved our understanding of immune responses by providing a framework in which different experimental models can be judged. However, it must also be emphasized that the extreme polarization upon which the model is based is not generally applicable, and multiple cytokine profiles have been reported in many ongoing immune reactions. The situation is further complicated when concomitant immune responses are occurring, and where no single factor appears responsible for skewing the helper T-cell response. While therapeutic suppression of Th2 responses in asthma and allergy is a worthy goal, the plethora of factors with the potential to bias the development of T-cell responses highlights the necessity to consider carefully the potential cytokine-network instability that may be induced.

## References

1. Parish CR. The relationship between humoral and cell-mediated immunity. Transplant Rev 1972;13:35–36
2. Mosmann TR, Cherwinski H, Bond MW, Gieldin MA, Coffman RL. Two types of murine helper T cell clone: I. Definition according to profiles of lymphokine activities and secreted proteins. J Immunol 1986;136:2348–2357.
3. Cherwinski HM, Schumacher JH, Brown KD, Mosmann TR. Two types of mouse helper T cell clone. III. Further differences in lymphokine synthesis between Th1 and Th2 clones revealed by RNA hybridization, functionally monospecific bioassays, and monoclonal antibodies. J Exp Med 1987;166:1229–1244.
4. Mosmann TR, Coffman RL. TH1 and TH2 cells: different patterns of lymphokine secretion lead to different functional properties. Annu Rev Immunol 1989;7:145–173.
5. Mosmann TR, Sad S. The expanding universe of T-cell subsets: Th1, Th2 and more. Immunol Today 1996;17:138–146.
6. Salgame P, Abrams JS, Clayberger C, Goldstein H, Convit J, Modlin RJ, Bloom BR. Differing lymphokine profiles of functional subsets of CD4 and CD8 T cell clones. Science 1991;254:279–282.
7. Maggi E, Biswas P, Del Prete G, Parronchi P, Macchia D, Simonelli C, Emmi L, De Carli M, Tiri A, Ricci M, Romagnani S. Accumulation of TH2-like helper T cells in the conjunctiva of patients with vernal conjuctivitis. J Immunol 1991;146:1169–1174.
8. Hsieh C-S, Macatonia SE, Tripp CA, Wolf SF, O'Garra A, Murphy KM. Development of Th1 $CD4^+$ T cells through IL-12 produced by *Listeria*-induced macrophages. Science 1993;260:547–549.
9. Le Gros G, Ben-Sasson SZ, Seder R, Finkelman FD, Paul WE. Generation of interleukin-4 (IL-4) producing cells in vitro and in vivo: IL-2 and IL-4 are required for in vitro generation of IL-4 producing cells. J Exp Med 1990;172:921–929.
10. Kopf M, Le Gros G, Bachmann M, Lamers MC, Bleuthmann H, Kohler G. Disruption of the murine IL-4 gene blocks Th2 cytokine responses. Nature 1993;362:245–248.
11. Constant S, Pfeiffer C, Pasqualini T, Bottomly K. Extent of T cell receptor ligation can determine the functional differentiation of naive CD4+ T cells. J Exp Med 1995;182:1591–1596.
12. Bretscher BA, Wu G, Menon N, Ohman H. Establishment of stable cell-mediated immunity that makes susceptible mice resistant to *Leishmania major*. Science 1992;257:539–542.
13. Biron CA, Gazzinelli RT. Effects of IL-12 on immune responses to microbial infections: a key mediator in regulating disease outcome. Curr Opin Immunol 1995;7:485–496.

14. Yoshimoto T, Paul WE. CD4pos, NK1.1pos T cells promptly produce interleukin 4 in response to in vivo challenge with anti-CD3. J Exp Med 1994;179:1285–1295.
15. Zhang Y, Rogers KH, Lewis DB. Beta 2-microglobulin-dependent T cells are dispensible for allergen-induced T helper 2 cells responses. J Exp Med 1996;184:1507–1512.
16. Brown DR, Fowell DJ, Corry DB, Wynn TA, Moskowitz NH, Cheever AW, Locksley RM, Reiner SL. β2-microglobulin-dependent NK1.1+ T cells are not essential for T helper cell 2 immune responses. J Exp Med 1996;184:1295–1304.
17. Yoshimoto T, Bedalac A, Watson C, Hu-Li J, Paul WE. Role of NK1.1+ T cells in a TH2 response and in immunoglobulin E production. Science 1995;270:1845–1847.
18. Schmitz J, Thiel A, Kuhn R, Rajewsky K, Muller W, Assenmacher M, Radbruch A. Induction of interleukin 4 (IL-4) expression in T helper (Th) cells is not dependent on IL-4 from non-Th cells. J Exp Med 1994;179:1349–1353.
19. Rincon M, Anguita J, Nakamura T, Fikrig E, Flavell RA. IL-6 directs the differentiation of IL-4-producing CD4+ T cells. J Exp Med 1997;185:461–469.
20. Burd PR, Thompson WC, Max EE, Mills FC. Activated mast cells produce interleukin 13. J Exp Med 1995;181:1373–1380.
21. Gordon JR, Burd PR, Galli SJ. Mast cells as a source of multifunctional cytokines. Immunol Today 1990;11:458–464.
22. Sabin EA, Kopf MA, Pearce EJ. *Schistosoma mansoni* egg-induced early IL-4 production is dependent upon IL-5 and eosinophils. J Exp Med 1996;184:1871–1878.
23. Pernis A, Gupta S, Gollob KJ, Garfein E, Coffman RL, Schindler C, Rothman P. Lack of interferon γ receptor β chain and the prevention of interferon γ signaling in Th1 cells. Science 1995;269:245–247.
24. Szabo SJ, Dighe AS, Gubler U, Murphy KM. Regulation of the interleukin (IL)-12Rβ2 subunit expression in developing T helper 1 (Th1) and Th2 cells. J Exp Med 1997;185:817–824.
25. Rogge L, Barberis-Maino L, Biffi M, Passini N, Presky DH, Gubler U, Sinigaglia S. Selective expression of an interleukin-12 receptor component by human T helper 1 cells. J Exp Med 1997;185:825–831.
26. Szabo SJ, Jacobsen NG, Dighe AS, Gubler U, Murphy KM. Developmental commitment to the Th2 lineage by extinction of IL-12 signalling. Immunity 1994;2:665–675.
27. Kuchroo VK, Prabhu Das M, Brown JA., Ranger AM, Zamvil SS, Sobel RA, Weiner HL, Nabavi N, Glimcher LH. B7-1 and B7-1 costimulatory molecules activate differentially the Th1/Th2 developmental pathways: application to autoimmune disease therapy. Cell 1995;80:707–718.
28. Borriello F, Sethna MP, Boyd SD, Schweitzer AN, Tivol EA, Jacoby D, Strom TB, Simpson EM, Freeman GJ, Sharpe AH. B7-1 and B7-2 have overlapping, critical roles in immunoglobulin class switching and germinal center formation. Immunity 1997;6:303–313.
29. Sanderson CJ. IL-5, eosinophils, and disease. Blood 1992;79:3101–3109.
30. Brown KD, Zurawski SM, Mosmann TR, Zurawski G. A family of small inducible proteins secreted by leukocytes are members of a new superfamily that includes

leukocyte and fibroblast-derived inflammatory agents, growth factors, and indicators of various activation processes. J Immunol 1989;142:679–687.
31. Minty A, Chalon P, Derocq J-M, Dumont X, Guillemot J-C, Kaghad K, Labit C, Leplatois P, Liauzun P, Miloux B, Minty C, Casellas P, Loison G, Lupker J, Shire D, Ferrara P, Caput D. Interleukin-13: a novel human lymphokine regulating inflammatory and immune responses. Nature 1993;362:248–250.
32. McKenzie ANJ, Culpepper JA, de Waal Malefyt R, Briere F, Punonnen J, Aversa G, Sato A, Dang W, Cocks BG, Menon S, de Vries JE, Banchereau J, Zurawski G. Interleukin-13, a novel T cell-derived cytokine that regulates human monocyte and B cell function. Proc Natl Acad Sci USA 1993;90:3735–3739.
33. Punnonen J, Aversa G, Cocks BG, McKenzie ANJ, Menon S, Zurawski G, de Waal Malefyt R, de Vries JE. Interleukin 13 induces interleukin 4-independent IgG4 and IgE synthesis and CD23 expression by human B cells. Proc Natl Acad Sci USA 1993;90:3730–3734.
34. Zurawski G, de Vries JE. Interleukin 13, an interleukin 4-like cytokine that acts on monocytes and B cells but not on T cells. Immunol Today 1994;15:19–26.
35. McKenzie ANJ, Li X, Largaespada DA, Sato A, Kaneda A, Zurawski SM, Doyle EL, Milatovich A, Francke U, Copeland NG, Jenkins NA, Zurawski G. Structural comparison and chromosomal localization of the human and mouse IL-13 genes. J Immunol 1993;150:5436–5444.
36. Willman CL, Sever CE, Pallavicini MG, Harada H, Tanaka N, Slovak ML, Yamamoto H, Harada K, Meeker TC, List AF, Taniguchi T. Deletion of IRF-1, mapping to chromosome 5q31.1, in human leukemia and preleukemic myelodysplasia. Science 1993;259:968–971.
37. Morgan JG, Dolganov GM, Robbins SE, Hinton LM, Lovett M. The selective isolation of novel cDNAs encoded by the regions surrounding the human interleukin 4 and 5 genes. Nucleic Acids Res 1992;20:5173–5179.
38. Chandrasekharappa SC, Rebelsky MS, Firak TA, Le Beau MM, Westbrook CA. A long-range restriction map of the interleukin-4 and interleukin-5 linkage group on chromosome 5. Genomics 1990;6:94–99.
39. Lee JS, Campbell HD, Kozak CA, Young, IG. The IL-4 and IL-5 genes are closely linked and are part of a cytokine gene cluster on mouse chromosome 11. Somat Cell Mol Genet 1989;15:143–152.
40. Le Beau MM, Lemons RS, Espinosa R, Larson RA, Arai N, Rowley JD. Interleukin-4 and interleukin-5 map to chromosome 5 in a region encoding growth factors and receptors and are deleted in myeloid leukemias with a del(5q). Blood 1989;73:647–650.
41. Vercelli D, Jabara HH, Lee B-L, Woodland N, Geha RS, Leung DYM. Human recombinant interleukin-4 induces FcεR/CD23 on normal human monocytes. J Exp Med 1988;167:1406–1416.
42. Cocks BG, de Waal Malefyt R, Galizzi J-P, de Vries JE, Aversa G. IL-13 induces proliferation and differentiation on human B cells activated by the CD40 ligand. Int Immunol 1993;5:657–663.
43. Defrance T, Carayon P, Billian G, Guillemot J-C, Minty A, Caput D, Ferrara P. Interleukin-13 is a B cell stimulating factor. J Exp Med 1994;179:135–143.

44. Kühn R, Rajewsky K, Müller W. Generation and analysis of interleukin-4 deficient mice. Science 1991;254:707–710.
45. Van der Weld T, Kopf M, Köhler G, Langhorne J. The immune response to *Plasmodium chabaudi* malaria in interleukin-4-deficient mice. Eur J Immunol 1994;24:2285–2293.
46. Morawetz RA, Gabriele L, Rizzo LV, Noben-Trauth N, Kuhn R, Rajewsky K, Muller W, Doherty TM, Finkelman F, Coffman RL, Morse HC III. Interleukin (IL)-4-independent immunoglobulin class switch to immunoglobulin (Ig)E in the mouse. J Exp Med 1996;184:1651–1661.
47. Gauchat J-F, Henchoz S, Mazzei G, Aubry J-P, Brunner T, Blasey H, Life P, Talabot D, Fores-Romo L, Thompson J, Kishi K, Butterfield J, Dahinden C, Bonnefoy J-Y. Induction of human IgE synthesis in B cells by mast cells and basophils. Nature 1993;365:340–343.
48. Jacobsen SEW, Okkenhaug C, Veiby OP, Caput D, Ferrara P, Minty, A. Interleukin-13: novel role in direct regulation of proliferation and differentiation of primitive hematopoietic progenitor cells. J Exp Med 1994;180:75–82.
49. de Waal Malefyt R, Figdor C, Huijbens R, Mohan-Peterson S, Bennett B, Culpepper J, Dang W, Zurawski G, de Vriew JE. Effects of IL-13 on phenotype, cytokine production, and cytotoxic function of human monocytes. J Immunol 1993;151:6370–6381.
50. Muzio M, Re F, Sironi M, Polentarutti N, Minty A, Caput D, Ferrara P, Mantovani A, Colotta, F. Interleukin-13 induces the production of interleukin-1 receptor antagonist (IL-1ra) and the expression of the mRNA for the intracellular (keratinocyte) form of IL-1ra in human myelomonocytic cells. Blood 1994;83:1738–1743.
51. Colotta F, Re F, Muzio M, Polentarutti N, Minty A, Caput D, Ferrara P, Mantovani A. Interleukin-13 induces expression and release of interleukin-1 decoy receptor in human polymorphonuclear cells. J Biol Chem 1994;269:12403–12406.
52. Doherty TM, Kastelein R, Menon S, Andrade S, Coffman RL. Modulation of murine macrophage function by interleukin-13. J Immunol 1993;151:7151–7160.
53. Doyle AG, Herbein G, Montaner LJ, Minty A, Caput D, Ferrara P, Gordon S. Interleukin-13 alters the activation state of murine macrophages in vitro: comparison with interleukin-4 and interferon-γ. Eur J Immunol 1994;24:1441–1445.
54. Sironi M, Sciacca FL, Matteucci C, Conni M, Vecchi A, Bernasconi S, Minty A, Caput D, Ferrara P, Colotta F. Regulation of endothelial and mesothelial cell function by interleukin-13: selective induction of vascular cell adhesion molecule-1 and amplification of interleukin-6 production. Blood 1994;84:1913–1921.
55. Montanier LJ, Doyle AG, Collin M, Herbein G, Illei P, James W, Minty A, Caput D, Ferrara P, Gordon S. Interleukin-13 inhibits human immunodeficiency virus type 1 production in primary blood-derived human macrophages in vitro. J Exp Med 1993;178:743–747.
56. Brewer JM, Conacher M, Satoskar A, Bluethmann H, Alexander J. In interleukin-4-deficient mice, alum not only generates T helper 1 responses equivalent to Freund's complete adjuvant, but continues to induce T helper 2 cytokine production. Eur J Immunol 1996;26:2062–2066.
57. Van der Pouw Kraan TC, Boieje LC, Troon JT, Rutschmann SK, Wijdenes J,

Aarden LA. Human IL-13 production is negatively influenced by CD3 engagement. J Immunol 1996;156:1818–1823.
58. Zurawski SM, Vega F Jr, Huyghe B, Zurawski G. Receptors for interleukin-13 and interleukin-4 are complex and share a novel component that functions in signal transduction. EMBO J 1993;12:3899–3905.
59. Zurawski SM, Chomarat P, Djousso O, Bidaud C, McKenzie ANJ, Miossec P, Banchereau J, Zurawski G. The primary binding subunit of the interleukin-4 receptor is also a component of the interleukin-13 receptor. J Biol Chem 1995;270:13869–13878.
60. Smerz-Bertling C, Duschl AL. Both interleukin 4 and interleukin 13 induce tyrosine phosphorylation of the 140-kDa subunit of the interleukin 4 receptor. J Biol Chem 1995;270:966–970.
61. Hilton DJ, Zhang J-G, Metcalf D, Alexander WS, Nicola NA, Willson TA. Cloning and characterization of a binding subunit of the interleukin 13 receptor that is also a component of the interleukin 4 receptor. Proc Natl Acad Sci USA 1996;93:497–501.
62. Caput D, Laurent P, Kaghad M, Lelias J-M, Lefort S, Vita N, Ferrara P. Cloning and characterization of a specific interleukin (IL)-13 binding protein structurally related to the IL-5 receptor $\alpha$ chain. J Biol Chem 1996;271:16921–16926.
63. Aman MJ, Tayebi N, Obiri NI, Puri RK, Modi WS, Leonard WJ. cDNA cloning and characterization of the human interleukin 13 receptor $\alpha$ chain. J Biol Chem 1996;271:29265–29270.
64. Gauchat J-F, Schlagenhauf E, Feng N-P, Moser R, Yamage M, Jeannin P, Alouani S, Elson G, Notarangelo LD, Wells T, Eugster H-P, Bonnefoy J-Y. A novel 4-kb interleukin-13 receptor $\alpha$ mRNA expressed in human B, T, and endothelial cells encoding an alternate type-II interleukin-4/interleukin-13 receptor. Eur J Immunol 1997;27:971–978.
65. Miloux B, Laurent P, Bonnin O, Lupker J, Caput D, Vita N, Ferrara P. Cloning of the human IL-13R$\alpha$1 chain and reconstitution with the IL-4R$\alpha$ of a functional IL-4/IL-13 receptor complex. FEBS Lett 1997;401:163–166.
66. Kondo M, Takeshita T, Ishii N, Nakamura M, Watanabe S, Arai K, Sugaamura K. Sharing of the interleukin-2 (IL-2) receptor $\gamma$ chain between receptors for IL-2 and IL-4. Science 1993;262:1874–1877.
67. Russell SM, Keegan AD, Harada N, Nakamura Y, Noguchi M, Leland P, Friedmann FC, Miyajima A, Puri RK, Paul WE, Leonard WJ. Interleukin-2 receptor $\gamma$ chain: a functional component of the interleukin-4 receptor. Science 1993;262:1880–1883.
68. He Y-W, Malek TR. The IL-2 receptor $\gamma$c chain does not function as a subunit shared by the IL-4 and IL-13 receptors: implication for the structure of the IL-4 receptor. J Immunol 1995;155:9–12.
69. Lin J-X, Migone T-S, Tsang M, Friedman M, Weatherbee JA, Zhou L, Yamauchi A, Bloom ET, Mietz J, John S, Leonard WJ. The role of shared receptor motifs and common stat proteins in the generation of cytokine pleiotropy and redundancy by IL-2, IL-4, IL-7, IL-13, and IL-15. Immunity 1995;2:331–339.
70. Jinquan T, Deleuran B, Gesser B, Maare H, Deleuran M, Gronhoj Larsen C,

Thestrup-Pedersen K. Regulation of human T lymphocyte chemotaxis in vitro by T cell-derived cytokines IL-2, IFNγ, IL-4, IL-10, and IL-13. J Immunol 1995;154:3742–3752.
71. Takeda T, Tanaka T, Shi W, Matsumoto M, Minami M, Kashiwamura S, Nakanishi K, Yoshida N, Kishimoto T, Akira S. Essential role of Stat6 in IL-4 signalling. Nature 1996;380:627–630.
72. Shimoda K, van Deursen J, Sangster MY, Sarawar SR, Carson RT, Tripp RA, Chu C, Quelle FW, Nosaka T, Vignali DAA, Doherty PC, Grosveld G, Paul WE, Ihle JN. Lack of IL-4-induced Th2 response and IgE class switching in mice with disrupted Stat6 gene. Nature 1996;380:630–633.
73. Kaplan MH, Schindler U, Smiley ST, Grusby MJ. Stat6 is required for mediating responses to IL-4 and for the development of Th2 cells. Immunity 1996;4:313–319.
74. Lederer JA, Perez VL, DesRoches L, Kim SM, Abbas AK, Lichtman AH. Cytokine transcriptional events during helper T cell subset differentiation. J Exp Med 1996;184:397–406.
75. Kotanides H, Reich NC. Interleukin-4-induced STAT6 recognizes and activates a target site in the promoter of the interleukin-4 receptor gene. J Biol Chem 1996;271:25555–25561.

# 9

# Interactions Between Interleukin-5 and the Eosinophil-Selective Chemokine Eotaxin: Potential Relevance in Allergic Disease

**PAUL D. COLLINS and TIMOTHY J. WILLIAMS**

Imperial College School of Medicine
London, England

## I. Introduction

Eosinophil accumulation is a characteristic feature of certain inflammatory diseases, particularly allergic conditions. There is evidence that the eosinophil is a major effector cell underlying tissue damage in both allergic and nonallergic asthma. Thus there is considerable interest in analyzing the mechanisms involved in eosinophil recruitment in pursuit of new targets for potential therapeutic intervention. In this chapter we will focus on the synergistic interaction between IL-5 and the recently described eosinophil-selective chemokine, eotaxin, to cause eosinophil accumulation and discuss the potential relevance of this interaction in allergic diseases and the development of a therapeutic strategy.

Eosinophils are thought to have evolved as part of the host defense system against helminth and other parasite infections. Immune reactions develop to worms and their products and allergy may be an unfortunate misdirection of this response triggered by otherwise innocuous agents. Thus, in its host defense role, the eosinophil needs to be recruited to the infected tissues where it adheres to the surface of the worm and releases its toxic granular contents. Similarly, in allergic conditions such as asthma, a regulated eosinophil infiltration into the tissue occurs, toxic granule components are released, and the associated tissue damage contributes to the pathology of the disease (this is covered in more detail in chapters 1 and 2). The suggestion that specific factors are responsible for the blood and tissue eosinophilia that occurs in response to allergen challenge of sensitized individuals was investigated as long ago as 1953 by Samter et al. (1). In elegant studies, ovalbumin-sensitized guinea pigs were challenged with ovalbumin and, following anaphylactic shock, a piece of lung tissue was transferred into the peritoneal cavity of naive animals. Over 24 hr animals receiving shocked lung developed a pronounced blood eosinophilia that did not occur following the transfer of normal or sensitized/sham challenged tissue. In prophetic statements they suggested that "an eosinotactic factor develops in the peribronchial tissue of guinea pigs subsequent to antigen-antibody reactions," and "the normal bone marrow is capable of releasing mature eosinophils without prolonged incubation."

Over the intervening years the emergence of soluble factors (chemoattractants) that induce activation and chemotaxis of leukocytes in vitro and their local tissue accumulation in vivo supported the supposition of Samter et al. (1). None of these molecules, however, appeared to mediate the selective eosinophil response seen in allergic reactions and helminth infections. The discovery in 1985 (2) of a murine cytokine, eosinophil differentiation factor (EDF), which also stimulated the selective proliferation, differentiation, and function of human eosinophils led rapidly to the identification of a human molecule with similar properties, interleukin-5 (IL-5) (3,4). Apart from its effects on eosinophil hematopoiesis and survival (5–8), IL-5 has been shown to induce eosinophil chemokinesis, chemotaxis, adhesion, and priming in vitro (7,9–16).

IL-5 quickly became established as a central cytokine involved in the regulation of local eosinophil recruitment in allergic diseases. Elevated levels of IL-5 protein and message are found in the bronchial mucosa of asthmatic individuals (17–21). Elevated serum IL-5 levels have also been detected (22). In a number of animal models of allergic inflammation and parasitic infection neutralizing anti-IL-5 antibodies effectively inhibit the eosinophil accumulation (23–30) and in models of allergic disease this can lead to an attenuation of the associated lung tissue damage and/or bronchial hyperreactivity (27,28,30). More recently, using transgenic animal technology it has been demonstrated that IL-5-deficient, and IL-5 receptor-deficient, mice are unable to mount an efficient eosinophil response in allergy and parasite infection models (31,32). Conversely, mice that overexpress IL-5 constitutively exhibit a pronounced blood and tissue eosinophilia (33,34).

## II. Discovery of Eotaxin

Despite the evident importance of IL-5 in the process of infiltration of eosinophils into tissues, the mechanism by which this occurs has remained controversial. This is due to the conflicting data regarding the ability of IL-5 to act as a direct eosinophil chemoattractant (10,14,15,35,36). Furthermore, IL-5 transgenic mice have a profound lung eosinophilia without any of the symptoms of allergic airways disease (33). This led our group to investigate the possible existence of other soluble eosinophil-selective chemoattractants.

We used a well-established in vivo model of allergic airways inflammation in the guinea pig where ovalbumin-sensitized animals were exposed to an aerosol of ovalbumin (under antihistamine cover to prevent fatal analphylaxis) and at various times following challenge bronchoalveolar lavage (BAL) was performed (37). The BAL fluid was injected intradermally into the shaved dorsal skin of naive recipient guinea pigs previously injected intravenously with $^{111}$In-labeled eosinophils (38) and the local accumulation of these radiolabeled cells quantified in response to the BAL fluid. Time course studies revealed the appearance of a selective eosinophil chemoattractant in BAL fluid within 30 min of antigen challenge of sensitized animals which peaked in 3–6 hr BAL fluid and was undetectable in BAL fluid obtained after 24 hr (little activity was found in BAL fluid from sensitized/sham-challenged or sham-sensitized/challenged animals) (37).

On the basis of these observations 3 hr BAL fluid was pooled from a large number of animals and subjected to a purification strategy based on sequential ion exchange, size exclusion, and reverse-phase HPLC. Eosinophil chemoattractant activity was detected in three fractions at the final stage of purification and amino acid sequencing revealed them to contain a CC chemokine with a novel sequence of 73 amino acids (37). The purified protein caused eosinophil but not neutrophil accumulation in guinea pig skin (37). Following aerosolization of the protein in guinea pigs there was a selective eosinophil infiltration into BAL fluid (39). In vitro the protein induced a transient intracellular calcium flux in guinea pig (39) and human eosinophils (37) but not neutrophils. Based on this biological profile we named the protein eotaxin. Further analysis suggested that eotaxin existed in at least three different glycosylated forms on the same protein backbone (37).

The chemokine family comprises over 30 different proteins which are divided into 4 groups based on the relative positions of the N-terminal cysteines which form disulfide bonds with cysteines toward the C terminus of the protein (there are several excellent general reviews covering this area) (40,41). The C, or $\gamma$-chemokine, and the $CX_3C$ chemokine groups each contain a single member active on lymphocytes and NK cells/monocytes, respectively (42,43). CC- or $\alpha$-chemokines, where there are two cysteines separated by an intervening amino acid, are predominantly neutrophil activators and chemoattractants which also have important effects on angiogenesis. Members of this group include interleukin-8 (IL-8), neutrophil activating protein-2 (NAP-2), and growth-related oncogene/melanoma growth stimulating activity (GRO/MGSA). CC- or β-chemokines of which eotaxin is a member, have two adjacent N-terminal cysteines and have a range of specificities for different leukocyte populations including eosinophils, monocytes, and lymphocyte subsets. Members of this group include monocyte chemotactic proteins 1–5 (MCP1–5), regulated on activation normal T-cell expressed and secreted (RANTES), and macrophage inflammatory protein-1α (MIP-1α).

Our original observation that guinea pig eotaxin was active on human eosinophils implied the existence of a human equivalent chemokine and a human eotaxin receptor. Using primers based on our guinea pig eotaxin sequence (37,44), human (45–47) and murine (48) eotaxins have now been cloned and sequenced, and the expressed proteins show the same high degree of eosinophil selectivity as the guinea pig protein. The selectivity of eotaxin for eosinophils can be attributed to the restricted expression of the eotaxin receptor (CCR3) (49,50). There are currently 10 CC-chemokine receptors designated CCR1–10 (51–54). CCR3 is highly expressed on eosinophils. More recently, expression has also been reported in brain microglial cells and basophils (55). Apart from eotaxin, other CCR3 ligands include RANTES, MCP-3, and MCP-4. While these latter chemokines are eosinophil chemoattractants, they all interact with at least one other CCR found on other leukocytes and hence do not have the selectivity of eotaxin which exclusively signals via CCR3.

### A. Synergism Between IL-5 and Eotaxin

Clearly the local generation of eotaxin and other eosinophil active chemokines could account for the selective accumulation of eosinophils which is characteristic of allergic disease. Experimental observations, however, suggest the existence of a more complex process. For example, in the guinea pig model of allergic airways inflammation an anti-IL-5 antibody inhibits eosinophil accumulation in the lung tissue and the BAL fluid without affecting the generation of eotaxin (56). This implies a synergistic cooperation between IL-5 and eotaxin to induce eosinophil infiltration. To investigate this possibility we injected eotaxin intradermally into guinea pig skin and measured the accumulation of endogenous eosinophils (36). This was achieved by quantifying the levels of the eosinophil granule constituent eosinophil peroxidase (EPO) in tissue extracts. As shown in Figure 1 we found that the eosinophil accumulation over 2 hr in response to locally injected eotaxin was markedly enhanced in a synergistic fashion if the animals were pretreated intravenously for 1 hr with a low dose of IL-5 (18 pmol/kg). In parallel experiments, no eosinophil accumulation was seen in response to intradermal IL-5 regardless of the absence or presence of an intravenous IL-5 pretreatment. Analysis of circulating eosinophil levels revealed that intravenous IL-5 induced a rapid blood eosinophilia within 15 to 30 min so that after 1 hr, when eotaxin was injected intradermally, there was a 15-fold elevation in circulating eosinophil numbers that was maintained throughout the experiment.

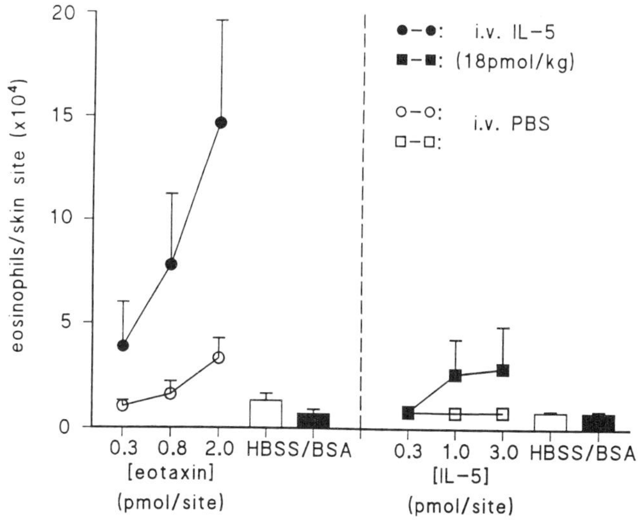


**Figure 1** Potentiation of eotaxin-induced eosinophil accumulation by IL-5. Interleukin-5 (18 pmol/kg) or vehicle (PBS) was administered intravenously in guinea pigs. IL-5 induced a rapid (within 30 min) blood eosinophilia by stimulating the release of a mobilizable pool of bone marrow cells. After 1 hr when circulating eosinophil numbers were elevated 15-fold, guinea pig eotaxin was injected intradermally and 2 hr later the number of migrated eosinophils determined by measurement of the granule constituent eosinophil peroxidase. The local eosinophil accumulation in response to intradermal eotaxin was significantly enhanced in animals pretreated with IL-5. In contrast, intradermal IL-5 induced no significant eosinophil accumulation in either the untreated group or in the group pretreated with intravenous interleukin-5. [Reproduced in a modified form with permission from J Exp Med 1995;182:1169–1174 © The Rockefeller University Press].

We established that a rapidly mobilizable pool of bone marrow eosinophils was responsible for the blood eosinophilia as there was a significant reduction in bone marrow eosinophil numbers 1 hr after intravenous IL-5 (36).

### B. IL-5, Eotaxin, and Asthma

Asthma is a complex inflammatory condition of the lungs characterized by an acute bronchoconstriction associated with mast cell degranulation and a later phase of bronchoconstriction and airway hyperresponsiveness accompanied by the infiltration of the lung tissue by eosinophils. The observations that IL-5 and eosinophil chemoattractants such as eotaxin cooperate in the regulation of eosinophil egress from the bone marrow, and accumulation in tissue has evolved into studies of the interactions between these mediators in asthma.

Following on from the original discovery of eotaxin in the BAL fluid obtained from challenged/sensitized guinea pigs (37) detailed analysis of eotaxin generation in animal models of allergic airways inflammation has been carried out. Elevated eotaxin mRNA expression has been detected within 3 hr of allergen challenge in guinea pigs (44,57) and mice (58). This precedes the appearance of eotaxin protein in the lung and BAL fluid, which is maximal 6 hr after challenge (56). At this point lung tissue eosinophilia is prominant. A delayed accumulation of eosinophils occurs in the lumen of the airways after 12 hr, which may reflect differential rates of clearance or metabolism of eotaxin in the tissue versus the mucus lining of the alveolar spaces (56). Other approaches used to dissect the role of eotaxin in eosinophil recruitment in allergic airways inflammation have included the use of anti-eotaxin antibodies (58) and the development of eotaxin knockout mice (59). In both cases a substantial but not complete abrogation of eosinophil accumulation was achieved.

Some studies using the allergen challenge model have also focused on the relationship between IL-5, tissue eosinophilia, and the eosinophil profile in the bone marrow and the blood. Humbles et al. (56) have demonstrated that following challenge of sensitized guinea pigs there is a rapid blood eosinophilia within 3 to 6 hr, which parallels the accumulation of eosinophils in the lung. Analysis of the bone marrow revealed a concomittant drop in the number of stromal eosinophils, indicating the bone marrow pool of eosinophils had been mobilized. In the same experiments the use of a neutralizing anti-IL-5 antibody (TRFK-5) effectively prevented the lung and BAL eosinophilia seen after allergen challenge and prevented the release of the bone marrow pool of eosinophils.

In mice, Kung et al. (30) similarly showed that allergen challenge following sensitization resulted in the characteristic lung damage that occurs in allergic disease and this was associated with a blood, lung tissue, and BAL fluid eosinophilia. Using a different approach Foster et al. (31) demonstrated that in challenged/sensitized IL-5 knockout mice the eosinophilia in all compartments was inhibited and the lung damage markedly reduced. Reconstitution of IL-5 using a recombinant vaccinia virus expressing IL-5 restored the inflammatory profile following challenge.

Two intriguing observations have also been made implying that eotaxin may play an important role in the homeostatic maintainance of circulating eosinophil levels. In eotaxin knockout mice, Rothenberg et al. (59) observed that basal circulating eosinophil levels were reduced although there was no effect on eosinophil numbers in the bone marrow. In contrast, Mould et al. (60) found that intravenous injection of eotaxin in normal (or IL-5 knockout) mice resulted in a rapid but transient blood eosinophilia. Surprisingly, this did not appear to be associated with a decrease in the bone marrow pool of eosinophils.

Taking all of this information as a whole, it becomes clear that a coordinated sequence of events can be hypothesized to account for the selective eosinophil accumulation observed in allergic diseases such as asthma (see Fig. 2). Allergen exposure of a sensitized individual initiates a rapid local production of IL-5 from T lymphocytes and/or mast cells, and eotaxin from some or all of the following cellular sources: bronchial epithelial cells, bronchial smooth muscle cells, alveolar macrophages, and endothelial cells. IL-5 diffuses into the blood and travels from its site of generation in the lung to the bone marrow. There it induces the rapid release (within minutes) of a mobilizable pool of bone marrow eosinophils into the circulation. Over the longer term (days to weeks) IL-5 promotes eosinophilopoiesis to replenish the mobilizable pool of cells. In the

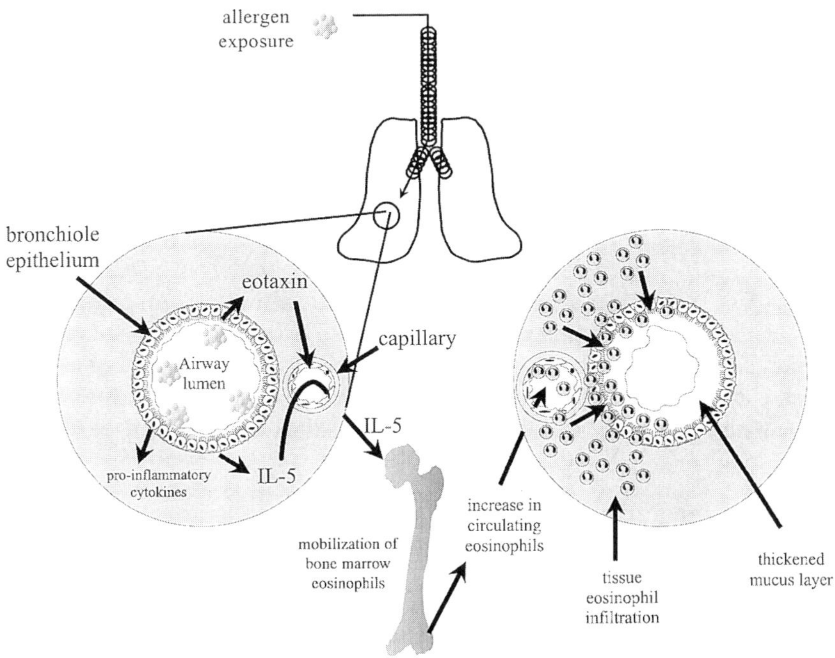


**Figure 2** Schematic representation of the potential cooperation between eotaxin and IL-5 that leads to esoinophil infiltration of the lung associated with allergic diseases such as asthma. Following allergen exposure of a sensitized individual, eotaxin and IL-5 are generated in the lung tissue. Eotaxin acts locally in the lung to cause eosinophil migration from the microvasculature. This is potentiated by IL-5 which enters the blood, travels to the bone marrow, and rapidly releases the mobilizable pool of eosinophils. In addition, IL-5 will induce eosinophilopoiesis in the bone marrow, prime eosinophil function, and enhance eosinophil survival in the tissue.

lung, eotaxin stimulates adhesive interactions between eosinophils and the microvascular wall, and induces eosinophil extravasation. IL-5 may facilitate this process by priming circulating cells. If the generation of eotaxin is sufficient it may reach physiologically active levels in the circulation and contribute circulation to the blood eosinophilia. Once in the lung the eosinophils will come under the influence of other locally generated mediators that control the release of toxic granule constituents, thus contributing to the tissue damage. IL-5 present in the lung tissue may also promote survival of tissue eosinophils.

## III. Conclusions

The observations discussed in this chapter have opened up possibilities for the design of novel antiasthmatic compounds targeted specifically on the eosinophil. Clearly IL-5 is an important target in itself, as discussed in other chapters. Eotaxin and its receptor, CCR3, provide a second target that is very attractive because successful blockade of CCR3 with a small molecule antagonist may provide an effective means of preventing eosinophil accumulation in a tissue and the associated pathology. Since the discovery of eotaxin and its receptor it is now known that other CC chemokines, with varying potency and selectivity, have chemoattractant activity for eosinophils. Fortuitously these other chemokines, for example, MCP-4, also signal eosinophils through CCR3. Thus different CC chemokines may be important in different phases or types of allergic and nonallergic eosinophilic inflammation. However, successful blockade of CCR3 would be expected to render the circulating eosinophil insensitive to such chemoattractants. This would be the acid test of the proposed relationship between eosinophils and tissue damage in asthma and allergy.

## Acknowledgments

The authors are indebted to the Wellcome Trust, UK, and the National Asthma Campaign, UK, for financial support.

## References

1. Samter M, Kofoed MA, Pieper W. A factor in lungs of anaphylactically shocked guinea pigs which can induce eosinophilia in normal animals. Blood 1953;8:1078–1090.
2. Sanderson CJ, Warren DG, Strath M. Identification of a lymphokine that stimulates eosinophil differentiation in vitro. Its relationship to interleukin 3, and functional properties of eosinophils produced in cultures. J Exp Med 1985;162:60–74.

3. Azuma C, Tanabe T, Konishi M, Kinashi T, Noma T, Matsuda F, Yaoita Y, Takatsu L, Hammarstrom L, Smith CIE, Severinson E, Honjo T. Cloning of cDNA for human T-cell replacing factor (interleukin-5) and comparison with the murine homologue. Nucleic Acids Res 1986;14:9149–9158.
4. Campbell HD, Tucker WQJ, Hort Y, Martinson ME, Mayo G, Clutterbuck EJ, Sanderson CJ, Young IG. Molecular cloning and expression of the gene encoding human eosinophil differentiation factor (interleukin-5). Proc Natl Acad Sci USA 1987;84:6629-6633.
5. Yamaguchi Y, Suda T, Suda J, Eguchi M, Miura Y, Harada N, Tominaga A, Takatsu K. Purified interleukin 5 supports the terminal differentiation and proliferation of murine eosinophilic precursors. J Exp Med 1988;167:43–56.
6. Clutterbuck EJ, Sanderson CJ. Human eosinophil hematopoiesis studied in vitro by means of murine eosinophil differentiation factor (IL-5): production of functionally active eosinophils from normal human bone marrow. Blood 1988;71:646–651.
7. Yamaguchi Y, Hayashi Y, Sugama Y, Miura Y, Kasahara T, Kitamura S, Torisu M, Mita S, Tominaga A, Takatsu K, Suda T. Highly purified murine interleukin 5 (IL-5) stimulates eosinophil function and prolongs *in vitro* survival. IL-5 as an eosinophil chemotactic factor. J Exp Med 1988;167:1737–1742.
8. Tai PC, Sun L, Spry CJF. Effects of IL-5, granulocyte/macrophage colony-stimulating factor (GM-CSF) and IL-3 on the survival of human blood eosinophils *in vitro*. Clin Exp Immunol 1991;85:312–316.
9. Lopez AF, Sanderson CJ, Gamble JR, Campbell HD, Young IG, Vadas MA. Recombinant human interleukin 5 is a selective activator of human eosinophil function. J Exp Med 1988;167:219–224.
10. Sehmi R, Wardlaw AJ, Cromwell O, Kurihara K, Waltmann P, Kay AB. Interleukin-5 selectively enhances the chemotactic response of eosinophils obtained from normal but not eosinophilic subjects. Blood 1992;79:2952–2959.
11. Warringa RAJ, Mengelers HJJ, Kuijper PHM, Raaijmakers JAM, Bruijnzeel PLB, Koenderman L. In vivo priming of platelet-activating factor-induced eosinophil chemotaxis in allergic asthmatic individuals. Blood 1992;79:1836–1841.
12. Coeffier E, Joseph D, Vargaftig BB. Activation of guinea pig eosinophils by human recombinant IL-5. Selective priming to platelet-activating factor-acether and interference of its antagonists. J Immunol 1991;147:2595–2602.
13. Walsh GM, Hartnell A, Wardlaw AJ, Kurihara K, Sanderson CJ, Kay AB. IL-5 enhances the in vitro adhesion of human eosinophils, but not neutrophils, in a leucocyte integrin (CD11/18)-dependent manner. Immunology 1990;71:258–265.
14. Schweizer RC, van Kessel-Welmers BAC, Warringa RAJ, Maikoe T, Raaijmakers JAM, Lammers JJ, Koenderman L. Mechanisms involved in eosinophil migration. Platelet-activating factor-induced chemotaxis and interleukin-5-induced chemokinesis are mediated by different signals. J Leuk Biol 1996;59:347–356.
15. Ebisawa M, Liu MC, Yamada T, Kato M, Lichtenstein LM, Bochner BS, Schleimer RP. Eosinophil transendothelial migration induced by cytokines II. Potentiation of eosinophil transendothelial migration by eosinophil-active cytokines. J Immunol 1994;152:4590–4596.

16. Ebisawa M, Yamada T, Bickel C, Klunk D, Schleimer RP. Eosinophil transendothelial migration induced by cytokines III. Effect of the chemokine RANTES. J Immunol 1994;153:2153-2160.
17. Hamid Q, Azzawi M, Ying S, Moqbel R, Wardlaw AJ, Corrigan CJ, Bradley B, Durham SR, Collins JV, Jeffery PK, Quint DJ, Kay AB. Expression of mRNA for interleukin-5 in mucosal bronchial biopsies from asthma. J Clin Invest 1991;87:1541–1546.
18. Broide DH, Paine MM, Firestein GS. Eosinophils express interleukin 5 and granulocyte macrophage-colony-stimulating factor mRNA at sites of allergic inflammation in asthmatics. J Clin Invest 1992;90:1414–1424.
19. Bradding P, Roberts JA, Britten KM, Montefort S, Djukanovic R, Meuller R, Heusser CH, Howarth PH, Holgate ST. Interleukin-4,-5,and -6 and tumor necrosis factor-α in normal and asthmatic airways: evidence for the human mast cell as a source of these cytokines. Am J Respir Cell Mol Biol 1994;10:471–480.
20. Krishnaswamy G, Liu MC, Su S, Kumai M, Xiao H, Marsh DG, Huang S. Analysis of cytokine transcripts in the bronchoalveolar lavage cells of patients with asthma. Am J Respir Cell Mol Biol 1993;9:279–286.
21. Hoshi H, Ohno I, Honma M, Tanno Y, Yamauchi K, Tamura G, Shirato K. IL-5, IL-8 and GM-CSF immunostaining of sputum cells in bronchial asthma and chronic bronchitis. Clin Exp Allergy 1995;25:720–728.
22. Corrigan CJ, Haczku A, Gemou-Engesaeth V, Doi S, Kikuchi Y, Takatsu K, Durham SR, Kay AB. CD4 T-lymphocytes activation in asthma is accompanied by increased serum concentrations of interleukin-5. Am Rev Respir Dis 1993;147:540–547.
23. Nagai H, Yamaguchi S, Inagaki N, Tsuruoka N, Hitoshi Y, Takatsu K. Effect of anti-IL-5 monoclonal antibody on allergic bronchial eosinophilia and airway hyperresponsiveness in mice. Life Sci 1993;53:243–247.
24. Chand N, Harrison JE, Rooney S, Pillar J, Jakubicki R, Nolan K, Diamantis W, Sofia RD. Anti-IL-5 monoclonal antibody inhibits allergic late phase bronchial eosinophilia in guinea pigs: a therapeutic approach. Eur J Pharmacol 1992;211:121–123.
25. Kaneko M, Kitoshi Y, Takatsu K, Matsumoto S. Role of interleukin-5 in local accumulation of eosinophils in mouse allergic peritonitis. Int Archs Allergy Appl Immunol 1991;96:41–45.
26. Coffman RL, Seymore BWP, Hudak S, Jackson J, Rennick D. Antibody to interleukin-5 inhibits helminth-induced eosinophilia in mice. Science 1989;245:308–310.
27. Van Oosterhout AJM, Ladenius RS, Savelkoul HFJ, Van Ark I, Delsman KC, Nijkamp FP. Effect of anti-IL-5 and IL-5 on airway hyperreactivity and eosinophils in guinea pigs. Am Rev Respir Dis 1993;147:548–552.
28. Mauser PJ, Pitman A, Witt A, Fernandez X, Zurcher J, Kung T, Jones H, Watnick AS, Egan RW, Kreutner W, Adams KG. Inhibitory effect of the TRFK-5 anti-IL-5 antibody in a guinea pig model of asthma. Am Rev Respir Dis 1993;148:1623–1627.
29. Gulbenkian AR, Egan RW, Fernandez X, Jones H, Kreutner W, Kung T, Payvandi

F, Sullivan L, Zurcher JA, Watnick AS. Interleukin-5 modulates eosinophil accumulation in allergic guinea pig lung. Am Rev Respir Dis 1992;146:263–265.

30. Kung TT, Stelts DM, Zurcher JA, Adams GK III, Egan RW, Kreutner W, Watnick AS, Jones H, Chapman RW. Involvement of IL-5 in a murine model of allergic pulmonary inflammation: prophylactic and therapeutic effect of an anti-IL-5 antibody. Am J Respir Cell Mol Biol 1995;13:360–365.
31. Foster PS, Hogan SP, Ramsay AJ, Matthaei KI, Young IG. Interleukin 5 deficiency abolishes eosinophilia, airways hyperreactivity, and lung damage in a mouse asthma model. J Exp Med 1996;183:195–201.
32. Yoshida T, Ikuta K, Sugaya H, Maki K, Takagi M, Kanazawa H, Sunaga S, Kinashi T, Yoshimura K, Miyazaki J, Takaki S, Takatsu K. Defective B-1 cell development and impaired immunity against *Angiostrongylus cantonensis* in IL-5Rα-deficient mice. Immunity 1996:4:483–494.
33. Dent LA, Strath M, Mellor AL, Sanderson CJ. Eosinophilia in transgenic mice expressing interleukin 5. J Exp Med 1990;172:1425–1431.
34. Lee JJ, McGarry MP, Farmer SC, Denzler KL, Larson KA, Carrigan PE, Brenneise IE, Horton MA, Haczku A, Gelfand EW, Leikauf GD, Lee NA. Interleukin-5 expression in the lung epithelium of transgenic mice leads to pulmonary changes pathognomonic of asthma. J Exp Med 1997;185:2143–2156.
35. Wang JM, Rambaldi A, Biondi A, Chen ZG, Sanderson CJ, Mantovani A. Recombinant human interleukin 5 is a selective eosinophil chemoattractant. Eur J Immunol 1989;19:701–705.
36. Collins PD, Marleau S, Griffiths-Johnson DA, Jose PJ, Williams TJ. Co-operation between interleukin-5 and the chemokine, eotaxin, to induce eosinophil accumulation *in vivo*. J Exp Med 1995;182:1169–1174.
37. Jose PJ, Griffiths-Johnson DA, Collins PD, Walsh DT, Moqbel R, Totty NF, Truong O, Hsuan JJ, Williams TJ. Eotaxin: a potent eosinophil chemoattractant cytokine detected in a guinea-pig model of allergic airways inflammation. J Exp Med 1994;179:881–887.
38. Faccioli LH, Nourshargh S, Moqbel R, Williams FM, Sehmi R, Kay AB, Williams TJ. The accumulation of $^{111}$In-eosinophils induced by inflammatory mediators in vivo. Immunology 1991;73:222–227.
39. Griffiths-Johnson DA, Collins PD, Rossi AG, Jose PJ, Williams TJ. The chemokine, eotaxin, activates guinea-pig eosinophils in vitro, and causes their accumulation into the lung in vivo. Biochem Biophys Res Commun 1993;197:1167–1172.
40. Baggiolini M, Dahinden CA. CC Chemokines in allergic inflammation. Immunol Today 1994;15:127–133.
41. Baggiolini M, Dewald B, Moser B. Interleukin-8 and related chemotactic cytokines—CXC and CC chemokines. Adv Immunol 1994;55:97–179.
42. Kelner GS, Kennedy J, Bacon KB, Kleyensteuber S, Largaespada DA, Jenkins NA, Copeland NA, Bazan JF, Moore KW, Schall TJ, Zlotnik A. Lymphotactin: a cytokine that represents a new class of chemokine. Science 1994;266:1395–1399.
43. Bazan JF, Bacon KB, Hardiman G, Wang W, Greaves DR, Zlotnik A, Schall TJ.

A new class of membrane-bound chemokine with a $CX_3C$ motif. Nature 1997;385:640–644.
44. Jose PJ, Adcock IM, Griffiths-Johnson DA, Berkman N, Wells TNC, Williams TJ, Power CA. Eotaxin: cloning of an eosinophil chemoattractant cytokine and increased mRNA expression in allergen-challenged guinea-pig lungs. Biochem Biophys Res Commun 1994;205:788–794.
45. Ponath PD, Qin S, Ringler DJ, Clark-Lewis I, Wang J, Kassam N, Smith H, Shi X, Gonzalo J, Newman W, Gutierrez-Ramos J, Mackay CR. Cloning of the human eosinophil chemoattractant, eotaxin. Expression, receptor binding and functional properties suggest a mechanism for the selective recruitment of eosinophils. J Clin Invest 1996;97:604–612.
46. Kitaura M, Nakajima T, Imai T, Harada S, Combadiere C, Tiffany HL, Murphy PM, Yoshie O. Molecular cloning of human eotaxin, an eosinophil-selective CC chemokine, and identification of a specific eosinophil eotaxin receptor, CC chemokine receptor 3. J Biol Chem 1996;271:7725–7730.
47. Garcia-Zepeda EA, Rothenberg ME, Ownbey RT, Celestin J, Leder P, Luster AD. Human eotaxin is a specific chemoattractant for eosinophil cells and provides a new mechanism to explain tissue eosinophilia. Nature Med 1996;2:449–456.
48. Rothenberg ME, Luster AD, Leder P. Murine eotaxin: an eosinophil chemoattractant inducible in endothelial cells and in interleukin 4-induced tumor suppression. Proc Natl Acad Sci USA 1995;92:8960–8964.
49. Ponath PD, Qin S, Post TW, Wang J, Wu L, Gerard NP, Newman W, Gerard C, Mackay CR. Molecular cloning and characterization of a human eotaxin receptor expressed selectively on eosinophils. J Exp Med 1996;183:2437–2448.
50. Daugherty BL, Siciliano SJ, DeMartino J, Malkowitz L, Sirontino A, Springer MS. Cloning, expression and characterization of the human eosinophil eotaxin receptor. J Exp Med 1996;183:2349–2354.
51. Murphy PM. Chemokine receptors: structure, function and role in microbial pathogenesis. Cyt Growth Factor Rev 1996;7:47–64.
52. Tiffany HL, Lautens LL, Gao J, Pease J, Locati M, Combadiere C, Modi W, Bonner TI, Murphy PM. Identification of CCR8: a human monocyte and thymus receptor for the CC chemokine I-309. J Exp Med 1997;186:165–170.
53. Baba M, Imai T, Nishimura M, Kakizaki MM, Takagi S, Hieshima K, Nomiyama H, Yoshie O. Identification of CCR6, the specific receptor for a novel lymphocyte-directed CC chemokine LARC. J Biol Chem 1997;272:14893–14898.
54. Yoshida R, Imai T, Hieshima K, Kusada J, Baba M, Kitaura M, Nishimura M, Kakizaki M, Nomiyama H, Yoshie O. Molecular cloning of a novel human CC chemokine EBI1-ligand chemokine that is a specific functional ligand for EBI1, CCR7. J Biol Chem 1997;272:13803–13809.
55. He J, Chen Y, Farzan M, Choe H, Ohagen A, Gartner S, et al. CCR3 and CCR5 are co-receptors for HIV-1 infection of microglia. Nature 1997;385:645–649.
56. Humbles AA, Conroy DM, Marleau S, Rankin SM, Palframan RT, Proudfoot AEI, Wells TNC, Dechun L, Jeffery PK, Griffiths-Johnson DA, Williams TJ, Jose PJ. Kinetics of eotaxin generation and its relationship to eosinophil accumulation in allergic airways disease: analysis in a guinea pig model *in vivo*. J Exp Med 1997;186:601–612.

57. Rothenberg ME, Luster AD, Lilly CM, Drazen JM, Leder P. Constitutive and allergen-induced expression of eotaxin mRNA in the guinea pig lung. J Exp Med 1995;181:1211–1216.
58. Gonzalo J, Jia G, Aguirre V, Friend D, Coyle AJ, Jenkins NA, Lin G, Katz H, Lichtman A, Copeland N, Kopf M, Gutierrez-Ramos J. Mouse eotaxin expression parallels eosinophil accumulation during lung allergic inflammation but it is not restricted to a Th2-type response. Immunity 1996;4:1–14.
59. Rothenberg ME, MacLean JA, Pearlman E, Luster AD, Leder P. Targeted disruption of the chemokine eotaxin partially reduces antigen-induced tissue eosinophilia. J Exp Med 1997;4:785–790.
60. Mould AW, Matthaei KI, Young IG, Foster PS. Relationship between interleukin-5 and eotaxin in regulating blood and tissue eosinophilia in mice. J Clin Invest 1997;5:1064–1071.

# 10

# Structure of Interleukin-5

**IRWIN M. CHAIKEN**

University of Pennsylvania School of Medicine
Philadelphia, Pennsylvania

**AMANDA E. I. PROUDFOOT***

Glaxo Wellcome Research and Development
Geneva, Switzerland

## I. Introduction

Interleukin-5 (IL-5) is a four-helix bundle growth factor protein of the immune system (1–7). It is the key cytokine responsible for the production, differentiation, and activation of eosinophils. It also has been shown in the mouse to be a B-cell growth factor. IL-5 acts by binding to a heterodimeric receptor, which is composed of an $\alpha$ chain specific for IL-5 uniquely and a common signaling chain $\beta_c$ that is also a component of the granulocyte-macrophage colony-stimulating factor (GM-CSF) and IL-3 receptors (8,9). Eosinophils bear 300 to 1000 such binding sites, to which IL-5 binds with a $K_d$ of 200 to 400 pM (10,11).

IL-5 and its receptor belong to a family of hematopoietic ligands and receptors that share significant genetic and structural homology. The structural homologies reveal a shared conformational motif in the growth factors and a similar subunit composition in their receptors. This finding evokes a central question of what driving forces derived from the intrinsic structural properties of these proteins as a class lead to specificity in the induction of cell regulation through receptor recognition and signal triggering.

**Current affiliation*: Serono Pharmaceutical Research Institute, Geneva, Switzerland.

The known human IL-5 structure, along with homologous structures of other growth factor proteins, have provided a starting point to investigate and map shared and unique receptor activation and signal triggering epitopes in the four-helix bundle framework. In this chapter we describe what is currently known about the IL-5 structure and the relationship between this structure and the function of IL-5 as a growth factor protein.

## II. Primary and Crystallographic Structure

Native IL-5 was isolated initially from murine T-cell supernatants and was shown to be a glycoprotein which exists as a homodimer (12). The protein was shown to have an apparent molecular mass of 45 kDa, but the subsequent cloning of the cDNA sequence indicated that the protein component is composed of two amino acid chains with a molecular mass of 13 kDa for each polypeptide monomer (13). The human IL-5 cDNA as well as the genomic DNA were subsequently cloned using the murine cDNA as a probe yielding a similar monomeric polypeptide which had 70% sequence similarity to the murine protein (14). Although the natural human protein has never been isolated, expression of the cDNA in eukaryotic systems (15) has shown that it is similarly a disulfide-linked homodimer with an apparent molecular mass of 40 to 50 kDa with O-linked glycosylation at Thr4 and N-linked glycosylation at Asn29 (16). However, the carbohydrate component does not appear to be essential for IL-5 activity, since the recombinant expression of the cDNA encoding the human sequence in the bacterial host *E. coli* produces fully active protein (17), as does the expression in baculovirus-infected *Sf9* cells in the presence of tunicamycin (15) or enzymic deglycosylation of IL-5 produced in *CHO* (18) and *Drosophila* (19) cells. The nonessentiality of glycosylation for biological activity is not unique to IL-5. Other examples of mammalian recombinant proteins that are fully active when produced in *E. coli* include GM-CSF, which is even more active as the unglycosylated protein than the glycosylated form (20). The role of glycosylation has been suggested to increase the stability of the protein (18), but the bacterially produced protein was active when administered in vivo and was shown capable of producing eosinophilia in mice (21).

When expressed in eukaryotic systems, the IL-5 polypeptide chain consists of 115 amino acids, with Ile20 of the IL-5 precursor as the amino terminal residue. In contrast, IL-5 constructed and produced in different laboratories has varied in exact sequence, in particular at the amino terminal end. For example, the synthetic gene used for bacterial expression was constructed to have Thr22 of the IL-5 precursor as the first residue (15) and retains the initiating methionine, giving rise to a 114 amino acid polypeptide. Varying constructions have led to differential numbering by laboratories describing mutagenesis studies. In this review we have chosen to use the numbering corresponding to the expected full-length wild-type protein as shown in Figure 1.

To date, IL-5 genes have been isolated from six species (Fig. 1). Alignments of their primary sequences show that they are highly conserved genes. The human protein shows 96 and 98% identity with two primate species, 73% with murine and rat, and 66% with bovine IL-5. Since the murine and human species were identified a decade ago, there are more data on their cross-reactivity. Briefly, both are equally active on human eosinophils (hence with human receptor), but human IL-5 is 100-fold less active on murine cells (with murine receptor). The region responsible for the species specificity was identified to be the carboxy terminal region using chimeric human/murine constructs, and it was found that changing only eight residues of human protein produced a protein that was fully active on murine cells (22).

An important feature of the IL-5 sequence is the pair of Cys residues which are involved in the formation of intermolecular disulfide bridges. These Cys residues appear to be essential for IL-5 function, since their removal by site-directed mutagenesis abolishes activity (22). Mutation of one or both of the Cys to Ala also prevents the refolding of bacterially expressed IL-5 from inclusion bodies (A. Proudfoot, unpublished results). The disulfide bond assignment of recombinant IL-5 showed that the intermolecular disulfide bonds linking the two subunits occur in a head-to-tail fashion where the Cys44 residue from each chain forms a disulfide with the Cys86 residue from the other (16,23).

Investigation of structure-function relationships in IL-5 progressed in a chronological order different from most proteins, in that the three-dimensional structure was solved prior to the accumulation of extensive mutagenesis data. The structure of IL-5 was first solved using the bacterially derived protein (24)

```
          1        10         20         30         40         50         60         70
Human     IPTEIPTSAL VKETLALLST HRTLLIANET LRIPVPVHKN HQLCTEEIFQ GIGTLESQTV QGGTVERLFK
Mangabey  IPTEIPTSAL VKETLTLLST HRTLLIGNET LRIPVPVHKH HQLCTEEIFQ GIGTLESQTL QGGTVERLFK
Macaque   IPTEIPASAL VKETLALLST HRTLLIANET LRIPVPVHKN HQLCTEEIFQ GIGTLESQTV QGGTVERLFK
Murine      MEIPMSTV VKETLTQLSA HRALLTSNET MRLPVPTHKN HQLCIGEIFQ GLDILKNQTV RGGTVEMLFQ
Rat         MEIPMSTV VKETLIQLST HRALLTSNET MRLPVPTHKN HQLCIGEIFQ GLDILKNQTV RGGTVEILFQ
Bovine      VESTMNRL VAETLTLLSS HRTLLIGDGN LMIPTPQHTN HQLCIEEVFQ GIDTLKNQTA QGDAVKKIFQ

                   80         90        100        110   115
Human     NLSLIKKYID GQKKKCGEER RRVNQFLDYL QEFLGVMNTE WIIES
Mangabey  NLSLIKKYID GQKKKCGEER RRVNQFLDYL QEFLGVMNTE WIIES
Macaque   NLSLIKKYIG GQKKKCGEER RRVNQFLDYL QEFLGVMNTE WIIES
Murine    NLSLIKKYID RQKEKCGEER RRTRQFLDYL QEFLGVMSTE WAMEG
Rat       NLSLIKKYID GQKEKCGEER RKTRHFLDYL QEFLGVMSTE WAMEV
Bovine    NLSLIKEYID LQKRKCGGER WRVKQFLDYL QVFLGVINTE WTMES
```

**Figure 1** Alignment of the amino acid sequences of the mature forms of the six IL-5 sequences cloned to date. Numbering is indicated for the human sequence. Highly conserved residues among the six species are shaded. The Cys residues that form the intermolecular disulfides are shown in bold.

and was subsequently solved for recombinant protein derived by expression from baculovirus infection of *Sf9* cells (25) and from *Drosophila* cells (19). The structure (Fig. 2) reveals a novel two-domain structure, with each domain consisting of a four-α-helix bundle. The latter conformational motif is characteristic of several members of the hematopoetic cytokine family. However, the four-helix bundles in IL-5 are composed of three helices from one subunit, with the fourth being provided by the other subunit, producing a dimerization organization which is unique to date to IL-5.

The dimeric structure of the two four-helix bundle domains forms an elongated ellipsoidal molecule. The packing of the two domains by the shared helices of each subunit is formed by an intimate dimerization interface involving a large number of covalent, hydrophobic and electrostatic interactions, suggesting that these multiple forces would suffice for the folding of the IL-5 dimer. Yet, without the Cys residues which form the intermolecular disulfides, the protein is unable to assemble from an unfolded state. Inspection of the three-dimensional structure shows that the surface area of each monomeric domain is 9300 Å$^2$, whereas the surface of the dimer is 11,500 Å$^2$. This indicates that a very large proportion of the monomer surface is involved in forming the dimerization interface. This suggests that a monomeric structure would be unstable. Interestingly though, monomeric IL-5 forms have been constructed and found to be stable enough to fold, though less so than wt IL-5 (see below).

IL-5 is not the only member of the cytokine family to exist in a well-defined aggregation state. Several unrelated cytokines are found to be dimers, including IFN-γ (26), TGF-β (27), and the chemokine family (28–30). Others such as TNF-α and CD40 ligand are trimeric (31). But IL-5 is the only member of the four-helix bundle cytokines that is a dimer. The cytokine fold that is shared by GM-CSF, M-CSF, and growth hormone, and that has been predicted for IL-3 and IL-6, belongs to the short-helix fold, while IL-2 and IL-4 belong to the long-helix family. The four-helix bundle fold of the cytokines differentiates them from other four-helix bundle proteins in two respects. First, the interhelical angles between the helices A and D′, and B and C′, are 20°, whereas the angles between the A/D′ and B/C pairs of helices are 40°, which is atypical for other four-helix bundle proteins. Second, the connectivity of the helices is up-up-down-down, whereas in four-helix bundle proteins not belonging to the cytokine family, the helices are connected up-down-up-down.

## III. Dynamics of IL-5 Interaction with Receptor α Chain

IL-5 can bind to the soluble extracellular domain of the receptor α subunit with comparatively high affinity versus full-length receptor. Optical biosensor kinetic analysis of wild-type human IL-5 interaction reveals a $K_d$ of 2 to 6 nM, and the value from isothermal titration calorimetry is 3.1 nM (Table 1). These values compare with 1 nM for the full-length α chain expressed on CTLL-2 or COS cells and with 0.3 to 0.5 nM for $\alpha/\beta_c$ together. The high affinity exhibited by soluble α chain has encouraged efforts to use this soluble form to investigate both the physical nature of receptor interaction and the topology of the receptor binding sites on the IL-5 structure. Topological studies will be described in sections 4 and 5. In this section we describe physical properties which have helped focus the structural investigations.

Observations have been made on stoichiometry and the possibility of conformational isomerization in the interaction of α chain with IL-5. The stoichiometry of IL-5 binding to shIL-5Rα has been found to be 1:1, that is, one α subunit per IL-5 dimer. This was first suggested by cross-linking and by quantitating the abundance of each component in a complex isolated by gel filtration chromatography (Fig. 3A) (36). The 1:1 stoichiometry has been measured rigorously by analytical ultracentrifugation (19) (Fig. 3B), and confirmatory evidence for a 1:1 stoichiometric ratio of human IL-5 and receptor α chain has been obtained by titration calorimetry (below) and cocrystallization (19). A 1:1 stoichiometry also is suggested to occur in cells, as judged by cross-linking results (10,25,37,38).

The above 1:1 stoichiometry is unexpected, since the IL-5 dimer has two four-helix bundle domains and each of them resembles the domain of four-helix bundle monomeric growth factor proteins, which as monomers would be expected to show stoichiometries of at least one molecule receptor per monomer. Indeed, human growth hormone is a monomeric four-helix bundle protein that has been shown crystallographically to bind two receptor chains (39–41). Explaining the structural basis for this 1:1 IL-5/receptor α chain stoichiometry has been a major focus of efforts to map the receptor recognition sites in IL-5 (see sections 4 and 5).

Titration microcalorimetric data initially were used to determine rigorous values for binding thermodynamics and to complement optical biosensor analysis of binding kinetics (19). Indeed, calorimetry data for the equilibrium binding reaction of hIL-5 with its soluble α receptor yielded $K_d$ values similar to those obtained with the biosensor and also fit to a stoichiometric ratio of $0.91 \pm 0.1$ mol IL-5 per mole receptor, in keeping with the absolute 1:1 stoichiometry discussed above.

Titration calorimetry measurements also have led to the prediction that conformational change may occur upon IL-5 interaction with shIL-5Rα. This has been deduced from the very large burial of residues that occurs in the interaction (19). The slope of the temperature dependence of the enthalpy change for the reaction of hIL-5 with shIL-5Rα is equal to the heat capacity change

**Table 1** Binding Affinities of IL-5 to Human IL-5 Receptor Measured with Isolated Receptor and in Cells

| hIL-5 form | Method | Isolated receptor: Dissociation constants (nM) | | | | Ref. | Receptor on cells: Dissociation constants (nM) and cell types | | | Ref. |
|---|---|---|---|---|---|---|---|---|---|---|
| | | | | | | | α | α/β | | |
| *Drosophila* | Biosensor | Immob α | 2.3 | Immob αFc | 5.7 | 32 | 6 | | *Drosophila* | 19 |
| | ITC | sol. α | 3.1 | | | 19 | 0.7 | 0.3–0.5 | CTLL-2 | 33 |
| | | | | | | | 0.9 | 0.5 | COS | 34 |
| *E. coli* | SPPA | Immob α | 1.0 (IC50) | | | 35 | | 0.25 | TF-1 | 35 |

ITC is isothermal titration calorimetry; SPPA is solid phase proximity assay. For cells, α is with α chain alone expressed, α/β are with both subunits coexpressed.

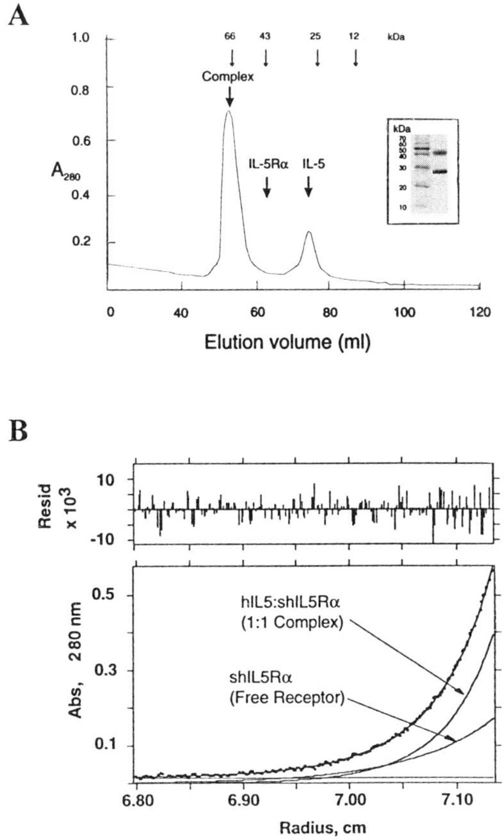


**Figure 3** IL-5 binds to the receptor α chain with 1:1 stoichiometry. (A) Gel filtration analysis, on a Superdex 200 column, of the receptor/ligand complex formed by mixing recombinant IL-5 and IL-5Rα in a molar ratio of 1.2:1. The elution volumes corresponding to the masses of the IL-5Rα and IL-5 proteins are indicated, which correspond to 43 kDa and 27 kDa, respectively. The complex elutes at a volume of 66 kDa corresponding to 1 mole of receptor and 1 mole of dimeric ligand, with the excess ligand eluting at the expected volume. The elution volumes of the proteins used to calibrate the column are indicated. Insert: SDS/PAGE analysis of the complex. (B) Equilibrium analytical ultracentrifuge data for a mixture of shIL-5Rα and hIL-5. Total protein concentration $\sim 10^{-5}$ M, 2:1 molar ratio of receptor to IL-5. A species analysis was used to fit the experimental data and showed that only terms for shIL-5Rα and the shIL-5Rα:hIL5 1:1 complex were needed for the fit. When terms for the other species, for example, hIL-5 and shIL-5Rα:hIL5 2:1 complex, were included, the fit did not converge. (Figure 3B adapted from reference 19.)

for the equilibrium reaction and is due in large part to changes in buried surface area of polar and apolar amino acid side chains. The amount of apolar and polar surface area buried when hIL-5 binds to shIL-5Rα was calculated as 2440 Å$^2$ and 1720 Å$^2$, respectively (19). Hence the total amount of buried surface was estimated as 4160 Å$^2$. An entire face of the IL-5 dimer exposes approximately 1900 Å$^2$. Hence, assuming that the entire face of hIL-5 is not involved directly in receptor interaction, the surface burial analysis suggests that some type of conformational change occurs upon hIL-5-receptor α chain interaction. Since the IL-5 dimer is an α-chain sharing two four-helix bundle structures without apparent hinge sites, large conformational changes in IL-5 seem unlikely. Rather, the receptor seems a more probable source of conformational change upon ligand interaction.

Cytokine receptor isomerization has been proposed for leukemia inhibitory factor (LIF), and multiple kinetic dissociation rates of LIF from its receptor as observed in a cell binding filter assay were proposed to reflect this isomerization (42). For the IL-5 receptor system, allosteric modification of IL-5 upon α chain binding has been hypothesized as a possible way to explain both the lack of binding to a second α chain and increased affinity for the $\beta_c$ chain (36). Such IL-5 allosterism, if it occurs, could involve subtle conformational change and might occur in addition to the conformational change of receptor proposed to occur upon ligand binding.

## IV. Alanine Scanning Mutagenesis with wtIL-5

The production of recombinant forms of IL-5 and receptor α-chain has enabled residues of both IL-5 and the IL-5 receptor α-chain required for receptor-ligand interaction to be mapped by mutagenesis studies. Several mutagenesis studies have been carried out by alanine scanning of wtIL-5 (25,32,35,43) mainly of charged and other exposed amino acids. Mutated proteins have been analyzed by binding assays to the isolated recombinant α chain as well as to the heterodimeric complex expressed on *TF-1* cells. The effects of mutations on bioactivity have been analyzed by proliferation of IL-5-dependent cell lines and, in one study, by the ability of IL-5 to induce eosinophil adhesion.

As was suggested from the construction of chimeric murine and human IL-5 proteins, where the specificity was found to reside in the carboxy terminal portion of the protein, the principal residues of IL-5 which bind the α chain are found on the fourth helix and on the β sheet preceding it. These residues are Glu89, Arg91, Glu110, and Trp111. Glu110 and Trp111 are situated toward the end of helix D, where Glu110 is exposed. In contrast, the Trp111 side chain is buried, and its role is therefore thought to be in maintaining correct packing of the D helix, rather than being directly involved in binding contact with the receptor. Mutation of this residue to Ala may affect the correct orientation of the important adjacent residue, Glu110. Trp111 can be substituted with larger hydrophobic residues such as Met with little effect on α chain affinity (32), consistent with a packing role for this residue. The importance of Trp111 in maintaining the correct structure of IL-5 is further supported by successive truncations of the amino terminal, where removal of this residue causes a significant loss of bioactivity and a concomitant loss of overall structure (44).

Alanine scanning mutagenesis of wtIL-5, when taken with the IL-5 structure, suggests the "pharmacophore" or binding site of the IL-5 protein. Glu89 and Arg91 are located on the second β sheet which joins the third helix to helix D. The distance between the side chains of these two charged residues is approximately 8 Å, and they are equidistant from Glu110, at a distance of approximately 26 Å. A second cluster of residues—His38, Lys39, and His41 (the numbering is that used for the *SF9* produced protein) on the loop connecting β-strand 1 to helix B—was found to have diminished binding to the α chain but did not have decreased biological activity. This indicates that a full biological response may be attained despite reduced receptor occupancy.

Although most of the mutant forms of IL-5 with changes at residues identified as being important in α-chain binding showed decreases in biological responses, they were able to attain maximal responses but at higher concentrations than the wild-type protein. However, a mutation on helix A, at Glu13 in the *E. coli* and *Sf9* proteins, led to only partial agonist activity. Mutation of Glu13 in the *E. coli* protein had no change in binding to the α chain (35), although a reduction in binding was observed with the *Sf9* protein (25). Taken together, these results identified this glutamic acid as playing a role in the activation of the $\beta_c$ chain. The two cytokines that share the $\beta_c$ chain similarly have a Glu on the first helix for $\beta_c$ activation: Glu21 for GM-CSF (45) and Glu22 for IL-3 (46). Mutating this acidic residue in the IL-5 protein to glutamine which is polar (25) or to the positively charged lysine (47) creates a mutein that is capable of antagonizing IL-5-induced cellular responses. Similarly, the mutation of Glu21 to arginine in GM-CSF (45) results in a protein antagonist which is able to bind the α chain but is unable to activate the signaling $\beta_c$ chain.

The results of wtIL-5 mutagenesis lead to a map of key residues in Figure 4. Analogous arrays of key residues have been identified in the homologous cytokines IL-3 and GM-CSF (Fig. 5). Since α chain binds to IL-5 with 1:1 stoichiometry (see above), the key residues for α chain binding likely function as one unit at any given time. This leads to the view of a single topologically distinct binding region for α-chain interaction as shown in Figure 6.

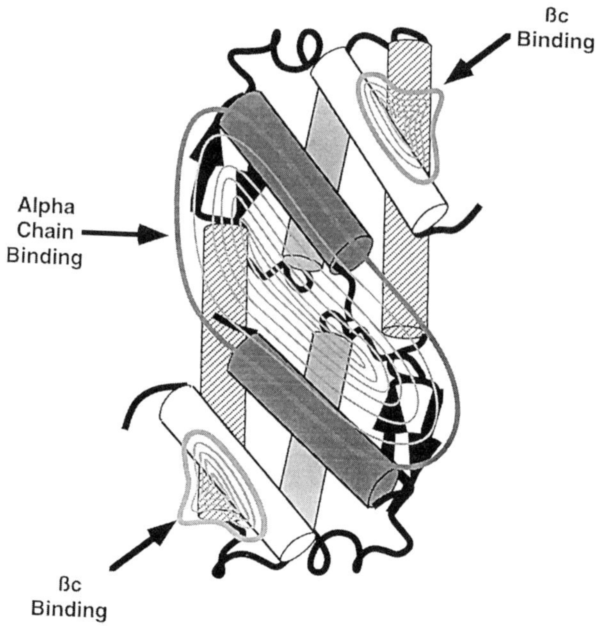


**Figure 6** Structural scheme of IL-5 depicting currently assigned locations of receptor $\alpha$ and $\beta_c$ binding sites on the cytokine surface. The helix bundle framework is as shown in Figure 2, with helices coded as A (open), B (light gray), C (cross-hatched), and D (dark gray). Separate binding sites are denoted by overlaid contours for $\alpha$ and $\beta_c$ subunits of receptor. (Figure adapted from reference 48.)

## V. Asymmetry in Receptor $\alpha$ and $\beta_c$ Recruitment by Symmetrically Dimeric IL-5

Mutagenesis of two types of reengineered IL-5 constructions, single-chain IL-5 (scIL-5) and monomeric IL-5 (monoIL-5), have led to the realization that the recruitment of $\alpha$ and $\beta_c$ subunits by IL-5 is asymmetric.

### A. Mutagenesis Studies with Single Chain IL-5

Determining the topography of receptor binding sites by mutagenesis of wtIL-5 (25,32,35) is impeded by the homodimeric nature of the protein. Because of this, a residue substitution inevitably results in symmetrical changes in side chains on both sides of the four-helix bundle interface. It is thus unclear from wtIL-5 mutagenesis whether one or both of the residues of a particular type found to be important, for example, Glu110, participate equally in receptor binding and, furthermore, whether the topology of binding is different for binding hIL-5Rα versus $\beta_c$. One way to overcome this limitation is asymmetric mutagenesis, that is, altering residues differentially in the two four-helix bundles related by the twofold symmetry axis.

Such asymmetric mutagenesis has proven possible with a redesigned version of IL-5 called single-chain IL-5 (scIL-5) (49,50). This form has allowed asymmetric substitution experiments, in which residues from one four-helix bundle can be replaced selectively without affecting the same residues on the other bundle. The gene of the scIL-5 was constructed by linking two hIL-5 genes in tandem separated by a spacer that encodes the dipeptide -Gly-Gly- (49) or a single Gly residue (50). The N-terminal half of the molecule is defined as (a), the C-terminal half as (b). Expression of these genes in COS cells or in *E. coli* yielded an scIL-5 protein having similar biological activity to that of wtIL-5, as judged by stimulation of human cell proliferation (see Table 2 and Fig. 7). Single-chain and wtIL-5 also had similar binding affinity for soluble IL-5 receptor α chain, the specificity subunit of the IL-5 receptor, as measured kinetically with an optical biosensor (Table 2).

Functionally active scIL-5 allows asymmetric mutagenesis of the symmetrical IL-5 molecule. Single site mutations in only one-half of scIL-5, at residues

**Table 2** Receptor Binding and Bioactivity Properties of wtIL-5 and scIL-5 Mutants

| IL-5 form | α Chain binding: $k_{on}$ (M/s × $10^5$) | α Chain binding: $k_{off}$ (M/s × $10^{-3}$) | α Chain binding: $K_d$ (nM) | Bioactivity *TF-1* $EC_{50}$ (pM) |
|---|---|---|---|---|
| wtIL-5 | 7.2 | 3.0 | 4.2 | 2 |
| R91A | 13.6 | 220 | 161 | 181 |
| W111A | 2.9 | 45.9 | 158 | 48 |
| E13A | 9.9 | 4.1 | 4.1 | 75 |
| scIL-5 | 7.9 | 1.8 | 2.3 | 3 |
| R91A(a) | 3.9 | 2.7 | 6.9 | 5 |
| R91A(b) | 5.1 | 2.3 | 4.5 | 6 |
| W111A(b) | 5.4 | 3.2 | 5.9 | 4 |
| R91A(a)W111A(b)[a] | 4.3 | 2.9 | 6.7 | 9 |
| R91A(b)W111A(b)[b] | 2.6 | 9.7 | 37 | 10 |

The rate constants $k_{on}$ and $k_{off}$ are from BIAcore optical biosensor assay of shIL-5Rα binding; the equilibrium dissociation constant $K_d$ is calculated from the ratio of $k_{off}/k_{on}$. Data were obtained from two individual experiments. *TF-1* activity is given as the concentration required for half maximal stimulation of *TF-1* cell proliferation. Asymmetric mutants contain denoted substitutions in either the amino terminal IL-5 domain of scIL-5 (a) or the carboxyl terminal IL-5 domain (b).

[a]The two substitutions were made in different four-helix bundle domains.

[b]The two substitutions were made in the same four-helix bundle domain. For wtIL-5 mutants, binding data are from IAsys biosensor assay. The mutants contain denoted substitutions on both chains of homodimeric IL-5. (Table adapted from Ref. 51.)

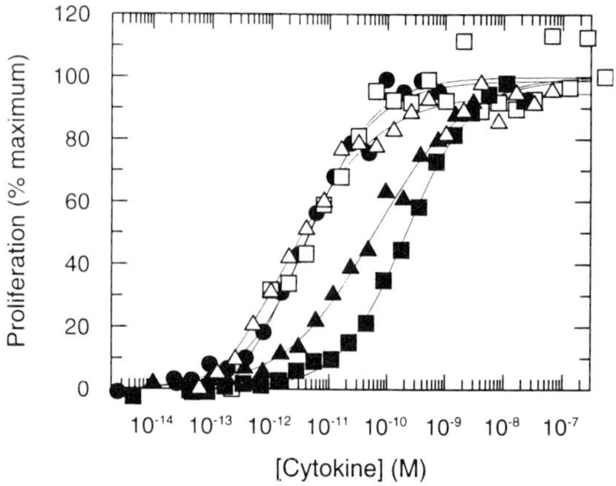


**Figure 7** Proliferation of the human erythroleukemic cell line *TF-1* by single-chain IL-5 (scIL-5) constructs containing the R91A and E110A single-copy mutations. The abilities of wtIL-5 (●), R91A in wtIL-5 (▲), E110A in wtIL-5 (■), R91A in scIL-5 (Δ), and E110A in scIL-5 (□) to cause proliferation of TF-1 cells. (Figure taken from reference 50.)

already shown to play a role in receptor α-chain binding, while having biological activity equivalent to the wtIL-5 protein, led to small but finite decreases (~50%) in shIL-5Rα binding affinity compared to wtIL-5. Such data show that the two four-helix bundle components of the α-chain binding site do not contribute equally. In contrast, data with multiple asymmetric mutations (49–51) do not fit well to a simple half-site binding model. For example, mutants with residues changed only in one four-helix bundle (such as R91A(b) and R91A(b)W111A(b)) did not have complete wild-type binding activity (Fig. 8 and Table 2).

Overall, the view emerging from asymmetric mutagenesis using scIL-5 is that the IL-5 receptor α-chain binding interaction is stabilized by contacts from both four-helix bundle surfaces but that one-half of the surface, corresponding to one-half of the whole IL-5 molecule, is sufficient for a functional interaction. This raises the question of how well a monomer of IL-5 might function as a mimetic of wtIL-5.

### B. Monomeric Constructions of IL-5

Based on the superposition of the high-resolution structures of GM-CSF and IL-5 as shown in Figure 9A, it was proposed that the IL-5 dimer might have been a monomer, and a loop deletion between helix C and D forced it instead to adopt an open D-helix swapped dimeric structure (52). This inferred that lengthening

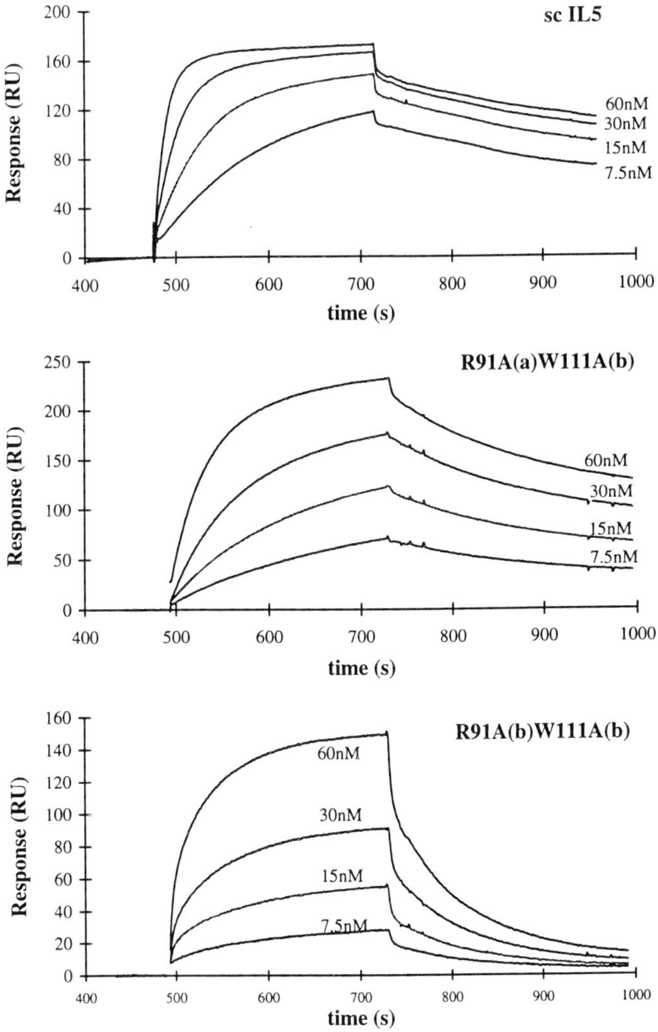


**Figure 8** Comparison of the binding kinetics of scIL-5, R91A(a)W111A(b), and R91A(b)W111A(b) in interacting with shIL-5Rα. Kinetic binding data were obtained with a BIAcore SPR biosensor. Overlays of sensorgrams showing binding of various concentrations of shIL-5Rα to IL-5 mutants were plotted. The marked numbers indicate the concentrations of shIL-5Rα. The increase in response shows the binding of shIL-5Rα. The decay represents the dissociation of bound shIL-5Rα. (Figure taken from Ref. 51.)

the CD loop could allow the IL-5 chain to fold into a monomer. The functional properties of such a monomer could yield further clues on the mechanism of receptor recruitment by IL-5.

Following from the original proposal by Bennett et al. (52), monomeric constructions of IL-5 have indeed been made by increasing the length of the CD loop (the chain between the C and D helices), as depicted in Figure 9B, to the length in GM-CSF (50,53,54). Furthermore, monomeric forms also have been formed by circular permutation of monoIL-5 (50,54). MonoIL-5 forms have been found to be significantly stable and active.

When the sequences of the dimeric hIL-5 with the monomeric hGM-CSF are compared structurally, the overlap of frameworks observed provide a basis to construct an IL-5 chain in which the CD loop is increased in length by eight residues, the length of the monomeric GM-CSF loop. IL-5 sequences have been constructed with either GM-CSF sequence (50,53) or de novo designed linkers (54) inserted between IL-5 residues in the CD loop. Permutated forms of IL-5 were formed in which one of the existing loops of wtIL-5 was clipped and a new loop was formed between helices A and D. The overall arrangement of protein sequences in these reengineered forms of IL-5 are shown in Figure 10.

CD loop expanded and circularly permuted forms of IL-5 have been characterized for conformational stability, receptor binding and cell proliferation activities (Table 3). The monomeric forms are reasonably stable, though less so than dimers, as judged by temperature dependence of helicity from circular dichroism measurements (50,54). Analysis of the unfolding curves shown in Figure 11 predicts that the dimer is 65,000-fold more stable than the monomers (54). The monomers also show significantly reduced receptor binding affinity

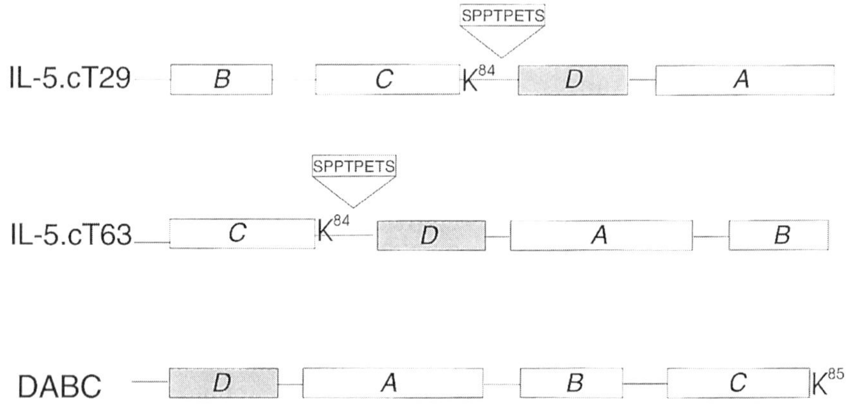


**Figure 10** Schematic representation of the permutated monomeric constructs. Helices *A*, *B*, and *C* are shown as open boxes, and helix *D* as a shaded box. The positions at which the loop has been introduced and their sequence are indicated.

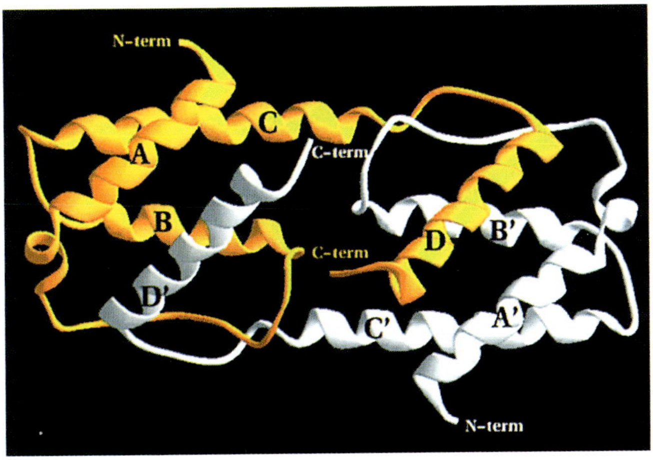


**Figure 10.2** The three-dimensional structure of human IL-5. The ribbon representation with one subunit in yellow and the other in white shows the novel dimeric topology of IL-5, where each four-helix bundle domain is formed by three helices from one monomer, the fourth being provided by the second subunit. (Adapted from reference 24.)

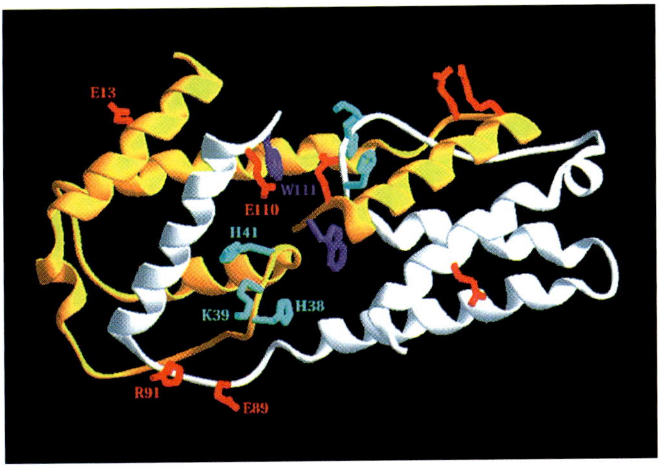


**Figure 10.4** The key residues involved in the interaction of IL-5 with its receptor. For clarity the residues are named on one domain only. The charged residues that affect both binding and function, and therefore compromise the functional pharmacophore, are shown in red, while those that have a small effect on binding but do not affect biological activity are shown in blue. Trp111 affects both binding and bioactivity, but since the side chain is buried, its mutation to Ala is thought to affect the positioning of the adjacent Glu110.

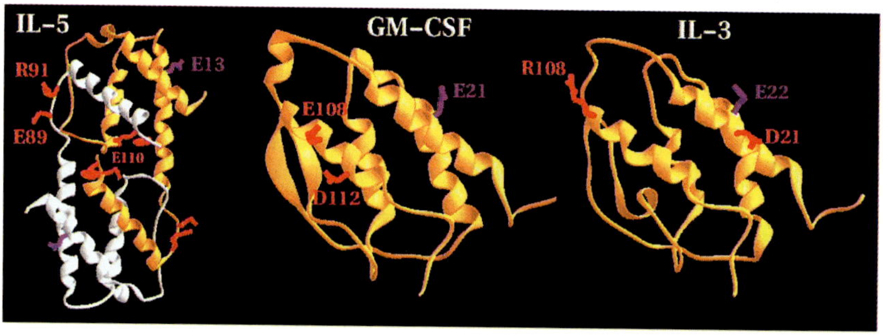


**Figure 10.5** Comparison of the functional epitopes of IL-5, GM-CSF, and IL-3. The structure of IL-3 was modeled using the automated model-building software ProMod (31). The key contact residue for $\beta_c$ through which these three proteins transmit signal is shown in magenta and is found in an equivalent position on the first helix. The key residues of IL-5, GM-CSF, and IL-3 that interact with their specific $\alpha$ chain are shown in red and are situated on the opposite side of the proteins to the $\beta_c$ contact residue, with the exception of Asp21 in IL-3.

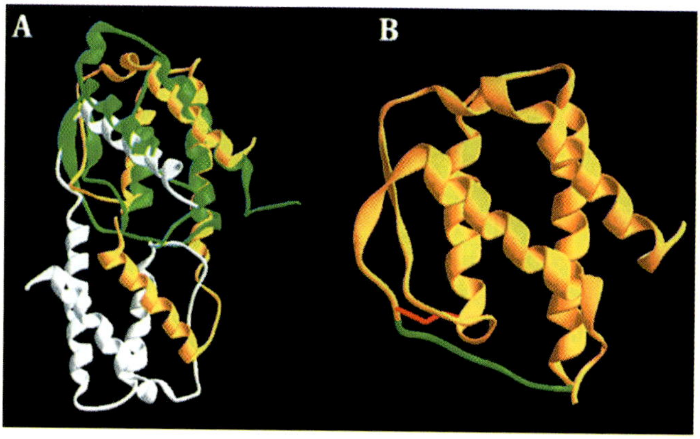


**Figure 10.9** Molecular models of IL-5, GM-CSF, and monomeric IL-5. (A) Superposition of GM-CSF onto one monomeric domain of IL-5. GM-CSF is depicted in green and the IL-5 subunits are shown in white and yellow. (B) Model of a monomeric IL-5 construct, with the eight amino acid loop (shown in green) inserted after Lys84 on the loop between helices C and D. The CD loop extension allows helix D to fold onto the parent monomer. The disulfide linking Cys44 to Cys86 is shown in red.

**Table 3** Receptor Binding, Bioactivity, and Stability of Monomeric Forms of IL-5

| IL-5 form | α Chain affinity (ratio of $K_d$) (wt:mutant) | Bioactivity (ratio of *TF-1*) $EC_{50}$ (wt:mutant) | Stability $\Delta T_m$ (°C) (mutant-wt) |
|---|---|---|---|
| wtIL-5 | (1) | (1) | (0) |
| GM1 IL-5 | $2.2 \times 10^{-2}$ | 0.125 | −4.1 |
| DABC IL-5 | $2.4 \times 10^{-2}$ | 0.25 | −8.2 |
| 5.3 | $7 \times 10^{-3}$ | 0.19 | −12.3 |
| 5.4 | $9 \times 10^{-4}$ | $5 \times 10^{-2}$ | −6.2 |
| T29 | $8 \times 10^{-4}$ | Partial agonist | −19.5 |
| T63 | $1 \times 10^{-3}$ | $3 \times 10^{-2}$ | −15.2 |
| DH1 | n.d. | $7 \times 10^{-2}$ | n.d. |

Data taken from Ref. 50 (for forms 5.3, 5.4, T29, T63), 53 (for form DH1), and 54 (for forms GM1 and DABC).

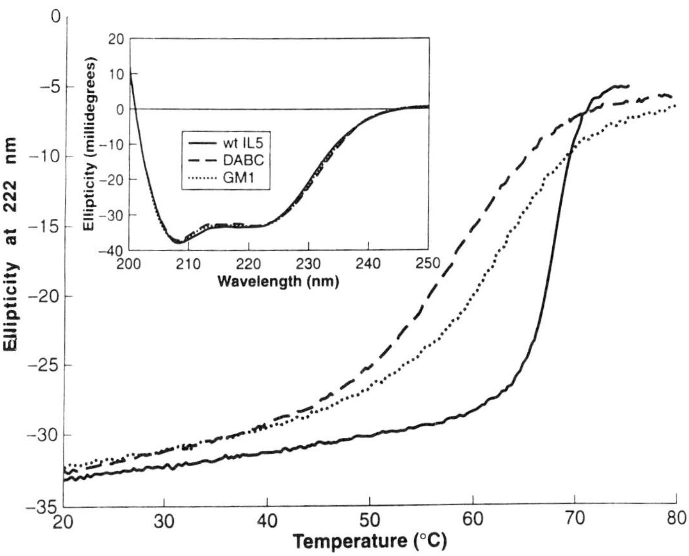


**Figure 11** Circular dichroism of wtIL-5 and two monomeric forms of IL-5, DABC and GM1. Thermal stability of IL-5 constructs was evaluated with a Jasco J-710 spectropolarimeter by monitoring the ellipticity at 222 nm in a 0.1 cm water-jacketed cuvette. Wild-type IL-5, solid line; DABC, dashed line; GM1, dotted line. Inset: Circular dichroism spectra at 25°C for the three forms of IL-5 as denoted in main figure. Conditions were the same as in the thermal stability measurements. Spectra shown are the average of three scans run at 50 nm/min with a 2 sec response time. (Figure taken from Ref. 54.)

versus wild-type, dimeric IL-5. Finally, most of the monomeric forms showed 5 to 20-fold reductions in biological activity, as judged by $EC_{50}$ values in TF-1 proliferation assays. The lowered receptor binding affinities and bioactivities of the monomers likely are due to loss of stabilizing contacts for receptor interaction and activation. This could arise from the reduced stabilities of the monomeric constructs compared to the dimeric protein as well as from loss of a full complement of receptor-interacting structural elements.

In spite of the lower activities and stabilities, the monomeric forms can be used as simplified versions of IL-5 for site-directed mutagenesis, since they have shown that a single domain is sufficient to achieve the biological activities attributed to IL-5. The mutation of the $\beta_c$ contact residue Glu13 to Lys in the circularly permutated constructs, IL-5.cT29 and IL-5.cT63, gave the unexpected result that these proteins were not inactive but retained partial agonist activity in both TF-1 proliferation and eosinophil adhesion (50). This result suggests that residues in addition to Glu13 likely comprise epitopes in IL-5 that play a direct role in receptor $\beta_c$ recruitment and signal triggering. Determining these other structural elements is a current need in IL-5 mechanism studies.

Overall the biological activity, receptor binding affinity and stability of monomeric forms of IL-5 establish these forms as tools for mutagenesis and mechanistic study. The IL-5 monomers can be compared directly with the naturally occurring monomeric cytokines GM-CSF and IL-3 in deducing features of receptor activation and signal triggering common to this family of cytokines. In addition, the viability of the monomers indicates that although the dimeric form of IL-5 may have arisen during evolution from a change in splicing pattern, the gene has continued to evolve to confer additional stability on the IL-5 protein.

### C. Working Model of Receptor Recruitment

Together scIL-5 mutagenesis and monoIL-5 constructions have shown that most of the energy for receptor α-chain interaction is derived from one of the four-helix bundles in wtIL-5, with the second bundle contributing fractionally (51). Furthermore, Glu13 mutagenesis in recently reported scIL-5 constructions has shown that either one of these residues in wtIL-5 can enable signaling through the $\beta_c$ chain (51). Hence wtIL-5 appears to contain two binding motifs for α and $\beta_c$ recruitment; but only one set of motifs, one for α centered around helix D and a second for $\beta_c$ centered around Glu13, need to function at a time [see Fig. 12 (left)]. Indeed, only one α-chain binding site is able to function at a time, as judged by the 1:1 stoichiometry described earlier. From these considerations and the viability of monomers to bind receptor and trigger a signal for bioactivity, a minimum pharmacophore for α-chain binding can be defined as shown in Figure 12 (right).

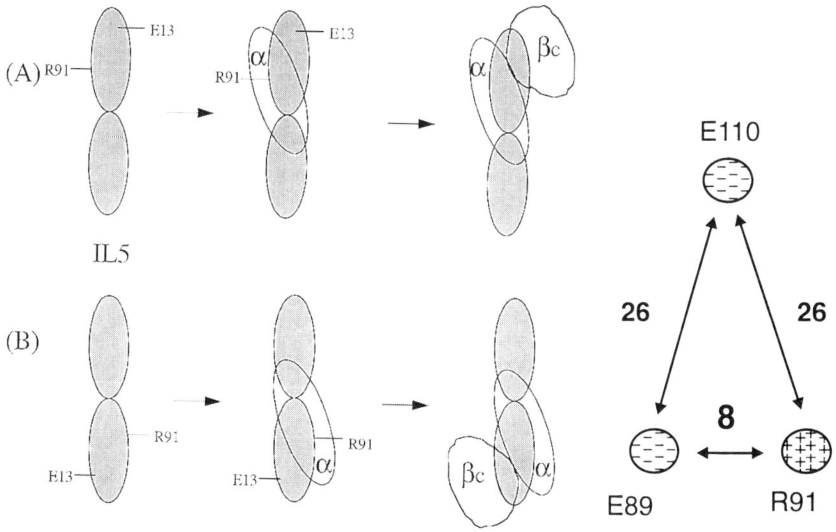


**Figure 12** (Left) Model for the mechanism of IL-5Rα binding and $\beta_c$ activation. IL-5 is represented in dark gray depicting the two four-helix bundle domains. Receptor α and $\beta_c$ chains are shown as unfilled structures. Part (A) depicts α chain binding stabilized mainly by one of the two four-helix bundle domains, part (B) by the other domain. Both α chain binding modes are identical with respect to stabilizing contacts on the IL-5 surface, since the two four-helix bundle domains of IL-5 are arranged symmetrically about the dyad axis. The positions of residues R91 and E13 are designated. Recruitment of $\beta_c$ is proposed to occur through E13 on the domain which predominates in stabilizing (including through R91) α chain recruitment. (Right) The minimal α chain binding pharmacophore required for biological activity. The distances are shown in angstroms, as deduced from the crystallographic three-dimensional structure, between the three residues found to be particularly important for α-chain binding and consequent functional activity. E89, R91, and E110 are all envisioned to come from the same protein chain. (Figure 12, left, taken from Ref. 51.)

## VI. The Future

Much has been learned about the structure of IL-5 and the topology of binding sites in the protein for subunits of the IL-5 receptor. Nonetheless, current research suggests that deeper mechanistic understanding of the structural involvement of IL-5 in receptor recruitment may be attainable. Crystallographic structure analysis of the IL-5 interface with receptor α chain looks promising. Small crystals of this complex have been obtained (19), and larger crystals recently obtained with *E. coli*-derived IL-5 diffract to 3.2 Å (A. Proudfoot et al., unpublished results). Furthermore, using structure as a guide, an expanded ability to investigate the role of different structural elements in conformational and receptor binding dynamics and bioactivity may be attainable by such molecular biological approaches as epitope randomization using filamentous phage display. Single-chain IL-5 has recently been displayed on phage with retention of receptor binding activity (I. M. Chaiken et al., unpublished results). It can be hoped that mechanistic investigation of receptor binding sites eventually will extend to receptor activation and signal triggering as early steps in the signal transduction cascade become amenable to experimental characterization. Hence the IL-5 system, including the array of reengineered forms and mutants, may well be a useful one with which to elucidate basic mechanisms of cytokine signal transduction. Finally, the elucidation of the topology of key receptor interaction sites in IL-5 can be expected to lead ultimately to the design of mimetics in general and receptor antagonists in particular. That the latter might provide tools for the design of the therapeutic agents of use in asthma and other eosinophilia-related diseases promises to further invigorate the investigation of IL-5 structure and function for some time to come.

## References

1. Sanderson CJ, Warren DJ, Strath M. Identification of a lymphokine that stimulates eosinophil differentiation in vitro. Its relationship to interleukin 3, and functional properties of eosinophils produced in cultures. J Exp Med 1985;162:60–74.
2. Warren DJ, Sanderson CJ. Production of a T-cell hybrid producing a lymphokine stimulating eosinophil differentiation. Immunology 1985;54:615–623.
3. Campbell HD, Tucker WQ, Hort Y, Martinson ME, Mayo G, Clutterbuck EJ, Sanderson CJ, Young IG. Molecular cloning, nucleotide sequence, and expression of the gene encoding human eosinophil differentiation factor (interleukin 5). Proc Natl Acad Sci USA 1987;84:6629–6633.
4. Clutterbuck E, Shields JG, Gordon J, Smith SH, Boyd A, Callard RE, Campbell HD, Young IG, Sanderson CJ. Recombinant human interleukin 5 is a eosinophil differentiation factor but has no activity in standard human B cell growth factor assays. Eur J Immunol 1987;17:1743–1750.
5. Lopez AF, Sanderson CJ, Gamble JR, Campbell HD, Young IG, Vadas MA. Recombinant human interleukin 5 is a selective activator of human eosinophil function. J Exp Med 1988;167:219–224.
6. Sanderson CJ. The biological role of interleukin 5 [review]. Int J Cell Cloning 1990;8(suppl 1):47–153; discussion 153–154.
7. McKenzie AN, Sanderson CJ. Interleukin-5 [review]. Chem Immunol 1992;51:135–152.
8. Murata Y, Takaki S, Migita M, Kikuchi Y, Tominaga A, Takatsu K. Molecular cloning and expression of the human interleukin 5 receptor. J Exp Med 1992;175:341–351.

9. Tavernier J, Devos R, Cornelis S, Tuypens T, Van der Heyden J, Fiers W, Plaetinck G. A human high affinity interleukin-5 receptor (IL5R) is composed of an IL5-specific alpha chain and a beta chain shared with the receptor for GM-CSF. Cell 1991;66:1175–1184.
10. Migita M, Yamaguchi N, Mita S, Higuchi S, Hitoshi Y, Yoshida Y, Tomonaga M, Matsuda I, Tominaga A, Takatsu K. Characterization of the human IL-5 receptors on eosinophils. Cell Immunol 1991;133:484–497.
11. Ingley E, Young IG. Characterization of a receptor for interleukin-5 on human eosinophils and the myeloid leukemia line HL-60. Blood 1991;78:339–344.
12. McKenzie DT, Filutowicz HI, Swain SL, Dutton RW. Purification and partial sequence analysis of murine B cell growth factor II (interleukin 5). J Immunol 1987;139:2661–2668.
13. Kinashi T, Harada N, Severinson E, Tanabe T, Sideras P, Konishi M, Azuma C, Tominaga A, Bergstedt-Lindqvist S, Takahashi M. Cloning of complementary DNA encoding T-cell replacing factor and identity with B-cell growth factor II. Nature 1986;324:70–73.
14. Azuma C, Tanabe T, Konishi M, Kinashi T, Noma T, Matsuda F, Yaoita Y, Takatsu K, Hammarstrom L, Smith CI, et al. Cloning of cDNA for human T-cell replacing factor (interleukin-5) and comparison with the murine homologue. Nucleic Acids Res 1986;14:9149–9158.
15. Tavernier J, Devos R, Van der Heyden J, Hauquier G, Bauden R, Fache I, Kawashima E, Vandekerckhove J, Contreras R, Fiers W. Expression of human and murine interleukin-5 in eukaryotic systems. DNA 1989;8:491–501.
16. Minamitake Y, Kodama S, Katayama T, Adachi H, Tanaka S, Tsujimoto M. Structure of recombinant human interleukin 5 produced by Chinese hamster ovary cells. J Biochem 1990;107:292–297.
17. Proudfoot AEI, Fattah D, Kawashima EH, Bernard A, Wingfield PT. Preparation and characterization of human interleukin-5 expressed in recombinant *Escherichia coli*. Biochem J 1990;270:357–361.
18. Kodama S, Tsujimoto M, Tsuruoka N, Sugo T, Endo T, Kobata A. Role of sugar chains in the in-vitro activity of recombinant human interleukin 5. Eur J Biochem 1993;211:903–908.
19. Johanson K, Appelbaum E, Doyle M, Hensley P, Zhao B, Abdel-Meguid SS, Young P, Cook R, Carr S, Matico R, Cusimano D, Dul E, Angelichio M, Brooks I, Winborne E, McDonnell P, Morton T, Bennett D, Sokoloski T, McNulty D, Rosenberg M, Chaiken I. Binding interactions of human interleukin 5 with its receptor alpha subunit. Large scale production, structural, and functional studies of *Drosophila*-expressed recombinant proteins. J Biol Chem 1995;270:9459–9471.
20. Burgess AW, Begley CG, Johnson GR, Lopez AF, Williamson DJ, Mermod JJ, Simpson RJ, Schmitz A, DeLamarter JF. Purification and properties of bacterially synthesized human granulocyte-macrophage colony stimulating factor. Blood 1987;69:43–51.
21. Van Oosterhout AJ, Fattah D, Van Ark I, Hofman G, Buckley TL, Nijkamp FP. Eosinophil infiltration precedes development of airway hyperreactivity and mucosal exudation after intranasal administration of interleukin-5 to mice. J Allergy Clin Immunol 1995;96:104–112.

22. McKenzie AN, Barry SC, Strath M, Sanderson CJ. Structure-function analysis of interleukin-5 utilizing mouse/human chimeric molecules. EMBO J 1991;10:1193–1199.
23. Proudfoot AEI, Davies JG, Turcatti G, Wingfield PT. Human interleukin-5 expressed in *Escherichia coli*: assignment of the disulfide bridges of the purified unglycosylated protein. FEBS Lett 1991;283:61–64.
24. Milburn MV, Hassell AM, Lambert MH, Jordan SR, Proudfoot AEI, Graber P, Wells TNC. A novel dimer configuration revealed by the crystal structure at 2.4 Å resolution of human interleukin-5. Nature 1993;363:172–176.
25. Tavernier J, Tuypens T, Verhee A, Plaetinck G, Devos R, Van der Heyden J, Guisez Y, Oefner C. Identification of receptor-binding domains on human interleukin 5 and design of an interleukin 5-derived receptor antagonist. Proc Natl Acad Sci USA 1995;92:5194–5198.
26. Rubin JR, Burton LE. Crystallization and preliminary X-ray diffraction studies of bovine recombinant immune interferon. J Mol Biol 1989;209:829–831.
27. Schlunegger MP, Grutter MG. An unusual feature revealed by the crystal structure at 2.2 Å resolution of human transforming growth factor-beta 2. Nature 1992;358:430–434.
28. Baldwin ET, Weber IT, St. Charles R, Xuan JC, Appella E, Yamada M, Matsushima K, Edwards BF, Clore GM, Gronenborn AM. Crystal structure of interleukin 8: symbiosis of NMR and crystallography. Proc Natl Acad Sci USA 1991;88:502-506.
29. Lodi PJ, Garrett DS, Kuszewski J, Tsang ML, Weatherbee JA, Leonard WJ, Gronenborn AM, Clore GM. High-resolution solution structure of the beta chemokine hMIP-1 beta by multidimensional NMR. Science 1994;263:1762–1767.
30. Chung CW, Cooke RM, Proudfoot AEI, Wells TNC. The three-dimensional solution structure of RANTES. Biochemistry 1995;34:9307–9314.
31. Peitsch MC, Jongeneel CV. A 3-D model for the CD40 ligands predicts that it is a compact trimer similar to the tumor necrosis factors. Int Immunol 1993;5:233–238.
32. Mortin T, Li J, Cook R, Chaiken I. Mutagenesis in the C-terminal region of human interleukin 5 reveals a central patch for receptor alpha chain recognition. Proc Natl Acad Sci USA 1995;92:10879–10883.
33. Takaki S, Murata Y, Kitamura T, Miyajima A, Tominaga A, Takatsu K. Reconstitution of the functional receptors for murine and human interleukin 5. J Exp Med 1993;177:1523–1529.
34. Tavernier J, Tuypens T, Plaetinck G, Verhee A, Fiers W, Devos R. Molecular basis of the membrane-anchored and two soluble isoforms of the human interleukin 5 receptor α subunit. Proc Natl Acad Sci USA 1992;89:7041–7045.
35. Graber P, Proudfoot AEI, Talabot F, Bernard A, McKinnon M, Banks M, Fattah D, Solari R, Peitsch MC, Wells TNC. Identification of key charged residues of human interleukin-5 in receptor binding and cellular activation. J Biol Chem 1995;270:15762–15769.
36. Devos R, Guisez Y, Cornelis S, Verhee A, Van der Heyden J, Manneberg M, Lahm HW, Fiers W, Tavernier J, Plaetinck G. Recombinant soluble human interleukin-

5 (hIL-5) receptor molecules. Cross-linking and stoichiometry of binding to IL-5. J Biol Chem 1993;268:6581–6587.

37. Mita S, Harada N, Naomi S, Hitoshi Y, Sakamoto K, Akagi M, Tominaga A, Takatsu K. Receptors for T cell-replacing factor/interleukin 5. Specificity, quantitation, and its implication. J Exp Med 1988;168:863–878.
38. Devos R, Plaetinck G, Van der Heyden J, Cornelis S, Vandekerckhove J, Fiers W, Tavernier J. Molecular basis of a high affinity murine interleukin-5 receptor. EMBO J 1991;10:2133–2137.
39. De Vos AM, Ultsch M, Kossiakoff AA. Human growth hormone and extracellular domain of its receptor: crystal structure of the complex. Science 1992;255:306–312.
40. Cunningham BC, Wells JA. Comparison of a structural and a functional epitope. J Mol Biol 1993;234:554–563.
41. Wells JA, De Vos AM. Structure and function of human growth hormone: implications for the hematopoietins [review]. Annu Rev Biophys Biomol Struct 1993;22:329–51.
42. Layton MJ, Lock P, Metcalf D, Nicola NA. Cross-species receptor binding characteristics of human and mouse leukemia inhibitory factor suggest a complex binding interaction. J Biol Chem 1994;269:17048–17055.
43. Cornelis S, Plaetinck G, Devos R, Van der Heyden J, Tavernier J, Sanderson CJ, Guisez Y, Fiers W. Detailed analysis of the IL-5-IL-5R alpha interaction: characterization of crucial residues on the ligand and the receptor. EMBO J 1995;14:3395–3402.
44. Proudfoot AEI, Brown SC, Graber P, Talabot F, Arod CY, Peitsch MC, Banks C, McKinnon M, Solari R, Wells TNC. The carboxy-terminal region of human interleukin-5 is essential for maintenance of tertiary structure but not for dimerization. J Prot Chem 1996;15:491–499.
45. Hercus TR, Bagley CJ, Cambareri B, Dottore M, Woodcock JM, Vadas MA, Shannon MF, Lopez AF. Specific human granulocyte-macrophage colony-stimulating factor antagonists. Proc Natl Acad Sci USA 1994;91:5838–5842.
46. Barry SC, Bagley CJ, Phillips J, Dottore M, Cambareri B, Moretti P, D'Andrea R, Goodall GJ, Shannon MF, Vadas MA, et al. Two contiguous residues in human interleukin-3, Asp21 and Glu22, selectively interact with the alpha- and beta-chains of its receptor and participate in function. J Biol Chem 1994;269:8488–8492.
47. McKinnon M, Page K, Uings IJ, Banks M, Fattah D, Proudfoot AEI, Graber P, Arod CY, Fish R, Wells TNC, Solari R. An interleukin-5 mutant distinguishes between two functional responses in human eosinophils. J Exp Med 1997;186:121–129.
48. Chaiken IM, Williams WV. Identifying structure-function relationships in 4-helix bundle cytokines: towards *de novo* mimetics design. Trends Biotechnol 1996;14:369–375.
49. Li J, Cook R, Dede K, Chaiken I. Single chain human interleukin 5 and its asymmetric mutagenesis for mapping receptor binding sites. J Biol Chem 1996;271:1817–1820.
50. Edgerton MD, Graber P, Willard D, Consler T, McKinnon M, Uings I, Arod CY,

Borlat F, Fish R, Peitsch M, Wells TNC, Proudfoot AEI. Spatial orientation of the $\alpha$ and $\beta_c$ receptor chain binding sites on monomeric human IL-5 constructs. J Biol Chem 1997; 272:20611–20618.
51. Li J, Cook R, Chaiken I, Cook R. Mutants of single chain interleukin 5 show asymmetric recruitment of receptor $\alpha$ and $\beta_c$ subunits. J Biol Chem 1996;271:31729–31734.
52. Bennett MJ, Schlunegger MP, Eisenberg D. 3D domain swapping: a mechanism for oligomer assembly [review]. Protein Sci 1995;4:2455–2468.
53. Dickason RR, Huston DP. Creation of a biologically active interleukin-5 monomer. Nature 1996;379:652–655.
54. Li J, Cook R, Hensley P, Doyle M, McNulty D, Chaiken I. Monomeric isomers of human interleukin 5 show that 1:1 receptor recruitment is sufficient for function. Proc Natl Acad Sci USA 1997;94:6694–6699.

# 11

# The Structural Basis for Interleukin-5 Receptor Assembly

**CHRISTOPHER J. BAGLEY, JOANNA M. WOODCOCK, FRANK C. STOMSKI, and ANGEL F. LÓPEZ**

Hanson Centre for Cancer Research
Adelaide, Australia

## I. Introduction

The biological activities of IL-5 are mediated by receptors expressed on the surface of target cells. The receptor is comprised of two chains: an α chain that binds IL-5 with moderate affinity ($K_d$ = 0.5 nM) but alone is unable to mediate signaling (1–3), and a β chain that represents the major signaling component of the receptor (2,4). The β chain is unable to bind IL-5 alone, but when expressed together with the IL-5 receptor α chain (IL-5Rα) it confers a modest two- to fivefold improvement in receptor affinity for IL-5 ($K_d$ = 0.1 nM) (2). The β chain is shared with the related receptors for granulocyte-macrophage colony-stimuating factor (GM-CSF) and IL-3 (2,4). In man these receptors are composed of ligand-specific α chains and the communal β chain, $\beta_c$ (5,6). A similar situation occurs in the mouse with the exception that there exists a second β chain specific for the mouse IL-3 receptor (7). We will focus our discussion here to the human receptors for IL-5, GM-CSF, and IL-3. These three cytokine receptors have been shown to share a high degree of similarity both structurally and functionally and we will therefore review the IL-5 receptor field with occasional reference to GM-CSF and IL-3 receptor literature.

## II. Receptor Structure

### A. The IL-5 Receptor α Chain

Normally expressed as a cell-surface glycoprotein, the 400 residue IL-5Rα possesses three extracellular domains, a transmembrane helix, and a small cytoplasmic domain. Two soluble isoforms that arise from alternative splicing of the IL-5Rα mRNA have also been reported (8). Based on sequence homology, the tertiary structure of IL-5Rα is thought to be similar to that of other class 1 cytokine receptors for which the three-dimensional structures are known from X-ray crystallography such as the growth hormone (GH) receptor (9), prolactin (Prl) receptor (10), and erythropoietin (Epo) receptor (11). These receptors are composed of two extracellular fibronectin type III (FnIII) domains that together constitute a cytokine receptor module (CRM) (12). Each structural domain is comprised of seven β strands, denoted A through G, arranged in a two-layer sandwich (9), and the two domains are oriented at approximately 90° with the cytokine binding site lying between them. The membrane-proximal pair of extracellular domains of IL-5Rα conform to the GHR paradigm and together constitute a CRM that may be recognized by both the presence of key motifs including two cysteine pairs and a Trp residue in the N-terminal domain and the so-called WSXWS (Trp-Ser-Xaa-Trp-Ser) motif in the C-terminal domain (13). The C-terminal domain contains an extra pair of Cys residues that are thought to form an additional disulfide bond (14). By both protein sequence and gene organizational criteria, the N-terminal domain of IL-5Rα is also thought to be an FnIII-like structure, related to the second domain of the CRM, although its similarity to other receptor domains including the equivalent domains of the GMRα and IL-3Rα chains is only weak (12). This domain has only one Cys residue and hence forms no intramolecular disulfide bonds.

### B. The Communal β-Chain of the IL-5, IL-3, and GM-CSF Receptors

The $\beta_c$ is a protein of nearly 900 amino acid residues comprising a 420 residue extracellular portion, a transmembrane helix, and a 430 amino acid cytoplasmic region. The extracellular portion of $\beta_c$ comprises four domains within two CRM (12). The membrane-proximal CRM (CRM2) more closely resembles the classical CRM than does the membrane-distal CRM (CRM1) in respect of disulfide pattern and possession of a true WSXWS sequence (WSEWS). CRM1 is only distantly related to CRM2 (15) and exhibits a variant WSXWS sequence (PSKWS) and also has supernumerary Cys residues in its N-terminal domain which may form additional disulfide bonds.

Based on the structure of the GH receptor, Lyne and coworkers modeled the membrane-proximal CRM of human $\beta_c$ (53). The contact sites for the ligands were predicted to include the B-C and F-G loops in the fourth domain of $\beta_c$ as demonstrated by mutagenesis studies (16,17), although the major role of Tyr residues in these loops in mediating ligand recognition, identified by mutagenesis, was not highlighted in the models of the IL-3 and GM-CSF receptor complexes. Of interest with respect to the receptor activation process is the observation of the formation of disulfide-linked IL-3R$\alpha$/$\beta$ receptor heterodimers upon binding of IL-3, leading to functional activation of these $\beta$ chains (18). The N-terminal domain of $\beta_c$ has seven cysteine residues and the second domain has one. The first two cysteine residues are encoded by one exon and probably form a conserved disulfide between the A and B strands. A second disulfide between the D and E strands is also predicted to occur, leaving three nonconserved cysteine residues, two of which (Cys$^{86}$ and Cys$^{91}$) lie in the C-D loop where they may either form an additional disulfide or be available for intermolecular disulfide formation (see below). The remaining cysteine residues (Cys$^{100}$ and Cys$^{234}$) are not present in the mouse $\beta$ chains and are thought not to play a role in intermolecular disulfide bond formation (54).

## III. Receptor-Ligand Interactions

### A. Receptor Studies

Activation of the IL-5 receptor is initiated by IL-5 binding to the receptor $\alpha$ chain followed by interaction of the $\beta$ chain, forming a high-affinity receptor complex. Although the $\beta$ chain does not detectably bind IL-5 in the absence of the $\alpha$ chain, cross-linking experiments with radio-iodinated IL-5 on cells expressing the IL-5 receptor show that IL-5 is in close proximity to both the $\alpha$ and $\beta$ chains (2,8,19–21). This being the case, structure-function studies have been carried out with both receptor chains to determine the receptor sites that contribute to IL-5 high-affinity binding.

The binding site for IL-5 interaction with its receptor $\alpha$ chain has been mapped to the N-terminal FnIII-like domain using a chimeric receptor approach (14). Within this domain three residues—Asp$^{55}$, Asp$^{56}$, and Tyr$^{57}$—in the proposed C-D loop (Fig. 1) were found to be important for IL-5 binding (14). Individual alanine substitution of these residues caused significant if not complete loss of IL-5 binding affinity (14). In an earlier study it was shown that isothiazolone derivatives were able to completely block IL-5 binding to the IL-5 receptor $\alpha$ chain, an effect mediated by the modification of sulfhydryl groups of cysteine residues. By protease cleavage analysis it was determined that cysteine residue modification occurred in the N-terminal domain that contains a single Cys at position 86. Mutagenesis of residue Cys$^{86}$ confirmed this to be the reactive site, highlighting the importance of the N-terminal domain in IL-5 binding (22). The N-terminal domains of GMR$\alpha$ and IL-3R$\alpha$ have also been shown to participate in ligand binding (23,24). Additionally, sites that corre-

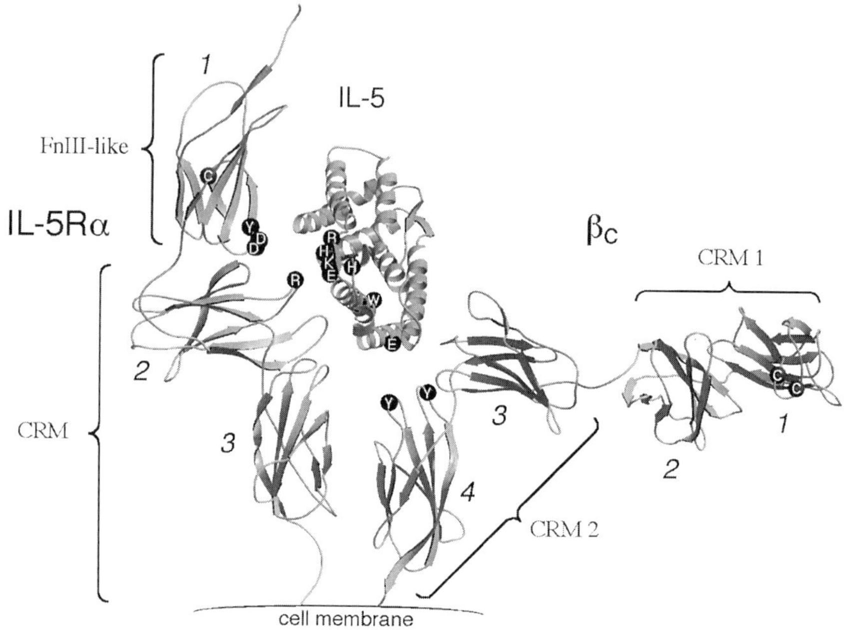


**Figure 1** Complex of IL-5 with its receptor. View of the IL-5 receptor complex based on the structure of the GHR (9). Residues implicated in receptor/ligand contact are highlighted in black, whereas Cys residues in the α and β chains of the receptor that are involved in intermolecular disulfides bonds are gray. Residues are identified by single-letter code. The relative orientation of the N-terminal domain of the IL-5Rα to the CRM is arbitrary but chosen to illustrate a potential mechanism of direct interaction with the IL-5. Similarly the angle between domains 2 and 3 of $\beta_c$ is only speculative. The figure was prepared using Molscript (51) and Raster3D (52).

spond to known ligand contact sites in growth hormone receptor have also been targeted for mutagenesis (14). By this approach a single residue, $Arg^{208}$, in the E-F loop of domain 1 of the CRM was found to be critical for IL-5 binding (Fig. 1). Alanine substitution of this residue alone led to greater than 100-fold loss in affinity for IL-5. Although the recognition of IL-5 by IL-5Rα is apparently shared between two domains (the FnIII-like domain and the first domain of the CRM), this does not seem to involve an interface region as seen for GHR binding of GH (9). Rather the sequence of the loop between the CRM and the N-terminal domain, containing conserved Gly and Pro residues, may favor a kinked structure that brings this domain into close proximity to the ligand as shown in Figure 1.

The communal β chain has also been examined for ligand contact sites. In the case of IL-5, this receptor chain has only a moderate effect on ligand binding, with a two- to fivefold increase in affinity over that of IL-5Rα alone. However, β chain has a more marked effect on the affinities of the GM-CSF and IL-3 receptor; the β chain confers a 20- to 50-fold and a 500- to 1000-fold improvement on the GM-CSF and IL-3 receptors, respectively. Thus $\beta_c$ is often referred to as the affinity converting subunit. Since the effect on IL-5 binding is marginal, ligand contact sites have been examined particularly in relation to GM-CSF and IL-3 where effects of mutation can be more easily ascertained. However, all mutations that had effects on GM-CSF and IL-3 binding were shown to also cause decreases in IL-5 binding, suggesting that the three ligands share a binding epitope.

Regions of β chain involved in GM-CSF, IL-3, and IL-5 binding were identified by mutagenesis (16,17,25). As with the IL-5Rα-chain studies, regions of β chain were targeted for mutagenesis on the basis of being analogous to known ligand contacts in GHR. A region of four residues was identified that is predicted to lie between the B and C strands in the membrane proximal domain of $\beta_c$. Alanine substitution of residues $Tyr^{365}$ / $Glu^{366}$ and $His^{367}$ / $Ile^{368}$ in this loop disrupted high-affinity binding of GM-CSF and IL-5, although cross-linking studies indicated that IL-5 still becomes associated with these $\beta_c$ mutants (16). Individual substitution of $Tyr^{365}$ alone was sufficient to completely abolish high-affinity binding of GM-CSF and IL-5 (16). A single tyrosine residue ($Tyr^{421}$) in the predicted F-G loop in this domain of $\beta_c$ was also found to be critical for high-affinity GM-CSF, IL-3, and IL-5 binding (17). Alanine substitution of this residue alone was sufficient to completely abolish high-affinity binding of all three cytokines. Significantly, alanine substitution of flanking residues in the predicted loop had little effect on ligand binding so long as $Tyr^{421}$ was retained (17). Hence it seems that, as with the GHR, hydrophobic residues play an important role in ligand binding in $\beta_c$.

### B. Ligand Studies

Human IL-5 exists as a glycosylated disulfide-linked homodimer of 25 to 40 kDa (26) with an antiparallel arrangement (27,28). Substitution of the Cys residues was found to result in inactive protein, suggesting the disulfides play a critical role in maintaining the IL-5 structure (27). The basis for the obligate formation of IL-5 dimers was revealed when the structure of human IL-5 produced in *E. coli* was determined by X-ray crystallography (29). IL-5 was found to exist as a dimer of four-helix bundles in which the D helix of one monomer is intertwined with the A, B, and C helices of the alternate monomer to form a four-helix bundle domain as shown in Figure 2. The individual domains were similar to the four-helix bundles of other cytokines of this family such as GM-CSF. In fact the structure of IL-5 can be viewed not simply as a disulfide-linked association of monomers but as two pseudo-monomers that are held together

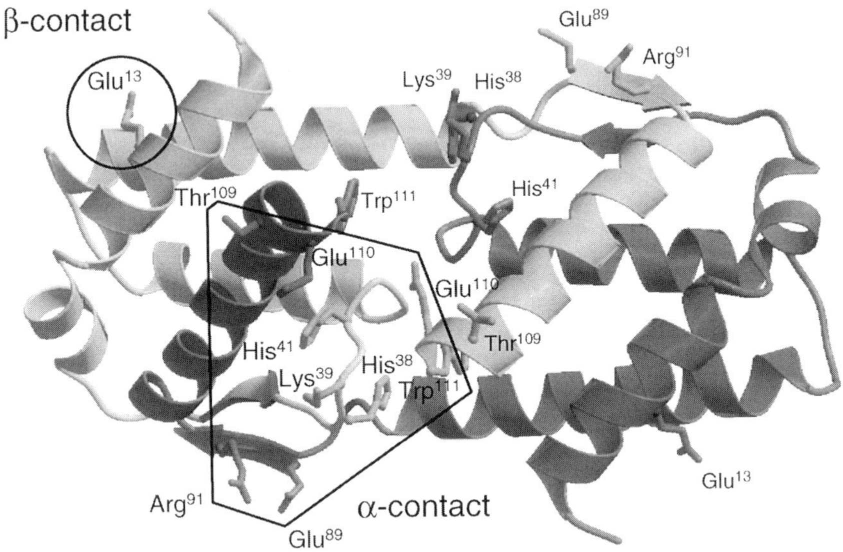


**Figure 2** Receptor-binding residues of IL-5. View of IL-5 with the helices represented as ribbons and the β strands as arrows. The side chains of residues proposed to contact the α and β chains of the receptor, as identified from mutagenesis studies, are indicated by sticks and labels. The figure was prepared using Molscript (51) and Raster3D (52).

intimately by the peptide backbone, hydrogen bonds, and hydrophobic packing as well as via intermolecular disulfides.

IL-5 from man and mouse exhibit unidirectional species cross-reactivity in that murine and human IL-5 are equipotent for binding to human receptors, whereas human IL-5 is 50-fold less potent than murine IL-5 for binding to murine receptors. This observation was exploited in early studies using mouse/human chimeras that demonstrated that binding determinants for the mouse receptor were located near the C terminus of the protein (30). More recently, systematic mutagenesis studies have identified clusters of residues—Glu$^{89}$, Glu$^{90}$, and Arg$^{91}$ and Thr$^{109}$, Glu$^{110}$, and Trp$^{111}$—in the C terminus (as well as His$^{38}$, Lys$^{39}$, and His$^{41}$) as being important for binding to the α chain of the receptor (31–33). Examination of the sites of receptor-binding residues in the context of the tertiary structure of IL-5 reveals that they lie close to the interface between the two four-helix bundle domains. This clustering suggested that the observation of an IL-5 dimer being able to bind only a single molecule of IL-5Rα (34) might be the result of steric hindrance but also raised the question as to whether residues from both domains and/or both chains contributed to IL-5Rα binding. Alternatively, the possibility of IL-5 undergoing conformational changes on binding to IL-5Rα has also been suggested (35).

Several approaches have been taken to dissect the contribution of the two IL-5 monomers to the activity of the IL-5 dimer. Chaiken and coworkers introduced a linker peptide between the C terminus of one monomer and the N terminus of the other, which lie close together in IL-5, allowing the generation of IL-5 analogs bearing single rather that duplicate substitutions (36). IL-5 was found to be highly tolerant of single substitutions within the motifs described above (36), suggesting that residues from both monomers do not contribute equally to the interaction with a single IL-5Rα. The individual substitutions E110A, R91A, and W111A cause only twofold reduction of affinity, whereas their double substitutions cause 12-, 40-, and 40-fold losses, respectively. Interestingly, the combination of R91A mutations in either domain with a single E110A mutation caused the same, additive reduction in affinity. In contrast, the double mutant of R91A and W111A in the same domain led to a greater than additive loss of affinity, whereas combining these substitutions in different domains had an effect no greater than those of the single mutations themselves. This suggests that $Arg^{91}$ cooperates functionally with $Trp^{111}$ of the opposing domain but with both $Glu^{110}$ residues to an equal extent, indicating that both domains are engaged simultaneously by IL-5Rα. Furthermore, by combining the α-chain-specific R91A mutation with the E13A substitution that selectively decreases receptor activation but not binding, Li et al. (37) showed that $Arg^{91}$ cooperates functionally with $Glu^{13}$ from the same domain. The relative locations of residues involved in association with IL-5Rα and $\beta_c$ are shown in Figure 2.

Understanding the structure of IL-5 has facilitated the design of single-domain IL-5 analogs with wild-type IL-5 (wtIL-5) properties. The ability of a single domain of IL-5 to function biologically was first demonstrated by introducing a linker peptide between the C and D helices of IL-5, which allowed the molecule to fold as a monomer rather than a dimer. This molecule was a full IL-5 agonist and exhibited only a 15-fold reduction in biopotency (38). A similar analog was found to exhibit only an eightfold reduced biopotency relative to wild type but a 40-fold reduced affinity for IL-5Rα (39). Another monomeric IL-5 analog, which was produced by a circular permutation created by introducing a new N terminus between helices C and D and joining the D and A helices by a diglycyl linker, also showed a 40-fold reduced affinity for IL-5Rα but only fourfold reduced potency for stimulating proliferation of human cells (39). Alternative circular permutations inserting the new N termini between the A and B or B and C helices and incorporating linker peptides between the C and D helices have been shown to exhibit 60- and 600-fold, respectively, reduced affinity for IL-5Rα (40). The reduced binding affinity of all the single-domain IL-5 analogs for IL-5Rα is consistent with the above observations that $Glu^{110}$ and $Trp^{111}$ of the opposing domain are also required for full binding and function. However, the impaired stability of the monomeric analogs and the likelihood of subtle alterations to their four-helix bundle structure have also been suggested to contribute to the poor activities of these analogs (39,40).

## IV. Mechanism of IL-5 Receptor Activation

The binding of IL-5 to both receptor subunits induces a series of molecular events in the receptor which lead ultimately to receptor activation. The nature and sequence of these events are only beginning to be understood. A key step in receptor activation in general is that of receptor dimerization (41). In the cytokine receptor subfamily comprising IL-5, IL-3, and GM-CSF, ligand has been shown to induce heterodimerization of each specific binding subunit with $\beta_c$ (18,42). Both IL-3 and GM-CSF induce a very rapid association ($<30$ sec) of their $\alpha$ chains with $\beta_c$ (15,18). This is analogous to the IL-6 and CNTF receptor systems where ligand induces association of the binding subunit to the signal transducer component, gp130 (43,44). The major difference, however, between the IL-5, IL-3, GM-CSF receptor subfamily and the IL-6 and growth hormone receptor families is that the latter rely on homodimerization of the signaling subunit, either gp130 or GHR, respectively, for receptor activation while the form requires the presence of the $\alpha$ chain in the dimerized/oligomerized complex. This is likely to reflect the participation of these $\alpha$ chains in function and is consistent with the lack of requirement of the cytoplasmic region of IL-6R$\alpha$ for IL-6 signaling but the absolute need for the cytoplasmic region of IL-5R$\alpha$ (45), GMR$\alpha$ (46), and IL-3R$\alpha$ (23) for receptor signaling.

An important recent observation in the IL-5, GM-CSF, and IL-3 receptor subfamily was the demonstration that binding of ligand induces both a noncovalent dimerization between the $\alpha$ chains and $\beta_c$ and a covalent interaction between the receptor subunits (18). The latter has been demonstrated by using iodoacetamide that alkylates the thiol groups of the free Cys residues in $\beta_c$ thus preventing disulfide bond formation (18), and more recently by mutational analysis of the relevant Cys residues (54). These studies examined several Cys residues in CRM1 of $\beta_c$ for their ability to form heterodimers with the receptor $\alpha$ chains. Of the five candidate Cys residues examined, Cys$^{86}$ and Cys$^{91}$ were found to be central to disulfide-linked IL-5, IL-3, and GM-CSF receptor dimerization. Interestingly, alignment of this region of $\beta_c$ to equivalent regions in other receptor subunits revealed that Cys$^{86}$ and Cys$^{91}$ represent a motif present in human $\beta_c$ and both mouse $\beta$ subunits but is absent from other receptor subunits. This motif illustrates the evolution of the IL-5, IL-3, and GM-CSF receptor subfamily to utilize a mechanism of receptor activation unique to this subfamily. It is interesting to note that the N-terminal domains of the IL-5R$\alpha$, IL-3R$\alpha$, and GMR$\alpha$ chains all have an odd number of Cys residues, suggesting that a free Cys is present to allow the formation of a disulfide bridge with either Cys$^{86}$ or Cys$^{91}$ in $\beta_c$. However, the identities of these Cys residues within

GMR$\alpha$ and IL-3$\alpha$ that form intermolecular disulfide bonds are not known, whereas IL-5R$\alpha$ possesses only a single eligible residue, Cys$^{86}$.

Whether IL-5R noncovalent and disulfide-linked dimers occur independently or are sequential steps in a single process is not yet clear. It is known, however, that disulfide-linked dimerization can be dissociated from high-affinity binding (18). On the other hand, disulfide-linked dimerization is necessary for receptor activation, at least in terms of phosphorylation of $\beta_c$ (54). These findings suggest a sequence of events where IL-5 binds initially to IL-5R$\alpha$ followed by recruitment of $\beta_c$ by the IL-5:IL-5R$\alpha$ complex. At this point it is not possible to separate high-affinity binding and noncovalent IL-5R dimerization, and in fact both may be different experimental measurements of the same process. In this model, contacting of $\beta_c$ by the conserved Glu residue in IL-5 (Glu$^{13}$), IL-3 (Glu$^{22}$), and GM-CSF (Glu$^{21}$) would actively promote the noncovalent dimerization of $\alpha$ and $\beta_c$ to form a ternary complex with a 1:1:1 stoichiometry. It would be interesting to test whether mutations in the ligand:receptor contact points either of the conserved Glu motif in the ligand or of the Tyr$^{421}$ in $\beta_c$ would impair $\alpha$:$\beta_c$ noncovalent dimerization.

Following high-affinity binding/noncovalent dimerization, it is likely that the complex undergoes conformational changes allowing disulfide-linked dimerization of one heterodimer with a second heterodimer to form a fully active complex consisting of a 2:2:2 stoichiometry. In this model, the $\alpha$ chain of the first heterodimer would form a disulfide bond with the $\beta_c$ (Cys$^{86}$ or Cys$^{91}$) in the second heterodimer and simultaneously the $\alpha$ chain of the second heterodimer may form a disulfide bond with the $\beta_c$ in the first heterodimer. The role of the disulfide bridging in bringing together two $\beta_c$ would not only stabilize the complex but also bring into close proximity the JAK-2 preassociated with $\beta_c$ leading to phosphorylation and full activation of the receptor (see Fig. 3).

Although disulfide bond formation has been shown to be essential for phosphorylation of $\beta_c$ on Tyr residues and, in the case of the IL-6 receptor family, tyrosine phosphorylation of gp130, it is not clear whether all cellular functions are dependent on this process. By using $\beta_c$ mutants in which Cys$^{86}$ or Cys$^{91}$ are substituted by Ala it may be possible to examine whether cellular functions may proceed after ligand binding and noncovalent dimerization in the absence of disulfide bond formation and $\beta_c$ phosphorylation. Antagonists of IL-5 may also be useful in examining this question. It is possible that IL-5 mutants in which Glu$^{13}$ is substituted by other amino acids, such as Gln, Lys, or Arg, act as antagonists because they prevent the formation of a disulfide bond while allowing noncovalent $\alpha$:$\beta_c$ interactions. This is consistent with the lack of tyrosine phosphorylation of $\beta_c$ by E13R (Fig. 4), the ability of $\beta_c$ to be cross-linked to and support the high-affinity binding of the antagonists E13Q (31) and E13K (47), and most interesting, the ability of E13K to support eosinophil survival (47).

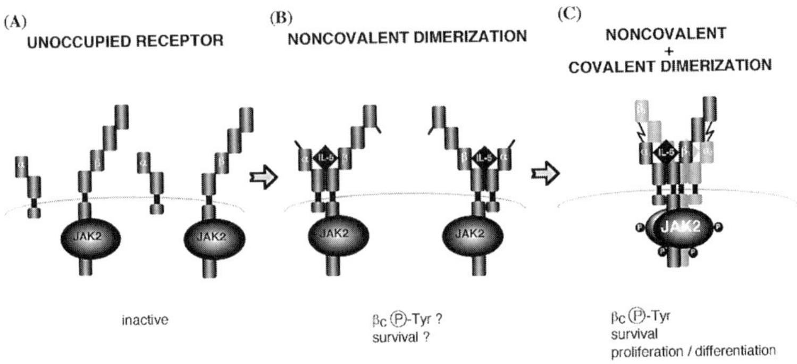


**Figure 3** Model for the sequential activation of the IL-5 receptor. A cartoon representing the possible sequence of events leading to IL-5 receptor activation. (A) The receptor $\alpha$ and $\beta_c$ chains in the absence of ligand. (B) The binding of IL-5 to $\alpha$ chain induces $\alpha:\beta_c$ heterodimerization giving rise to a trimer with an IL-5:$\alpha:\beta_c$ stoichiometry of 1:1:1 with high-affinity binding of IL-5. The free cysteine residues in the $\alpha$ and $\beta_c$ subunits are illustrated by dark lines. (C) The $\alpha$ subunit of receptor 1 forms a disulfide bond with $\beta_c$ of receptor 2, and the $\alpha$ subunit of receptor 2 forms a disulfide bond with $\beta_c$ of receptor 1, possibly as a result of conformational change in the receptor complex. This leads to a receptor complex of IL-5:$\alpha:\beta_c$ stoichiometry of 2:2:2. The disulfide bridges between the $\alpha$ and $\beta_c$ subunits are illustrated by lighting strikes. The bringing together of two $\beta_c$ with their associated JAK-2 molecules would then lead to receptor activation.

and most interesting, the ability of E13K to support eosinophil survival (47). These findings raise the possibility that noncovalent and covalent dimers forming 1:1:1 or 2:2:2 complexes, respectively, are coupled to different cellular functions. Similarly, they suggest that $\beta_c$ phosphorylation is not essential for all receptor functions. Whether disulfide-linked dimerization leading to $\beta_c$ tyrosine phosphorylation is required for activation of unique cellular functions, or acts as a potentiator of biochemical cascades that are already initiated, remains to be determined.

## V. The Future

Studies of receptor recognition by IL-5 has raised the possibility of designing specific peptide or nonpeptide molecules corresponding to the specific array of chemical functional groups required to bind to IL-5R$\alpha$, that is, the pharmacophore. These molecules might then be able to prevent activation of the IL-5

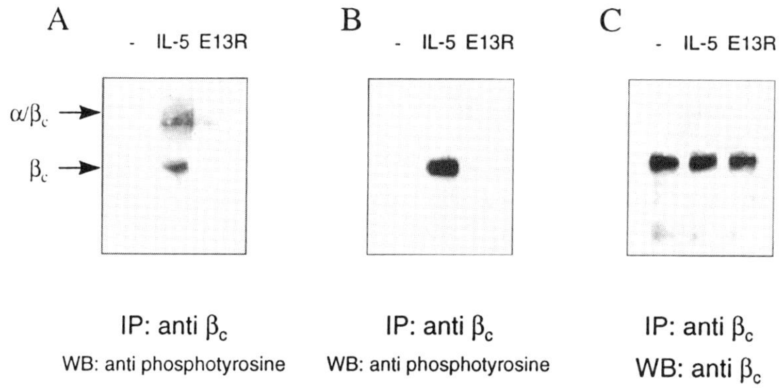


**Figure 4** An IL-5 antagonist, E13R, does not induce disulfide-linked receptor dimerization or phosphorylation of $\beta_c$. TF1.8 cells were either incubated with medium alone (–) or treated with medium containing 3.8 nM IL-5 (IL-5) or 192 nM IL-5 analog (E13R) for 5 min at 37°C. After cell lysis, protiens were immunoprecipitated with anti-$\beta_c$ MAb 8E4 and the immunoprecipitates were resolved either under nonreducing (A) or reducing (B,C) conditions on an SDS-7.5% polyacrylamide gel and transferred to nitrocellulose filters. The filters were then probed either with antiphosphotyrosine antibody 3-365-10 (A,B) or anti-$\beta_c$ MAb 1C1 (C).

receptor by binding specifically to IL-5Rα. This approach has been demonstrated for the EpoR (48) and thrombopoietin receptor (49) for which specific peptide agonists have been generated. Recently small molecules have been identified that associate irreversibly with IL-5Rα and prevent binding of IL-5 but also inhibit the GM-CSF and IL-3 receptors (50). The possibility exists to modify these lead compounds to improve their specificity for the IL-5Rα and reduce their nonspecific cytotoxicity. Targeting of $\beta_c$, on the other hand, by identifying agents that target the F-G loop of domain 4 or $Cys^{86}$ and $Cys^{91}$, may lead to general inhibitors of the IL-5, IL-3, and GM-CSF receptor family.

## Acknowledgments

Supported by grants from the National Health and Medical Research Council of Australia and the Anti-Cancer Foundation of the Universities of South Australia. C. J. Bagley is a Florey Research Fellow of the Royal Adelaide Hospital.

## References

1. Takaki S, Tominaga A, Hitoshi Y, Mita S, Sonoda E, Yamaguchi N, Takatsu K. Molecular cloning and expression of the murine interleukin-5 receptor. EMBO J 1990;9:4367–4374.
2. Tavernier J, Devos R, Cornelis S, Tuypens T, Van der Heyden J, Fiers W, Plaetinck G. A human high affinity interleukin-5 receptor (IL5R) is composed of an IL5-specific α chain and a β chain shared with the receptor for GM-CSF. Cell 1991;66:1175–1184.
3. Murata Y, Takaki S, Migita M, Kikuchi Y, Tominaga A, Takatsu K. Molecular cloning and expression of the human interleukin 5 receptor. J Exp Med 1992;175:341–351.
4. Takaki S, Mita S, Kitamura T, Tominaga A, Miyajima A, Takatsu K. Identification of the second subunit of the murine interleukin-5 receptor: interleukin-3 receptor-like protein, AIC2B is a component of the high affinity interleukin-5 receptor. EMBO J 1991;10:2833–2838.
5. Hayashida K, Kitamura T, Gorman DM, Arai K, Yokota T, Miyajima A. Molecular cloning of a second subunit of the receptor for human granulocyte-macrophage colony-stimulating factor (GM-CSF): reconstitution of a high-affinity GM-CSF receptor. Proc Natl Acad Sci USA 1990;87:9655–9659.
6. Kitamura T, Sato N, Arai K, Miyajima A. Expression cloning of the human IL-3 receptor cDNA reveals a shared β subunit for the human IL-3 and GM-CSF receptors. Cell 1991;66:1165–1174.
7. Itoh N, Yonehara S, Schreurs J, Gorman D, Maruyama K, Ishii A, Yahara I, Arai K-I, Miyajima A. Cloning of an interleukin-3 receptor gene: a member of a distinct receptor gene family. Science 1990;247:324–327.
8. Tavernier J, Tuypens T, Plaetinck G, Verhee A, Fiers W, Devos R. Molecular basis of the membrane-anchored and two soluble isoforms of the human interleukin 5 receptor alpha subunit. Proc Natl Acad Sci USA 1992;89:7041–7045.
9. De Vos AM, Ultsch M, Kossiakoff AA. Human growth hormone and extracellular domain of its receptor: crystal structure of the complex. Science 1992;255:306–312.
10. Somers W, Ultsch M, De Vos AM, Kossiakoff AA. The X-ray structure of a growth hormone-prolactin receptor complex. Nature 1994;372:478–481.
11. Livnah O, Stura EA, Johnson DL, Middleton SA, Mulcahy LS, Wrighton NC, Dower WJ, Joliffe LK, Wilson IA. Functional mimicry of a protein hormone by a peptide agonist: the EPO receptor complex at 2.8Å. Science 1996;273:464–471.
12. Goodall GJ, Bagley CJ, Vadas MA, Lopez AF. A model for the interaction of the GM-CSF, IL-3 and IL-5 receptors with their ligands. Growth Factors 1993;8:87–97.
13. Bazan JF. Structural design and molecular evolution of a cytokine receptor superfamily. Proc Natl Acad Sci USA 1990;87:6934–6938.
14. Cornelis S, Plaetinck G, Devos R, Van der Heyden J, Tavernier J, Sanderson CJ, Guisez Y, Fiers W. Detailed analysis of the IL-5-IL-5R alpha interaction: characterization of crucial residues on the ligand and the receptor. EMBO J 1995;14:3395–3402.

15. Bagley CJ, Woodcock JM, Stomski FC, Lopez AF. The structural and functional basis of cytokine receptor activation: lessons from the common β subunit of the granulocyte-macrophage colony-stimulating factor, interleukin-3 (IL-3) and IL-5 receptors. Blood 1997;89:1471–1482.
16. Woodcock JM, Zacharakis B, Plaetinck G, Bagley CJ, Qiyu S, Hercus TR, Tavernier J, Lopez AF. Three residues in the common β chain of the human GM-CSF, IL-3 and IL-5 receptors are essential for GM-CSF and IL-5 but not IL-3 high affinity binding and interact with $Glu^{21}$ of GM-CSF. EMBO J 1994;13:5176–5185.
17. Woodcock JM, Bagley CJ, Zacharakis B, Lopez AF. A single residue in the membrane proximal domain of the GM-CSF, IL-3 and IL-5 receptor common β chain is necessary and sufficient for high affinity binding and signalling by all three ligands. J Biol Chem 1996;271:25999–26006.
18. Stomski FC, Sun Q, Bagley CJ, Woodcock JM, Goodall GJ, Andrews RK, Berndt MC, Lopez AF. Human interleukin-3 (IL-3) induces disulphide-linked receptor α and β chain heterodimerization which is required for receptor activation but not high affinity binding. Mol Cell Biol 1996;16:3035–3046.
19. Plaetinck G, Van der Heyden J, Tavernier J, Fache I, Tuypens T, Fischkoff S, Fiers W, Devos R. Characterization of interleukin 5 receptors on eosinophilic sublines from human promyelocytic leukemia (HL-60) cells. J Exp Med 1990;172:683–691.
20. Lopez AF, Vadas MA, Woodcock JM, Milton SE, Lewis A, Elliott MJ, Gillis D, Ireland R, Olwell E, Park LS. Interleukin-5, interleukin-3, and granulocyte-macrophage colony-stimulating factor cross-compete for binding to cell surface receptors on human eosinophils. J Biol Chem 1991;266:24741–24747.
21. Takaki S, Murata Y, Kitamura T, Miyajima A, Tominaga A, Takatsu K. Reconstitution of the functional receptors for murine and human interleukin-5. J Exp Med 1993;177:1523–1529.
22. Devos R, Guisez Y, Plaetinck G, Cornelis S, Tavernier J, Van der Heyden J, Foley LH, Scheffler JE. Covalent modification of the interleukin-5 receptor by isothiazolones leads to inhibition of the binding of interleukin-5. Eur J Biochem 1994;225:635–640.
23. Rapoport AP, Luhowskyj S, Doshi P, DiPersio JF. Mutational analysis of the alpha subunit of the human interleukin-3 receptor. Blood 1996;87:112–122.
24. Barry SC, Korpelainen E, Sun Q, Stomski FC, Moretti PA, Wakao H, D'Andrea RJ, Vadas MA, Lopez AF, Goodall GJ. Roles of the N and C terminal domains of the interleukin-3 receptor alpha chain in receptor function. Blood 1997;89:842–852.
25. Lock P, Metcalf D, Nicola NA. Histidine-367 of the human common beta chain of the receptor is critical for high-affinity binding of human granulocyte-macrophage colony-stimulating factor. Proc Natl Acad Sci USA 1994;91:252–256.
26. Takatsu K, Tominaga A, Harada N, Mita S, Matsumoto M, Takahashi T, Kikuchi Y, Yamaguchi N. T cell-replacing factor (TRF)/interleukin 5 (IL-5): molecular and functional properties. Immunol Rev 1988;102:107–135.
27. McKenzie AN, Ely B, Sanderson CJ. Mutated interleukin-5 monomers are biologically inactive. Mol Immunol 1991;28:155–158.
28. Minamitake Y, Kodama S, Katayama T, Adachi H, Tanaka S, Tsujimoto M. Struc-

ture of recombinant human interleukin 5 produced by Chinese hamster ovary cells. J Biochem (Tokyo) 1990;107:292–297.
29. Milburn MV, Hassel AM, Lambert MH, Jordan SR, Proudfoot AEI, Graber P, Wells TNC. A novel dimer configuration revealed by the crystal structure at 2.4Å resolution of human interleukin-5. Nature 1993;363:172–176.
30. McKenzie AN, Barry SC, Strath M, Sanderson CJ. Structure-function analysis of interleukin-5 utilizing mouse/human chimeric molecules. EMBO J 1991;10:1193–1199.
31. Tavernier J, Tuypens T, Verhee A, Plaetinck G, Devos R, Van der Heyden J, Guisez Y, Oefner C. Identification of receptor-binding domains on human interleukin 5 and design of an interleukin 5-derived receptor antagonist. Proc Natl Acad Sci USA 1995;92:5194–5198.
32. Graber P, Proudfoot AE, Talabot F, Bernard A, McKinnon M, Banks M, Fattah D, Solari R, Peitsch MC, Wells TN. Identification of key charged residues of human interleukin-5 in receptor binding and cellular activation. J Biol Chem 1995;270:14762–15769.
33. Morton T, Li J, Cook R, Chaiken I. Mutagenesis in the C-terminal region of human interleukin 5 reveals a central patch for receptor alpha chain recognition. Proc Natl Acad Sci USA 1995;92:10879–10883.
34. Devos R, Guisez Y, Cornelis S, Verhee A, Van der Heyden J, Manneberg M, Lahm HW, Fiers W, Tavernier J, Plaetinck G. Recombinant soluble human interleukin-5 (hIL-5) receptor molecules. Cross-linking and stoichiometry of binding to IL-5. J Biol Chem 1993;268:6581–6587.
35. Devos R, Plaetinck G, Cornelis S, Guisez Y, Van der Heyden J, Tavernier J. Interleukin-5 and its receptor: a drug target for eosinophilia associated with chronic disease. J Leukoc Biol 1995;57:813–819.
36. Li J, Cook R, Dede K, Chaiken I. Single chain human interleukin 5 and its asymmetric mutagenesis for mapping receptor binding sites. J Biol Chem 1996;271:1817–1820.
37. Li J, Cook R, Chaiken I. Mutants of single chain interleukin 5 show asymmetric recruitment of receptor $\alpha$ and $\beta_c$ subunits. J Biol Chem 1996;271:31729–31734.
38. Dickson RR, Huston DP. Creation of a biologically active interleukin-5 monomer. Nature 1996;379:652–655.
39. Li J, Cook R, Doyle ML, Hensley P, McNulty DE, Chaiken I. Monomeric isomers of human interleukin 5 show that 1:1 receptor recruitment is sufficient for function. Proc Natl Acad Sci USA 1997;94:6694–6699.
40. Edgerton MD, Graber P, Willard D, Consler T, McKinnon M, Uings I, Arod CY, Borlat F, Fish R, Peitsch MC, Wells TNC, Proudfoot AEI. Spatial orientation of the $\alpha$ and $\beta_c$ receptor chain binding sites on monomeric human interleukin-5 constructs. J Biol Chem 1997;272:20611–20618.
41. Heldin C-H. Dimerization of cell surface receptors in signal transduction. Cell 1995;80:213–223.
42. Eder M, Ernst TJ, Ganser A, Jubinsky PT, Inhorn R, Hoelzer D, Griffin JD. A low affinity chimeric human alpha/beta-granulocyte-macrophage colony-stimulating factor receptor induces ligand-dependent proliferation in a murine cell line. J Biol Chem 1994;269:30173–30180.

43. Murakami M, Hibi M, Nakagawa N, Nakagawa T, Yasakawa K, Yamanishi K, Taga T, Kishimoto T. IL-6 induced homodimerisation of gp130 and associated activation of a tyrosine kinase. Science 1993;260:1808–1810.
44. Davis S, Aldrich TH, Stahl N, Pan L, Taga T, Kishimoto T, Ip NY, Yancopoulos GD. LIFRβ and gp130 as heterodimerizing signal transducers of the tripartite CNTF receptor. Science 1993;260:1805–1808.
45. Takaki S, Kanazawa H, Shiiba M, Takatsu K. A critical cytoplasmic domain of the interleukin-5 (IL-5) receptor alpha chain and its function in IL-5-mediated growth signal transduction. Mol Cell Biol 1994;14:7404–7413.
46. Watanabe S, Mui AL, Muto A, Chen JX, Hayashida K, Yokota T, Miyajima A, Arai K. Reconstituted human granulocyte-macrophage colony-stimulating factor receptor transduces growth-promoting signals in mouse NIH 3T3 cells: comparison with signalling in BA/F3 pro-B cells. Mol Cell Biol 1993;3:1440–1448.
47. McKinnon M, Page K, Uings IJ, Banks M, Fattah D, Proudfoot AE, Graber P, Arod C, Fish R, Wells TN, Solari R. An interleukin 5 mutant distinguishes between two functional responses in human eosinophils. J Exp Med 1997;186:121–129.
48. Wrighton NC, Farrell FX, Chang R, Kashyap AK, Barbone FP, Mulcahy LS, Johnson DL, Barrett RW, Joliffe LK, Dower WJ. Small peptides as potent mimetics of the protein hormone erythropoietin. Science 1996;273:458–463.
49. Cwirla SE, Balasubramanian P, Duffin DJ, Wagstrom CR, Gates CM, Singer SC, Davis AM, Tansik RL, Mattheakis LC, Boytos CM, Schatz PJ, Baccanari DP, Wrighton NC, Barrett RW, Dower WJ. Peptide agonist of the thrombopoietin receptor as potent as the natural cytokine. Science 1997;276:1696–1699.
50. Wiekowski M, Prosser D, Taremi S, Tsarbopoulos A, Jenh CH, Chou CC, Lundell D, Zavodny P, Narula S. Characterization of potential antagonists of human interleukin 5 demonstrates their cross-reactivity with receptors for interleukin 3 and granulocyte-macrophage colony-stimulating factor. Eur J Biochem 1997;246:625–632.
51. Kraulis P. MOLSCRIPT: a program to produce both detailed and schematic plots of protein structures. J Appl Cryst 1991;24:946–950.
52. Merritt EA, Murphy MEP. Raster3D version 2.0, a program for photorealistic molecular graphics. Acta Cryst Sect D 1994;50:869–873.
53. Lyne PD, Bamborough P, Duncan D, Richards WG. Molecular modeling of the GM-CSF and IL-3 receptor complexes. Protein Sci 1995; 4:2223–2233.
54. Stomski FC, Woodcock JM, Zacharakis B, Bagley CJ, Sun Q, López AF. Identification of a Cys motif in the common β chain of the interleukin-3, granulocyte-macrophage colony-stimulating factor, and interleukin-5 receptor essential for disulfide-linked receptor heterodimerization and activation of all three receptors. J Biol Chem 1998; 273:1192–1199.

# 12

# Analysis of the Expression Pattern of Human Interleukin-5 Receptor α Isoforms In Vitro

**JAN TAVERNIER, ANNICK VERHEE, JOËL VANDEKERCKHOVE, and XAVEER VAN OSTADE**

University of Ghent
Ghent, Belgium

**JOSÉ VAN DER HEYDEN**

Roche Research Ghent
Ghent, Belgium

## I. Introduction

The interleukin-5 receptor (IL-5R) is a complex consisting of α and β subunits. The α subunit is ligand specific, which it binds with intermediate affinity in man ($K_d$ of 500 pM to 1 nM) and low affinity in the mouse ($K_d$ of 5 to 10 nM). In both species, association with the β subunit leads to a high-affinity receptor complex ($K_d$ of approximately 150 pM). No binding of IL-5 could be observed to the β chain alone. The latter receptor component however is critical for signaling and is shared with the receptors for IL-3 and granulocyte-macrophage colony-stimulating factor (GM-CSF), which also have their own ligand-specific α subunits. For this reason, the β subunit is now often referred to as β-common or $\beta_c$. In contrast to the $\beta_c$ chain, which is ubiquitously expressed in the hematopoietic system, the α-receptor subunit is only expressed on eosinophils and the related basophils in man (and on the B1 subpopulation of B lymphocytes in the mouse). These expression patterns explain on the one hand why the function of IL-5 is limited to these cell types, and on the other hand why IL-3, IL-5, and GM-CSF have overlapping biological functions on cells which coexpress the specific α subunits. For recent reviews, we refer to references 1 to 3.

Despite the twofold symmetrical structure of homodimeric IL-5, which opens the possibility for two symmetrical receptor binding sites, association with only one α subunit is seen in solution (4). This suggests that either sterical hindrance or an induced fit in the IL-5 molecule prevent the binding of a second IL-5Rα chain. A full high-affinity complex including α and $\beta_c$ subunits cannot be reconstituted in solution. Moreover, no association can be detected between the soluble IL-5/IL-5Rα complex and the membrane-bound $\beta_c$ chain. This forms the basis for the antagonistic properties of the secreted IL-5Rα chain (see below).

The exact stoichiometry of the IL-5/IL-5R complex on a cell surface remains unclear. The simplest model of a signaling complex is the combination of one IL-5 dimer together with one α and one β subunit. On Cos1 cells, recent evidence using IL-5R-gp130 chimeras points to the existence of such a complex, capable of signaling (5). The presence of a single IL-5Rα chain in an active complex is also suggested by the observation neutralizing antibodies directed against IL-5 can potentiate signaling (J. Tavernier, manuscript in preparation). Likewise, chimeric GM-CSF receptors with the extracellular parts of the α and β subunits placed by the leucine zipper domains of the Fos and Jun molecules heterodimerize into signaling complexes (6). In contrast, several reports point to a dimerization of $\beta_c$ chains. Enforced clustering of $\beta_c$ cytoplasmic tails has been shown to be sufficient for mitotic signaling (7–11). Muto et al. (12) have described the presence of $\beta_c$ dimers on the cell surface, even in the absence of ligand. For a more detailed discussion on the relative contributions of α and $\beta_c$ chains in receptor complex formation, we refer to Bagley et al. (13).

Given the importance of the IL-5-eosinophil axis in allergic pathologies (see Chapter 10), efforts by several teams have focused on the development of IL-5 antagonists. One obvious target is the binding of IL-5 on its receptor. So far screening efforts for small molecular weight compounds capable of blocking this interaction were largely unsuccessful (14). Recent successes in the identification of peptide antagonists or agonists for cytokines such as IL-1 (15) or erythropoietin (16), respectively, have however pointed to the ultimate feasibility of these approaches.

Alternatively, protein-based antagonists have been developed including humanized monoclonal antibodies capable of neutralizing IL-5 bioactivity, IL-5 muteins with antagonistic properties (17, see also Chapter 10, this volume), and a secreted IL-5Rα subunit (18). In this contribution, we focus on this naturally occurring IL-5 antagonist.

## II. Secreted Receptors in the Cytokine Receptor Family

Gene cloning and biochemical experiments have revealed that most cytokine receptors can exist either as a membrane-anchored or as a secreted isoform. In case of receptors for the four α-helical bundle cytokines, alternative splicing appears to be the primary mechanism involved in the formation of a specific transcript encoding secreted receptor variants. Alternatively, proteolytic cleavage is used for the generation of soluble receptors for IL-1 (19), tumour necrosis factor (TNF) (20), macrophage-CSF (M-CSF), (21), platelet-derived growth factor (PDGF) (22), or nerve growth factor (NGF), (23). This functional dichotomy between cytokine receptor subfamilies certainly is not absolute: sIL-6Rα and sFas, for example, can be generated by shedding and by alternative splicing, respectively (24,25). The ciliary neurotrophic factor (CNTF) receptor is a unique case because it is shed from the cell surface by phospholipase C-mediated cleavage of its glycosyl phosphatidyl inositol linkage (26).

The precise physiological role of these secreted receptors is not well understood at present, but very likely will differ from case to case. Models in which the antagonistic effects prevail include surface receptor down-modulation and ligand capture. On the other hand, secreted receptors may bind ligand in circulation resulting in the prolongation of its serum half-life or may facilitate ligand-mediated signaling. These features are well illustrated in the IL-6 receptor family. The secreted IL-6R (sIL-6Rα), for example, binds IL-6 in solution and this resulting complex is still able to associate with and activate the gp130 signal transducer on the cell membrane. This signaling IL-6/sIL-6Rα complex can be detected in circulation, as well as a secreted variant of the gp130 signal transducer (27,28). This latter form however is able to antagonize the function of the IL-6/sIL-6Rα complex (and of other members of this family) (27). Hence the relative concentrations of circulating IL-6, sIL-6Rα, and sgp130 may in concert determine the final physiological effect. Variations in these expression levels have been observed in several human diseases (29 and references therein). In this cytokine family, which is centered around the shared use of gp130, secreted receptors may also serve to expand the biological repertoire of one family member. The CNTF/CNTFRα complex, for example, can activate cells outside the nervous system, which do not have the CNTFRα, provided they coexpress gp130 and the leukemia inhibitory factor (LIF) β receptor, which is the third component of the CNTF receptor complex (26).

## III. Expression Pattern of the IL-5Rα Chain

Human eosinophils express, through differential splicing, three different transcripts from the same IL-5Rα locus (18,30–32). This may lead to the synthesis of two secreted receptor variants in addition to the membrane-bound receptor isoform. Surprisingly, one of these transcripts is predominantly expressed (>95%) in eosinophilic cells differentiated from the HL60 C115 subclone, in circulating mature eosinophils and in eosinophils obtained from cord blood cultures. This transcript arises from splicing to a "soluble-specific" exon, which precedes the exon encoding the transmembrane region. The structure of the hIL-5Rα gene, which is located on chromosome 3p26, and the observed differential splicing patterns are shown in Figure 1 (adapted from reference 31).

Alternative splicing as a mechanism to generate secreted receptor variants is a common feature for receptors of the α-helical-bundle cytokines. The hIL-5Rα splicing pattern is however exceptional since, in most cases described, transcripts for the secreted isoforms arise by "transmembrane exon" skipping. The only other cases of genes containing soluble-specific exons described so far are the genes encoding IL-4 (33) and leukemia inhibitory factor (LIF) (34,35).

Interestingly, a different splice pattern is used for the generation of secreted variants in man or mouse, since in the latter case no evidence for a "soluble" exon has been obtained so far (36). It should be pointed out that it is unclear at present whether this represents an interspecies variation or a cell-type-dependent difference, since in the mouse, IL-5Rα transcripts have only been analyzed in B cells. Such evolutionary divergence is not uncommon in other members of this family, and in the case of growth hormone, different mechanisms are used in different species: the so-called growth hormone binding pro-

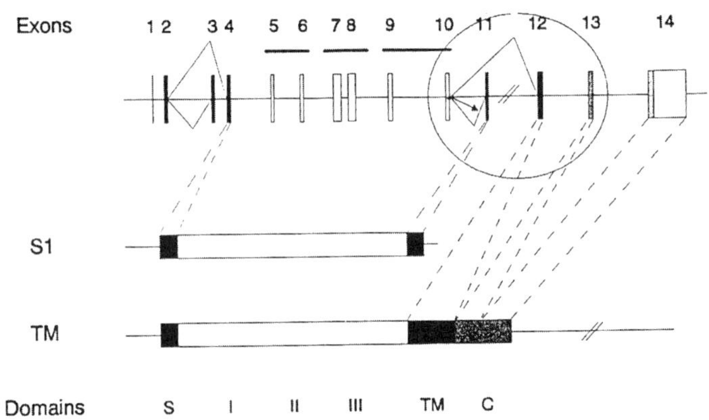


**Figure 1** The structure of the hIL-5Rα-subunit gene. On top, the gene organization is shown, with the exons numbered. Areas of alternative splicing are indicated; the encircled region is used in the generation of the minigene constructs (see Fig. 3). Thick lines on top refer to the domains of the extracellular part of the receptor. Dashed lines link the exon encoding the signal peptide, the soluble-specific exon and the exon containing the transmembrane region with the two cDNA types (S1 and TM correspond to the major soluble and the membrane anchored isoform, respectively; see references 30 and 31). Domains of the membrane-anchored receptor are shown below; S: signal peptide; TM: transmembrane region; C: cytoplasmic tail.

tein (GH-BP) is generated by alternative splicing in mice and rats and by proteolytic processing in rabbits and probably also in man (37,38).

The secreted human IL-5Rα subunit (sIL-5Rα) can function as an antagonist (18). Quite in contrast to the IL-6R family, truncation of the cytoplasmic tail of the membrane-bound IL-5Rα leads to complete abrogation of IL-5-dependent mitosis (39,40), indicating a critical role in signaling in addition to ligand capturing. Furthermore, the IL-5/sIL-5Rα complex is unable to associate and activate membrane-bound $\alpha_c$ chains. The antagonistic behavior of the secreted α receptor can be demonstrated in eosinophil differentiation assays as well as in proliferation assays using IL-5-responsive cell lines. Recombinant secreted α receptor can be produced in cell lines such as Cos1, CHO, or Sf9. However, while production in the former two cell types is marginal, high-level synthesis can be obtained in Sf9 cells using the baculovirus expression system.

Secreted hIL-5Rα has so far not been detected in serum nor in supernatants of cultured eosinophils. The reason underlying this observation is unclear at present. One possible explanation may be the thermolability of shIL-5Rα. As shown in Figure 2, prolonged incubation of recombinant soluble hIL-5Rα at 37°C results in loss of biological activity. We have found that such treatment leads to irreversible adsorption of this polypeptide to plastic supports, possibly by a conformational change leading to exposition of highly hydrophobic patches. This observation may help to explain the much better production

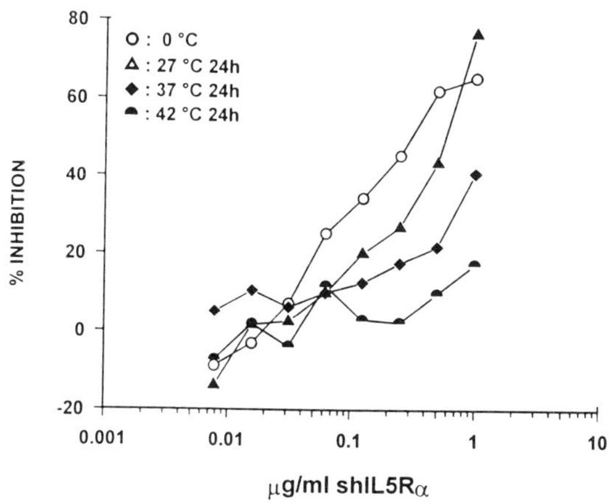


**Figure 2** Thermolability of recombinant soluble hIL-5Rα. Dilution series of recombinant soluble hIL-5Rα were incubated in RPMI 1640 medium, without serum added, for 24 hr at temperatures as indicated. Graphs represent the remaining inhibition by shIL-5Rα of IL-5-dependent proliferation of FDC-P1-CA1 cells. In all assay points, 2 U/ml hIL-5 was added.

level observed in Sf9 cells, which are cultured at 28°C. Importantly, this intrinsic behavior of the shIL-5Rα chain may also cause a significant loss of shIL-5Rα from serum samples by adherence to the collection vials. Illustrating this, treatment of $^{125}$I-shIL-5Rα at 42°C for 48 hr leads to an almost complete adherence to eppendorf tube walls, irrespective of the presence of human IL-5 (data not shown).

Another explanation may be that the shIL-5Rα is stored in eosinophilic granules, waiting for release upon the proper stimulus, for example, at the site of tissue inflammation. Finally, this differential splicing may also merely serve to down-modulate the cell-surface receptor isoform, rendering the cells irresponsive to IL-5.

## IV. Design of Minigene Constructs

Although the precise role of the secreted IL-5Rα isoform in vivo needs further clarification, this functional switch offers a potentially novel and important regulatory key to control eosinophil activation. For that purpose we have initiated an approach using so-called minigene constructs. In such minigenes, parts of the gene are replaced by cDNA segments as shown in Figure 3. The design of pSV-MINI-1 is such that functional hIL-5Rα receptors can be expressed. pSV-MINI-2 and -4 are derivatives characterized by the insertion of a unique restriction site in the intron separating the "soluble" and "transmembrane" exons, and the insertion of an additional SV40 polyadenylation site at that location to ensure mRNA stability, respectively. pSV-MINI-3 has most of the extracellular region of the hIL-5Rα replaced by human or mouse IL-6 (3h and 3m versions, not shown). This converts such minigene into a useful reporter system (see below).

All minigenes are assembled in the pSV-SPORT vector and are under control of the early SV40 promoter. Transcripts encoding the transmembrane isoform contain the SV40 polyadenylation signal from the vector. Since only part of the 3′ untranslated region from the hIL-5Rα cDNA is used, a transcript of around 2.7 kb is obtained instead of the 4.7 kb seen in eosinophils. The "soluble" exon has its own polyadenylation site, which is retained in the minigene, leading to a transcript identical to the natural situation.

To analyze the isoform expression pattern in different samples (both from cells transfected with the human minigene or from clinical origin), we have set up a sensitive, competitive reverse transcriptase polymerase chain reaction (RT-PCR) protocol (Fig. 4). In this approach, total RNA is converted into cDNA and is added in a PCR using three primers: one forward primer, which is shared by both receptor isoform transcripts, and two reverse primers, which are specific for either isoform (Fig. 4b). Since both reaction products can be separated

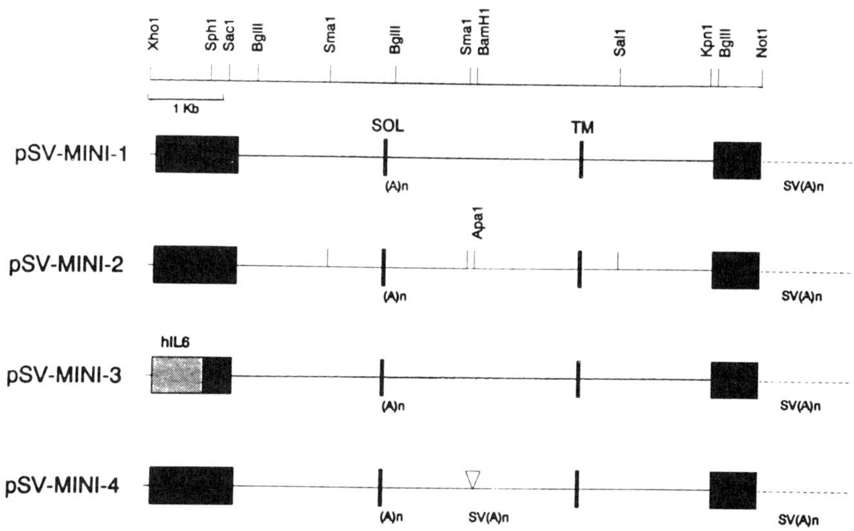


**Figure 3** Structure of minigenes encoding hIL-5Rα. The intron/exon structure of four minigenes is shown, with filled boxes corresponding to the coding sequences. A map with relevant restriction sites is shown on top. SOL and TM indicate the soluble-specific exon and the exon containing the membrane anchor, respectively. (A)n and SV(A)n show the positions of the polyadenylation sites of the SOL exon and coming from the pSV-SPORT vector, respectively. In pSV-MINI-3, the location of the IL-6 sequence is shown in gray.

by gel electrophoresis, comparison of band intensities allows rapid and easy estimation of the relative expression levels of both receptor variants. Experiments using model templates have indicated that a twofold difference in expression level between both receptor isoforms can readily be detected (Fig. 4b).

## V. Expression Pattern of Minigenes in Cos1 and FDC-P1 Cells

Here we describe the transcription pattern from minigenes transfected in two cell types: fibroblastoid Cos1 cells and hemopoietic FDC-P1 cells. All four minigenes were transiently expressed in Cos1 cells and mRNAs were analyzed by Northern blot analysis (Fig. 5a,b). In all cases, only transcripts for the membrane-anchored receptor were detected. No evidence for soluble-specific transcripts could be obtained, even by PCR analysis (not shown). Since in the pSV-MINI-4 construct an additional SV40 polyadenylation site is inserted downstream of the poly-A site of the "soluble" exon, it is unlikely that inability to recognize the latter underlies the absence of the soluble-specific transcript.

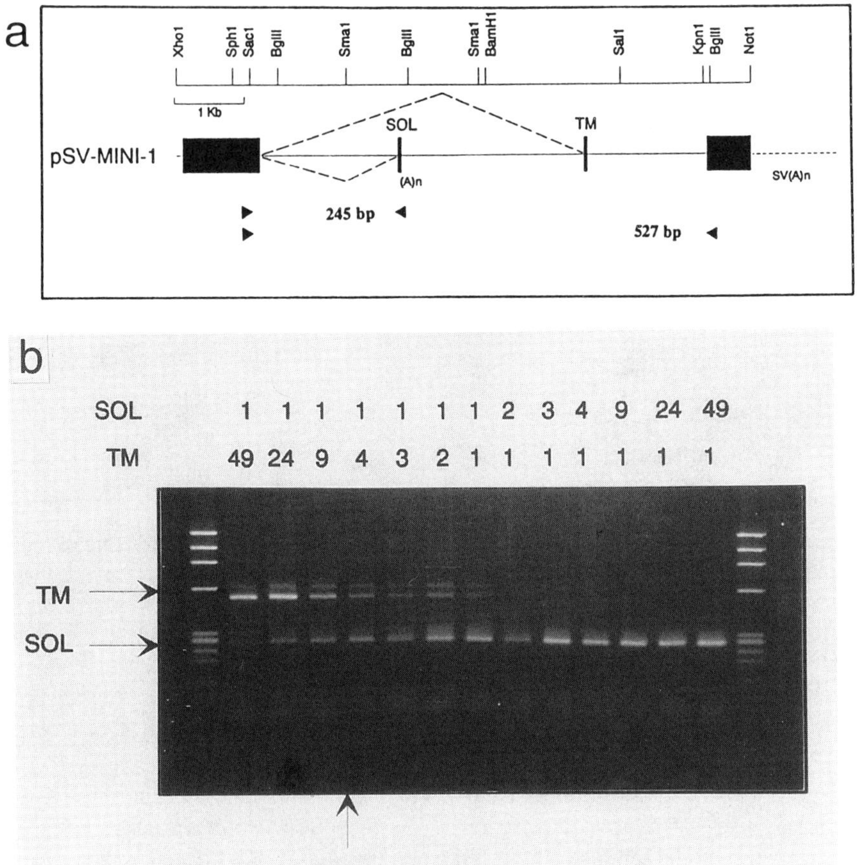


**Figure 4** Design of a competitive RT-PCR for hIL-5Rα isoform detection. (a) Structure of pSV-MINI-1, highlighting the alternative splicing pattern; SOL and TM represent the soluble-specific and transmembrane anchor exon, respectively. Filled triangles show the positions of forward and reverse primers used in the RT-PCR. The size of the amplified fragments is also indicated. (b) Agarose-gel electrophoretic separation of PCR products obtained using a dilution range of model templates for the SOL and TM isoforms. The ratios of both templates in each PCR reaction are shown on top. Arrows indicate the positions of reaction products corresponding to either isoform. Note the approximately fivefold bias in favor of the soluble-specific isoform (vertical arrow).

In FDC-P1 cells, a stable subclone was selected by cotransfection of pSV-MINI-1 with a puromycin resistance marker. In this cell line, a transcription pattern reminiscent of what is observed in mature human eosinophils is obtained (Fig. 5C).

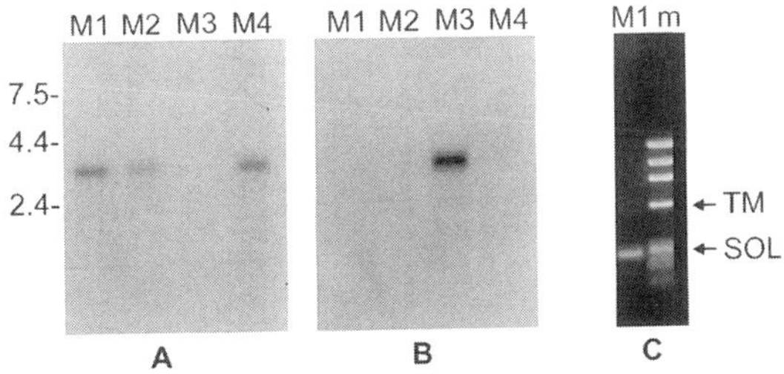


**Figure 5** Expression pattern of hIL-5Rα isoforms in Cos1 and FDC-P1 cells. Panels A and B show Northern blots of transcripts from Cos1 cells transiently transfected with minigene constructs as indicated. In panels A and B, probes correspond to the extracellular domain of hIL-5Rα and hIL-6, respectively. Panel C shows a competitive RT-PCR experiment using mRNA from the FDC-P1 clone, stabile transfected with pSV-MINI-1; SOL and TM indicate the positions of the amplicons derived from transcripts encoding the secreted and membrane-anchored isoforms, respectively.

Since the minigenes are designed to express functional receptor isoforms, we checked for IL-5 binding on the transfected Cos1 cells. As can be seen in Figure 6, all minigenes, with the exception of MINI-3 can direct the expression of a functional hIL-5Rα subunit on the Cos1 cell surface.

Importantly, these results imply that the minigenes used in this study contain the control elements required for the recognition and exon skipping of the "soluble" exon.

## VI. Design of a Minigene-Based Screening System

Such minigene approach can be turned into a screening system, for example, for the detection of regulators controlling the alternative splicing choice. It is well established that a combination of *cis*-elements and *trans*-factors are involved in the selection of one particular exon. It is also clear that in general the regulatory *cis*-elements are located close to the splice acceptor sites. Likewise, our data indicate that all relevant elements required for the recognition of the hIL-5Rα "soluble" exon appear to be contained within the minigenes.

Here we present one example of how derivatives of pSV-MINI-1 can be designed to yield a powerful screening system for splicing regulators/modifiers. In the pSV-MINI-3 constructs, the cDNA encoding most of the extracellular part of the hIL-5Rα has been replaced by a DNA segment encoding IL-6 (two versions have been made: human, hIL-6 and mouse, mIL-6). In parallel, control constructs were made wherein IL-6 was fused, in a similar way as in the minigenes, to hIL-5Rα cDNAs encoding either the secreted or the mem-

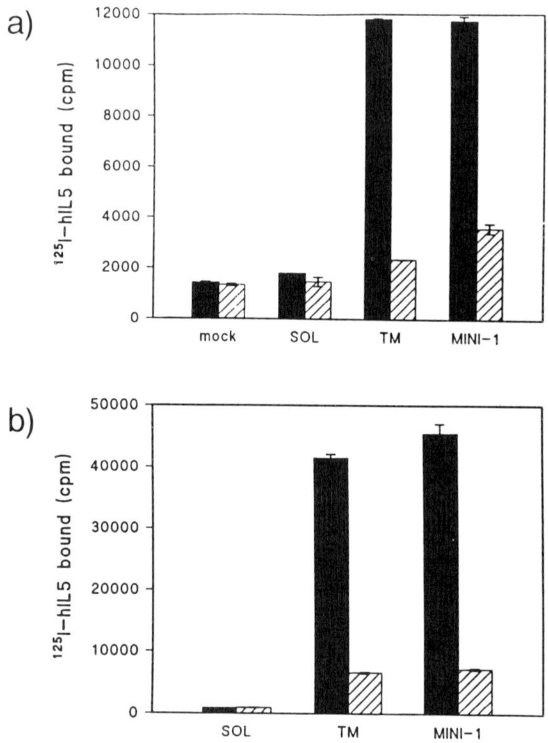


**Figure 6** Detection of minigene-derived hIL-5Rα on Cos1 cells. Panels a–d represent binding experiments using $^{125}$I-hIL-5 on Cos1 cells transfected as indicated; mock: vector only; SOL and TM: pCDM8-SOLhIL-5Rα and pCDM8-TMhIL-5Rα controls (from Refs. 18 and 30, respectively). The MINI series refers to the pSV-MINI vectors. For each experiment, 3 nM $^{125}$I-labeled hIL-5 was incubated with $3.10^5$ Cos1 cells for 45′ on ice. Filled and hatched bars indicate $^{125}$I-hIL-5 binding in the absence or presence of 100-fold excess unlabeled hIL-5.

brane-bound form. Results of transfection experiments in Cos1 cells are shown in Figure 7. IL-6 bioactivity present in Cos1 supernatants is measured by a proliferation assay using an IL-6-dependent cell line. Panel A shows Cos1 cells transfected with the hIL-6-shIL-6Rα control construct. This demonstrates that the IL-6-shIL-5Rα chimera is functional and that a background signal is present due to monkey IL-6 constitutively released by the Cos1 cells into the cell medium. To eliminate this background, we added the D3 monoclonal antibody (a gift from Dr. J Van Snick) which neutralizes hIL-6 and monkey IL-6, but not mIL-6 (Fig. 7, panels b–e). Since the pSV-MINI-3m construct leads to the ex-

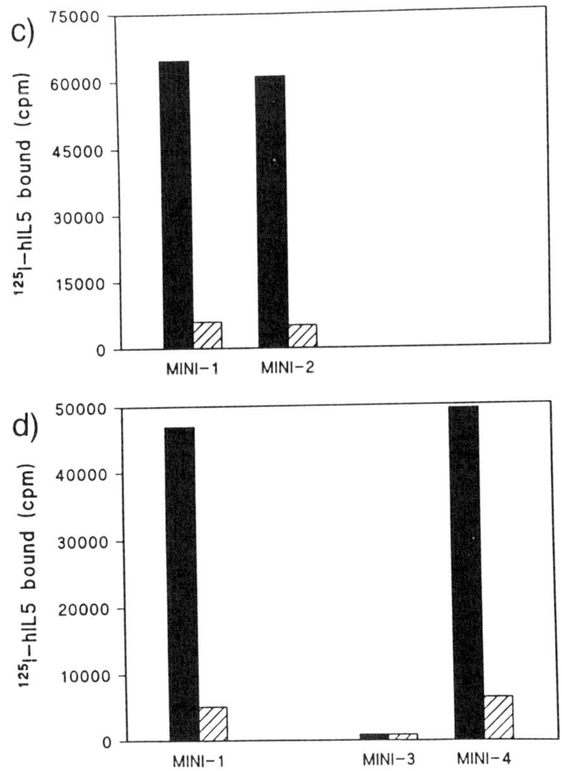


**Figure 6** Continued.

pression of a membrane-bound mIL-6-hIL-5Rα fusion protein, release of mIL-6 activity can hence be used to monitor alterations in the splicing pattern.

## VII. Conclusion

A biological stimulus is often the net result of a balance between agonistic and antagonistic molecules. A prime example of such balance is well illustrated in the developing early *Xenopus* embryo. The dorsoventral patterning and neural plate formation during gastrulation is under control of a signaling center called the Spemann organizer or dorsal lip (42). During the past few years it was found that several polypeptides secreted by this cell group play a dominant role in determining this differentiation pattern. Two of these, chordin and noggin, turned out to be able to capture mature bone morphogenetic protein 4 (BMP-4), hence

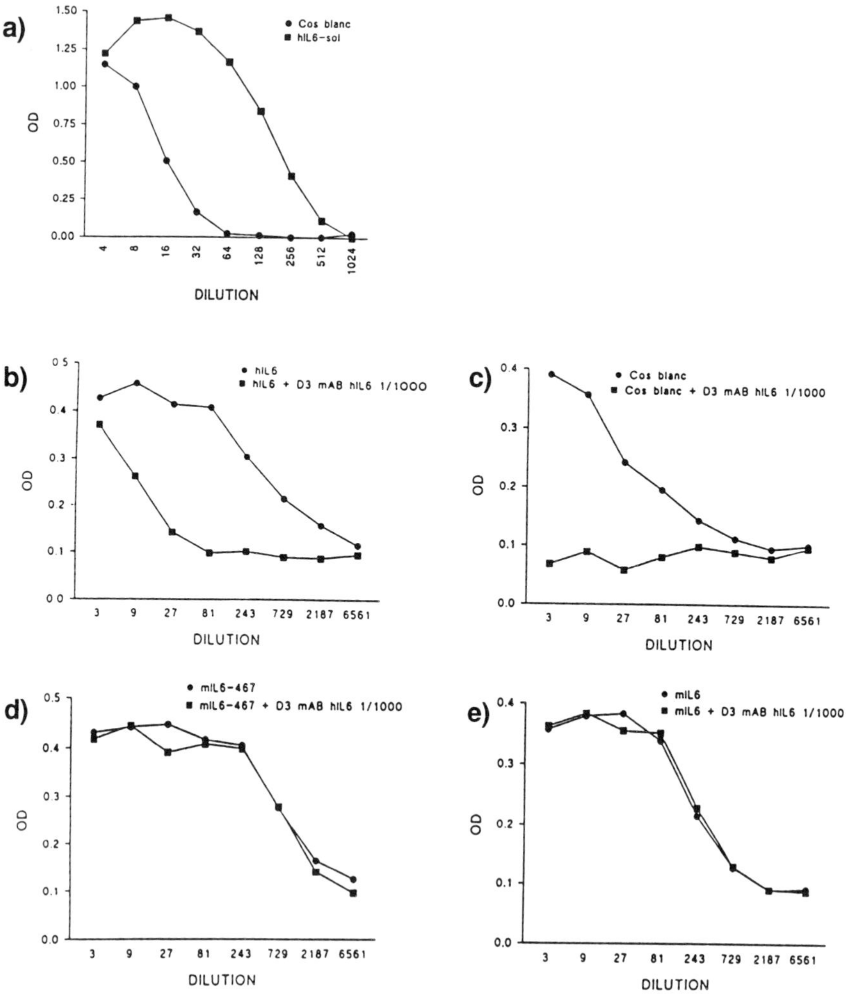


**Figure 7** Detection of IL-6 biological activity. Proliferation curves are shown, obtained using a colorimetric assay on the IL-6-responsive 7-TD1 cell line. Panels a and d show the growth response using supernatants of Cos1 cells transfected with vectors expressing a human or mouse IL-6/shIL-5Rα chimera, respectively (mIL6-467 refers to the mIL-6/shIL5Rα chimeric construct). Panels b and e illustrate the effect of the monoclonal antibody D3 on human and mouse IL-6-driven 7-TD1 proliferation, respectively. Panel c shows the neutralization of Cos1-derived monkey IL-6 by the same antibody.

preventing it from binding to and activating its receptor. Since BMP-4, which is produced in the animal cap and the ventrolateral marginal zone, but not in the Spemann organiser, promotes ventralization and prevents neuralization, the local balance between the diffusable chordin and noggin signals and BMP-4 may determine the final cell differentiation fate (43,44). The very conserved nature of this mechanism is illustrated by the fact that amphibian noggin has similar effects on the development of the *Drosophila* embryo (45). Other examples of such agonist/antagonist equilibria in development are activin/follistatin in mesoderm induction (46) and frzb-1/wnt-8, also in axial patterning (47,48).

In accordance with an important role for secreted cytokine receptors in antagonizing their cognate ligands is a mechanism by which several viruses escape the cellular and host defense machinery. Many larger viruses with more flexible genomes have learned to anticipate the antiviral defense by the acquisition of strategic cellular genes. In addition to virally encoded proteins interfering with the apoptotic cell response, a growing number of so-called viroceptors are being discovered. Genes encoding functional secreted IL-1R and TNFR homologues have been identified in the genomes of several Poxviruses, and their ability to modulate the host antiviral response has been demonstrated (49–52). Not unexpectedly, viral secreted variants of receptors belonging to the four-helical-bundle cytokine family have been described for the interferons (53–56).

Agonist/antagonist equilibria may also influence hematopoietic development: a recent example is the molecular cloning of osteoprotegerin (OPG) (57). OPG is a member of the TNFR family which appears to exist solely as a secreted protein. Transgenic mice expressing OPG were found to exhibit generalized osteopetrosis, associated with a dramatic decrease in osteoclast formation. It was found that osteoclast differentiation from hematopoietic progenitors was inhibited by OPG. The precise mechanism of action is unclear at present, but interference with the interaction of a so far unknown osteoclast differentiation/maturation factor with its receptor, either by ligand or receptor trapping is likely (57).

It is tempting to extrapolate these examples to the situation found with the four-helical-bundle cytokines and their receptors. The mere fact of evolutionary conservation of mechanisms leading to secreted receptor variants throughout the whole receptor family indicates their functional importance. As discussed in a previous section, it is however not always clear whether secreted cytokine receptors will antagonize or agonize the function of their cognate ligands. The net effect may often be concentration dependent, with low concentrations leading to potentiating effects by ligand stabilization or altered biodistribution and high concentrations leading to antagonism. This may be especially true for in vivo situations: administration of sIL-4R, for example, can, depending on the experimental design, both antagonize or superinduce IL-4-dependent IgE production in a murine model system (58). Further underscoring our poor understanding of the biological role of secreted receptor variants is the recent, unexpected finding that secreted TPO-R and G-CSF-R isoforms are able to synergize with steel factor (SF) or flt3/Flk2 ligand (FL) in supporting proliferation of hematopoietic progenitors (59). The molecular mechanism involved is unclear, but perhaps these effects may be explained by a joint action with an autocrine-produced ligand.

Nevertheless, in many cases, secreted receptor variants can function as potent antagonists. Dose-dependent inhibition of ligand binding and bioactivity has been reported for, for example, gp130 (see above) (27), LIFRβ (60), and in the $\beta_c$ group of cytokine receptors for GM-CSFRα (61) and the IL-5Rα (18). The latter case is particularly intriguing given the very high levels of soluble IL-5Rα-specific mRNA in circulating eosinophils. So far no evidence has been obtained for a regulatory in vivo role for the shIL-5Rα in eosinophilopoiesis. However, we recently demonstrated that regulation of the hIL-5Rα splicing pattern can occur in vivo (62). In this study, endobronchial biopsies taken from patients with stable, mild asthma and from control subjects were analyzed by in situ hybridization using isoform-specific probes. In the asthmatic subjects, both atopic and intrinsic, it was found that the number of eosinophils expressing mRNA for the membrane-bound hIL-5Rα isoform correlated inversely with the FEV-1, as a measure for airflow limitation. In contrast, in the same patients, a direct correlation was demonstrated between mRNA for the secreted isoform and the FEV-1, and comparison of the expression of both isoforms showed a significant inverse correlation. These results indicate that regulated expression of the hIL-5Rα isoforms may modulate the eosinophilic contribution to airway inflammation. As discussed before, such effect may be caused by reduced eosinophil activation due to a lower cell-surface hIL-5Rα expression level or by the release of antagonistic secreted hIL-5Rα at the site of inflammation. Little is known however about the intracellular mechanisms underlying the splicing control, nor about the external stimuli which may modulate this splicing pattern. For both these purposes, the in vitro minigene system described here may offer a straightforward strategy and may help to define novel regulatory levels controlling eosinophilic inflammation.

## Acknowledgments

We are greatly indebted to Dr. J. Van Snick for the D3 monoclonal antibody and the IL-6-dependent 7-TD1 cell line. We wish to thank Johan Bostoen and Wim Drijvers for their artwork. This work is supported by a grant from GOA 1205 1296; BOF 01193VEG–97.

## References

1. Singh AD, Sanderson CJ. The role of interleukin-5 in eosinophilia and allergy. In: Testa NG, Lord BI, DexterTM, eds. Hematopoietic Lineages in Health and Disease. New York: Marcel Dekker, Inc., 1997:161–188.
2. Hara T, Miyajima A. Function and signal transduction mediated by the interleukin 3 receptor system in haematopoiesis. Stem Cells 1996;14:605–618.
3. Tavernier J, Plaetinck G, Guisez Y, Van der Heyden J, Kips J, Peleman R, Devos R. The role of interleukin 5 in the production and function of eosinophils. In: Whetton AD, Gordon J, eds. Blood Cell Biochemistry, Vol. 7: Haematopoietic Cell Growth Factors and Their Receptors. New York: Plenum Press, 1996:321–361.
4. Devos R, Guisez Y, Cornelis S, Verhee A, Van der Heyden J, Manneberg M, Lahm H-W, Fiers W, Tavernier J, Plaetinck G. Recombinant soluble human interleukin-5 (hIL-5) receptor molecules. Cross-linking and stoichiometry of binding to IL-5. J Biol Chem 1993;268:6581–6587.
5. Behrmann I, Janzen C, Gerhartz C, Schmitz-Van de Leur H, Hermanns H, Heesel B, Graeve L, Horn F, Tavernier J, Heinrich P. A single STAT recruitment module in a chimeric cytokine receptor complex is sufficient for STAT activation. J Biol Chem 1997;272:5269–5274.
6. Patel N, Herrman JM, Timans JC, Kastelein RA. Functional replacement of cytokine receptor extracellular domains by leucine zippers. J Biol Chem 1996;27:30386–30391.
7. Zon LI, Moreau J-F, Mathey-Prevot B, D'Andrea A. The erythropoietin receptor transmembrane region is necessary for activation by the Friend virus gp55 glycoprotein. Mol Cell Biol 1992;12:2949–2957.
8. Takaki S, Kanazawa H, Shiba M, Takatsu K. A critical cytoplasmic domain of the interleukin-5 (IL-5) receptor alpha chain and its function in IL-5-mediated growth signal transduction. Mol Cell Biol 1994;14:7404–7413.
9. Jenkins BJ, D'Andrea R, Gonda T. Activating point mutations in the common beta subunit of the human GM-CSF, IL-3 and IL-5 receptors suggest the involvement of beta subunit dimerization and cell type-specific molecules in signalling. EMBO J 1995;14:4276–4287.
10. Hannemann J, Hara T, Kawai M, Miyajima A, Ostertag W, Stocking C. Sequential mutations in the interleukin-3 (IL3)/granulocyte-macrophage colony-stimulating factor/IL5 receptor beta-subunit genes are necessary for the complete conversion to growth autonomy mediated by a truncated beta c subunit. Mol Cell Biol 1995;15:2402–2412.
11. D'Andrea RJ, Barry SC, Moretti P, Jones K, Ellis S, Vadas M, Goodall GJ. Extracellular truncations of human beta c, the common signaling subunit for interleukin-3 (IL-3), granulocyte-macrophage colony-stimulating factor (GM-CSF), and IL-5, lead to ligand-independent activation. Blood 1996;87:2641–2648.
12. Muto A, Watanabe S, Miyajima A, Yokota T, Arai K. The beta subunit of human granulocyte-macrophage colony-stimulating factor receptor forms a homodimer and is activated via association with the alpha subunit. J Exp Med 1996;183:1911–1916.
13. Bagley CJ, Woodcock JM, Stomski FC, Lopez AF. The structural and functional basis of cytokine receptor activation: lessons from the common β subunit of the

granulocyte-macrophage colony-stimulating factor, interleukin 3 (IL-3), and IL-5 receptors. Blood 1997;89;1471–1482.

14. Devos R, Guisez Y, Plaetinck G, Cornelis S, Tavernier J, Van der Heyden J, Foley LH, Scheffler JE. Covalent modification of the interleukin 5 receptor by isothiazolones leads to inhibition of the binding of interleukin 5. Eur J Biochem 1994;225:635–640.
15. Yanofsky SD, Baldwin DN, Butler JH, Holden FR, Jacobs JW, Balasubramanian P, Chinn JP, Cwirla SE, Peters-Bhatt E, Whitehorn EA, Tate EH, Akeson A, Bowlin TL, Dower WJ, Barrett RW. High affinity type I interleukin 1 receptor antagonists discovered by screening recombinant peptide libraries. Proc Natl Acad Sci USA 1996;93:7381–7386.
16. Wrighton NC, Farrell FX, Chang R, Kashyap AK, Barbone FP, Mulcahy LS, Johnson DL, Barrett RW, Jolliffe LK, Dower WJ. Small peptides as potent mimetics of the protein hormone erythropoietin. Science 1996;273:458–463.
17. Tavernier J, Tuypens T, Verhee A, Plaetinck G, Devos R, Van der Heyden J, Guisez Y, Oefner C. Identification of receptor binding domains on human interleukin-5 (IL-5) and design of an IL-5-derived receptor antagonist. Proc Natl Acad Sci USA 1995;89:7041–7045.
18. Tavernier J, Devos R, Cornelis S, Tuypens T, Van der Heyden J, Fiers W, Plaetinck G. A human high affinity interleukin-5 receptor (IL5R) is composed of an IL5-specific alpha chain and a beta chain shared with the receptor for GM-CSF. Cell 1991;66:1175–1184.
19. Symons JA, Duff DW. A soluble form of the interleukin-1 receptor produced by a human B-cell line. FEBS Lett 1990;172:133–139.
20. Hwang C, Gatanaga M, Granger G, Gatanaga T. Mechanism of release of soluble forms of tumor necrosis factor/lymphotoxin receptors by phorbol myristate acetate-stimulated human THP-1 cells in vitro. J Immunol 1993;151:5631–5638.
21. Downing JR, Roussel MF, Sherr CJ. Ligand and protein kinase C down-modulate the colony-stimulating factor 1 receptor by independent mechanisms. Mol Cell Biol 1989;9:2890–2896.
22. Tiesman J, Hart CE. Identification of a soluble receptor for platelet-derived growth factor in cell-conditioned medium and human plasma. J Biol Chem 1993;268:9621–9628.
23. Barker PA, Miller FD, Large TH, Murphy RA. Generation of the truncated form of the nerve growth factor receptor by rat Schwann cells. Evidence for post-translational processing. J Biol Chem 1991;266:19113–19119.
24. Müllberg J, Schooltink H, Stoyan T, Gunther M, Graeve L, Buse G, Mackiewicz A, Heinrich PC, Rose-John S. The soluble interleukin-6 receptor is generated by shedding. Eur J Immunol 1993;23:473–480.
25. Hughes DPM, Crispe IN. A naturally occurring soluble isoform of murine Fas generated by alternative splicing. J Exp Med 1995;182:1395–1404.
26. Davis S, Aldrich TH, Ip NY, Stahl N, Scherer S, Farruggella T, DiStefano PS, Curtis R, Panayotatos N, Gascan H, Chevalier S, Yancopoulos GD. Released form of CNTF receptor α-component as a soluble mediator of CNTF responses. Science 1993;259:1736–1739.

27. Narazaki M, Yasukawa K, Saito T, Ohsugi Y, Fukui H, Koishihara Y, Yancopoulos G, Taga T, Kishimoto T. Soluble forms of the interleukin-6 signal-transducing receptor component gp130 in human serum possessing a potential to inhibit signals through membrane-anchored gp130. Blood 1993;82:1120–1126.
28. Frieling J, Sauerwein R, Wijdenes J, Hendriks T, van der Linden C. Soluble interleukin-6 receptor in biological fluids from human origin. Cytokine 1994;6:376–381.
29. Klein B, Brailly H. Cytokine-binding proteins: stimulating antagonists. Immunol Today 1995;16:216–220.
30. Tavernier J, Tuypens T, Plaetinck G, Verhee A, Fiers W, Devos R. Molecular basis of the membrane-anchored and two soluble isoforms of the human interleukin 5 receptor alpha subunit. Proc Natl Acad Sci USA 1992;89:7041–7045.
31. Tuypens T, Plaetinck G, Baker E, Sutherland G, Brusselle G, Fiers W, Devos R, Tavernier J. Organization and chromosomal localization of the human interleukin 5 receptor α-chain gene. Eur Cytok Netw 1992;3:451–459.
32. Murate Y, Takaki S, Migita M, Kikuchi Y, Tominaga A, Takatsu K. Molecular cloning and expression of the human interleukin 5 receptor. J Exp Med 1992;175:341–351.
33. Mosely B, Beckmann MP, March CJ, Idzerda RL, Gimpel SD, VandenBos T, Friend D, Alpert A, Anderson D, Jackson J, Wignall JM, Smith C, Gallis B, Sims JE, Urdal D, Widmer MB, Cosman D, Park LS. The murine interleukin-4 receptor: molecular cloning and characterization of secreted and membrane bound forms. Cell 1989;59:335–348.
34. Tomida M, Yamamoto-Yamaguchi Y, Hozumi M. Three different cDNAs encoding mouse D-factor/LIF receptor. J Biochem 1994;115:557–562.
35. Owczarek CM, Layton MJ, Robb LG, Nicola N, Begley CG. Molecular basis of the soluble and membrane-bound forms of the murine leukemia inhibitory factor receptor α-chain. J Biol Chem 1996;271:5495–5504.
36. Takaki S, Tominaga A, Hitoshi Y, Mita S, Sonada E, Yamaguchiu N, Takatsu K. Molecular cloning and expression of the murine interleukin-5 receptor. EMBO J 1990;9:4367–4373.
37. Baumbach WR, Horner DL, Logan JS. The growth hormone-binding protein in rat serum is an alternatively spliced form of the rat growth hormone receptor. Genes Dev 1989;3:1199–1205.
38. Sotiropoulos A, Goujon L, Simonin G, Kelly PA, Postel-Vinay MC, Finidori J. Evidence for generation of the growth hormone-binding protein through proteolysis of the growth hormone membrane receptor. Endocrinology 1993;132:1863–1865.
39. Cornelis S, Faché I, Van der Heyden J, Guisez Y, Tavernier J, Devos R, Fiers W. Characterization of critical residues in the cytoplasmic domain of the human interleukin-5 receptor α chain required for growth signal transduction. Eur J Immunol 1995;25:1857–1864.
40. Takaki S, Murata Y, Kitamura T, Miyajima A, Tominaga A, Takatsu K. Reconstitution of the functional receptors for murine and human interleukin 5. J Exp Med 1993;177:1523–1529.

41. Wang J, Manley JL. Regulation of pre-mRNA splicing in *Metazoa*. Curr Opin Gen Dev 1997;7:205–211.
42. Spemann H, Mangold H. Uber induktion von embryonalanlagen durch implantation artfremder organisatoren. Roux's Arch Entw Mech 1924;100:599–638.
43. Piccolo S, Sasai Y, Lu B, De Robertis EM. Dorsoventral patterning in *Xenopus*: inhibition of ventral signals by direct binding of chordin to BMP-4. Cell 1996;86:589–598.
44. Zimmerman LB, De Jseu-Escobar JM, Harland RM. The Spemann organizer signal noggin binds and inactivates bone morphogenetic protein 4. Cell 1996;86:599–606.
45. Holley SA, Neul JL, Attisano L, Wrana JL, Sasai Y, O'Connor MB, De Robertis EM, Ferguson EL. The *Xenopus* dorsalizing factor noggin ventralizes *Drosophila* embryos by preventing dpp from activating its receptor. Cell 1996;86:607–617.
46. Schneyer AL, Rzucidlo DA, Sluss PM, Crowley WF Jr. Characterization of unique binding kinetics of follistatin and activin or inhibin in serum. Endocrinology 1994;135:667–674.
47. Leyns L, Bouwmeester T, Kim S-H, Piccolo S, De Robertis EM. Frzb-1 is a secreted antagonist of wnt signaling expressed in the Spemann organizer. Cell 1997;88:747–756.
48. Wang S, Krinks M, Lin K, Luyten FP, Moos M Jr. Frzb, a secreted protein expressed in the Spemann organizer, binds and inhibits wnt-8. Cell 1997;88:757–766.
49. Spriggs MK, Hruby DE, Maliszewski CR, Pickup DJ, Sims JE, Buller RML, VanSlyke J. Vaccinia and Cowpox viruses encode a novel secreted interleukin-1 binding protein. Cell 1992;71:145–152.
50. Alcami A, Smith GL. A soluble receptor for interleukin 1β encoded by Vaccinia virus: a novel mechanism of virus modulation of the host response to infection. Cell 1992;71:153–167.
51. Smith CA, Hu FQ, Smith TD, Richards CL, Smolak P, Goodwin RG, Pickup DJ. Cowpox virus genome encodes a second soluble homologue of cellular TNF receptors, distinct from CrmB, that binds TNF but not LT alpha. Virology 1996;223:132–147.
52. Schreiber M, Rajarathnam K, McFadden G. Myxoma virus T2 protein, a tumor necrosis factor (TNF) receptor homolog, is secreted as a monomer and dimer that each bind rabbit TNFα, but the dimer is a more potent TNF inhibitor. J Biol Chem 1996;271:13333–13341.
53. Symons J, Alcami A, Smith GL. Vaccinia virus encodes a soluble type I interferon receptor of novel structure and broad species specificity. Cell 1995;81:551–560.
54. Colamonici OR, Domanski P, Sweitzer SM, Larner A, Buller RM. Vaccinia virus B18R gene encodes a type I interferon-binding protein that blocks interferon alpha transmembrane signaling. J Biol Chem 1995;270:15974–15978.
55. Upton C, Mossman K, McFadden G. Encoding of a homolog of the IFN-gamma receptor by myxoma virus. Science 1992;258:1369–1372.
56. Mossman K, Upton C, McFadden G. The myxoma virus-soluble interferon-gamma receptor homolog, M-T7, inhibits interferon-gamma in a species-specific manner. J Biol Chem 1995;270:3031–3038.

57. Simonet WS, Lacey DL, Dunstan CRJ, Kelley M, Chang MS, Luthy R, Nguyen HQ, Wooden S, Bennett L, Boone T, Shimamoto G, DeRose M, Elliott R, Colombero A, Tan HL, Trail G, Sullivan J, Davy E, Bucay N, Renshaw-Gegg L, Hughes TM, Hill D, Pattison W, Campbell P, Sander S, Van G, Tarpley J, Derby P, Lee R, Boyle WJ. Osteoprotegerin: a novel secreted protein involved in the regulation of bone density. Cell 1997;89:309–319.
58. Sato TA, Widmer MB, Finkelman FD, Madani H, Jacobs CA, Grabstein KH, Maliszewski CR. Recombinant soluble murine IL-4 receptor can inhibit or enhance IgE responses in vivo. J Immunol 1993;150:2717–2723.
59. Ku H, Kirayama F, Kato T, Miyazaki H, Aritomi M, Ota Y, D'Andrea AD, Lyman SD, Ogawa M. Soluble thrombopoietin receptor (Mp1) and granulocyte colony-stimulating factor receptor directly stimulate proliferation of primitive hematopoietic progenitors of mice in synergy with steel factor or the ligand for Flt3/Flk2. Blood 1996;88:4124–4143.
60. Layton ML, Cross BA, Metcalf D, Ward LD, Simpson RJ, Nicola NA. A major binding protein for leukemia inhibitor factor in normal mouse serum: identification as a soluble form of the cellular receptor. Proc Natl Acad Sci USA 1992;89:8616–8620.
61. Brown C, Beaudry P, Laing TD, Shoemaker S, Kaushansky K. In vitro characterization of the human recombinant soluble granulocyte-macrophage colony-stimulating factor receptor. Blood 1995;85:1488–1495.
62. Yasruel Z, Humbert M, Kotsimbos TC, Ploysongsang Y, Minshall E, Durham SR, Pfister R, Menz G, Tavernier J, Kay AB, Hamid Q. Membrane-bound and soluble alpha IL-5 receptor mRNA in the bronchial mucosa of atopic and nonatopic asthmatics. Am J Respir Crit Care Med 1997;155:1413–1418.

# 13

# Role of the Common β Subunit of the Interleukin-3, Interleukin-5, and Granulocyte Macrophage-Colony Stimulating Factor Receptors

**ATSUSHI MIYAJIMA, TAISEI KINOSHITA, and TAKAHIKO HARA**

University of Tokyo
Tokyo, Japan

## I. Introduction

Hematopoiesis is regulated constitutively and inducibly by stroma cells as well as various cytokines. IL-3, IL-5, and GM-CSF are genetically, structurally, and functionally related to each other and are mainly produced by activated T cells and mast cells, but the production by bone marrow stroma cells is minimum if any. Thus it has been hypothesized that these cytokines play a major role in hematopoiesis in an emergency situation such as inflammation (1). IL-3 and GM-CSF act on broad hematopoietic progenitors and thereby exhibit a number of different biological activities, whereas IL-5 responsive cells are restricted to eosinophils, basophils, and some mouse B cells. However, IL-3, GM-CSF, and IL-5 exhibit almost identical biological activities when they act on the same target cells, such as eosinophilic progenitors.

Molecular cloning of the receptor subunits and reconstitution experiments have revealed that the IL-3, IL-5, and GM-CSF receptors are composed of a cytokine-specific α subunit and a common β subunit, $\beta_c$ (2). Thus the functional overlap among IL-3, GM-CSF, and IL-5 can be explained by this shared receptor subunit. On the other hand, molecular cloning of the receptors indicate that there is only one specific receptor for each cytokine except for murine IL-3, which has two distinct receptors, and therefore the pleiotropic function of a cytokine must be explained by the differential intracellular signaling events depending on the target cells (3). Therefore to study the mechanism of signal transduction by cytokines is important for understanding their function. This chapter describes recent findings on function and signal transduction of the IL-3, IL-5, and GM-CSF receptors.

## II. Structure of the IL-3, IL-5, and GM-CSF Receptors

The high-affinity receptors for IL-3, GM-CSF, and IL-5 consist of a cytokine-specific $\alpha$ subunit and a common $\beta$ subunit, $\beta_c$ (2) (Fig. 1). Both are members of the class I cytokine receptor superfamily. The $\alpha$ subunits are glycoproteins of 60 to 70 kDa with a small cytoplasmic domain of about 50 amino acid residues and bind their specific ligand with low affinity. The shared $\beta_c$ is a glycoprotein of 120 to 130 kDa with two repeats of a conserved motif of the class I cytokine receptors in the extracellular domain. Its large cytoplasmic domain contains two motifs known as box-1 and box-2 which are conserved in members of the class I cytokine receptors with signaling function, such as gp130,

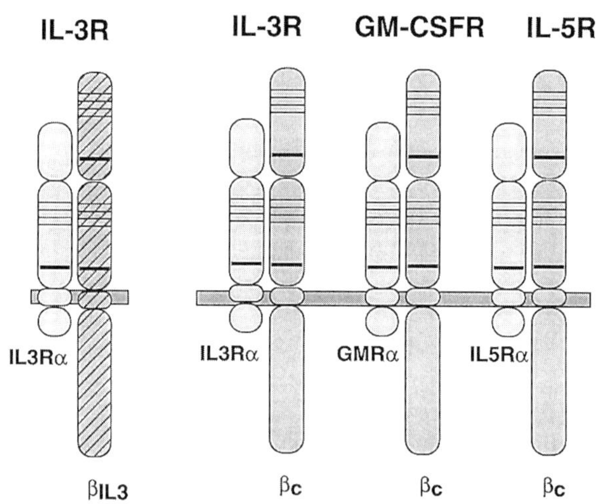


**Figure 1** Structure of the murine GM-CSF, IL-3, and IL-5 receptors. The IL-3, IL-5, and GM-CSF receptors, consist of a cytokine-specific $\alpha$ subunit and the common $\beta$ subunit, $\beta_c$. The IL-3 receptor $\alpha$ subunit forms another high-affinity receptor with the IL-3-specific $\beta$ subunit, $\beta_{IL3}$ which is homologous to $\beta_c$ and is present in the mouse but not in the human.

G-CSF receptor (G-CSFR), IL-2 receptor β (IL-2Rβ), and erythropoietin receptor (EPOR). The $\beta_c$ does not bind any cytokine by itself, but is required for the formation of a high-affinity receptor with any of the three α subunits, IL-3 receptor α (IL-3Rα), GM-CSF receptor α (GM-CSFRα), and IL-5 receptor α (IL-5Rα).

Like receptor tyrosine kinases, dimerization of the receptor subunits is a key step for activation of the class I cytokine receptors. Although the cytoplasmic domains of both α and $\beta_c$ are required for signaling, the $\beta_c$ cytoplasmic domain plays a major role in signal transduction. This is supported by experiments using chimeric receptors that are forced to form a dimer, for example, the chimeric receptors which consists of the $\beta_c$ cytoplasmic domain and the extracellular domain of homodimerizing EPOR-induced full growth signals in response to EPO (4), whereas similar chimeric receptors with a cytoplasmic domain of the α subunits failed to induce any signals (5,6). Thus the α subunits provide the cytokine specificity and $\beta_c$ induces common signals. This model well explains the functional overlap among the three cytokines.

Curiously, in the mouse, there are two homologous β subunits, $\beta_c$ and the IL-3-specific β subunit, $\beta_{IL\text{-}3}$, which binds IL-3 with low affinity and forms a high-affinity receptor with only IL-3Rα (7) (Fig. 1). No functional differences have been found between the two high-affinity mIL-3Rs which consist of either $\beta_c$ or $\beta_{IL\text{-}3}$. There is no evidence that $\beta_{IL\text{-}3}$ exists in the human.

## III. Expression of the Receptor Subunits

Expression of α and β subunits of the IL-3/GM-CSF/IL-5 receptors is mainly restricted to hematopoietic cells (8), while some expression is also found in nonhematopoietic tissues such as testis, placenta, and brain (9–11). The $\beta_c$ and $\beta_{IL\text{-}3}$ are expressed in various myeloid progenitor cells, macrophages, mast cells, $CD5^+$ B cells, and some endothelial cells, but not in erythroblasts, mature T cells, and fibroblasts (12). The expression of the α subunits is more restricted to each cytokine-response cell that is, for example IL-3Rα, but not GM-CSFRα and IL-5Rα, and is expressed in mast cells and multipotential progenitor cells which form CFU mix. In contrast, IL-5Rα is predominantly expressed in eosinophils and a subset of B cells and IL-5 is a major cytokine for eosinophils, but not other hematopoietic cells (13).

Although IL-3 and GM-CSF exhibit a broad spectrum of biological function, IL-5 function is restricted to mainly eosinophils (1). This may be due to the restricted expression of the α subunits. Alternatively, each α subunit may play an active role in inducing cytokine-specific functions. To distinguish these possibilities, we generated a transgenic mouse strain that expresses IL-5Rα ubiquitously by using the constitutive promoter derived from the phosphoglycerokinase-1 (PGK-1) gene (14). Bone marrow cells of the transgenic mice formed colonies of multiple lineages in response to IL-5 in a manner similar to IL-3, indicating that the limited activity of IL-5 is due to the restricted expression of IL-5R$\alpha$ and that IL-5R$\alpha$ is functionally equivalent to IL-3R$\alpha$. The results further suggest that hematopoietic cells have their own differentiation program that is not affected by the $\alpha$ subunits.

It has been a subject of dispute for many years whether or not cytokines are actively involved in the commitment of differentiation. Erythroid differentiation may be a typical example. Epo is a major cytokine for erythroid differentiation and was shown to induce globin expression in IL-3-dependent BaF3 cells when the Epo receptor (EpoR) was ectopically expressed, while IL-3 had no such activity (15,16). This indicates that EpoR delivers a specific signal for differentiation. However, in the transgenic mice expressing the human GM-CSFR, human GM-CSF induced formation of erythroid colonies in the absence of Epo (17). The results clearly indicate that GM-CSF can substitute the effect of Epo if the receptor is expressed. Likewise, an erythroid cell line, SKT6, differentiated in response to Epo and this differentiation was induced by prolactin when the prolactin receptor was ectopically expressed in this cell line (18). Conversely, Epo stimulated multiple hematopoietic cell lineages when EpoR was expressed in hematopoietic progenitors by retrovirus (19). While some difference is found between Epo and IL-3 in BaF3 cells (15,16), the current results rather suggest that hematopoietic cells differentiate by their own program and no specific signals induced by a particular cytokine are necessary for differentiation. Expression of the cytokine receptor is thus crucial for specific function of cytokines. Since IL-5 is the major cytokine for eosinophil development and the expression of the IL-5R$\alpha$ is rather restricted to eosinophils, it is interesting to study the regulation of the receptor in eosinophils. This is also important for development of drugs to control eosinophils.

## IV. Mice Devoid of the IL-3, GM-CSF, and IL-5 Function

The receptor model predicts that $\beta_c$ is crucial for IL-5 and GM-CSF, whereas $\beta_{IL-3}$ may be dispensable since there are two IL-3 receptors (2). To test the role of each $\beta$ subunit, mice devoid of either one of the $\beta$ subunits were generated (20). As predicted, the mice deficient in $\beta_{IL-3}$ showed no apparent phenotype and no hematopoietic defect was found. In contrast, bone marrow cells of the $\beta_c$-deficient mice did not form a colony in the presence of either GM-CSF or IL-5, while IL-3 stimulated colony formation normally, indicating that $\beta_c$ is essential for the function of GM-CSF and IL-5. A significant reduction of the number of eosinophils in the peripheral blood was noticed in the $\beta_c$-deficient mouse, consistent with the idea that IL-5 is the major cytokine for eosinophil development (13).

The $\beta_c$-deficient mice exhibited lung abnormalities, including accumulation of proteinous material in the alveolar spaces and peribronchovascular lymphocytic infiltration. These observations are probably attributable to the deficiency of GM-CSF function since the same phenotype was observed in GM-CSF-deficient mice (21). Alveolar macrophages may play a role in lung homeostasis by clearing surfactacnt and other debris from alveolar space and the function of these macrophages may be impaired in such mice.

The apparently normal hematopoiesis other than a reduced number of eosinophils in $\beta_c$-deficient mice may be due to the presence of the functional IL-3 receptor composed of $\beta_{IL-3}$. Therefore it is interesting to make double knockout mice lacking both β subunits. However, because two β subunit genes are tightly linked on chromosome 15, it is difficult to generate a double knockout mouse line by mating two mutant mice. As IL-3 knockout mouse was generated and was apparently normal, we crossed the IL-3 ligand knockout mouse and the $\beta_c$ knockout mouse to generate the mouse line lacking the entire function of IL-3, GM-CSF, and IL-5 (22). To our surprise, the mice developed normally and were fertile. Hematopoiesis in these mice was similar to the $\beta_c$ knockout. While the eosinophil number was reduced and the lung disease was developed in the double knockout mice, the severity was not changed compared to that of $\beta_c$ mutant mice. Thus the entire function of IL-3, GM-CSF, and IL-5 is dispensable for hematopoiesis in normal life.

The generation of mice devoid of the entire function of the three cytokines may not be too surprising since the major source of these cytokines is activated T cells and basal levels of these cytokines are almost negligible in the normal bone marrow. In fact, it has been hypothesized that the major role of these cytokines is to promote hematopoiesis in an emergency situation such as inflammation (1). To address the question whether these cytokines are essential for emergency hematopoiesis, the mutant mice were infected with parasites and bacteria. However, there was no significant difference in the sensitivity between the normal and mutant mice, indicating that IL-3, GM-CSF, and IL-5 are dispensable even in emergency situations and the defects can be compensated by other unknown cytokines (22). These results indicate a remarkable functional redundancy of cytokines to maintain the hematopoiesis.

The results that knocking out the $\beta_c$ subunit results in no major defect suggest that $\beta_c$ can be a reasonable target for developing new drugs for eosinophil-mediated allergy.

## V. Signal Transduction

Unlike tyrosine kinase receptors, neither α nor β subunit has an intrinsic tyrosine kinase; however, IL-3, GM-CSF, and IL-5 induce rapid tyrosine phosphorylation of various cellular proteins including the β subunit, PI-3 kinase, Vav, Shc, and PTP-1D (2,23). Much effort has been made to identify a tyrosine kinase that associates with the β subunits or that is immediately activated upon cytokine stimulation. Lyn and Fyn, members of the Src family of tyrosine kinase, were shown to be involved in certain cell types (24). However, since some cells lacking these tyrosine kinases are able to respond to IL-3/GM-CSF, the role of these kinases in IL-3/GM-CSF signaling remains unknown. Btk is a member of a structurally distinct family of tyrosine kinases and has been implicated in IL-5 signaling in B cells (25), however, whether a similar type of tyrosine kinase is involved in IL-3/GM-CSF signaling in myeloid cells remains unclear.

In contrast, JAK kinases are now believed to play the most critical role in cytokine signaling (26). The JAK kinase family, which includes JAK-1, JAK-2, JAK-3, and TYK-2, are cytoplasmic proteins of approximately 130 kDa and possess a characteristic structure of conserved regions at the N termini followed by a kinase-like domain and a tyrosine kinase domain at the C terminus. JAK kinases were originally found to be a critical molecule in interferon-mediated signaling and were subsequently shown to be involved in signal transduction by most of the class I and class II cytokine receptors. Jaks are bound to cytokine receptors in the absence of a ligand and are activated by cytokine-induced receptor dimerization. The activated Jaks then phosphorylate tyrosine residues of the receptor itself. The tyrosine phosphorylated sites are used to recruit various signaling molecules with an SH2 domain, which are subsequently activated by the JAKs. Among many signaling molecules activated by cytokines, Shc and Grb2 are adapter molecules that transduce the signal to Ras. Activation of Ras leads to the activation of various signaling pathways including the Raf/Map kinase cascade and PI-3 kinase (27,28). These signaling pathways transduce signals to the nucleus through various signal transducing molecules. In contrast, STAT-mediated signaling pathways link the receptor to the genes directly. Currently, seven members of STAT (signal transducer and activator of transcription) genes have been identified (29). STATs are DNA binding proteins of approximately 90 kDa with an SH2 domain and a tyrosine phosphorylation site at the C-terminal part. The tyrosine phosphorylated STATs then form a homo- or a heterodimer and translocate to the nucleus where they bind to their specific DNA elements.

Conserved motifs among various cytokine receptors known as box-1 and box-2 are present in the membrane proximal regions of the receptors and are responsible for binding and activation of JAKs (26). Deletion analysis of the β subunit revealed that the membrane proximal region (between 455 and 544) including the box-1 region is necessary and sufficient for activation of Jak2 and STAT-5 in response to IL-3 and GM-CSF (30) (Fig. 2). This region is also

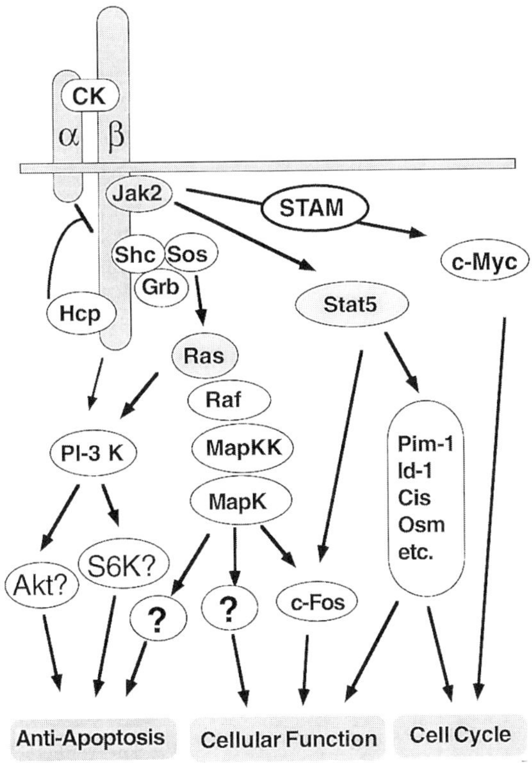


**Figure 2** Signal transduction pathways from the IL-3, IL-5, and GM-CSF receptors. JAK-2 kinase is associated with the β subunit and is activated by cytokine binding to the receptor. JAK-2 then phosphorylates STAT-5 which induces several cytokine-inducible genes. Ras is activated through SOS and transduces signals to downstream molecules, Raf, and PI-3 kinase, which also transmit the signals to their target molecules.

responsible for induction of several cytokine-inducible genes including c-myc. The more distal portion (544 to 626) is required for activation of Ras, Raf, Map kinase, and PI-3 kinase as well as induction of c-fos and c-jun (23,31). The C-terminal portion (763 to the C terminus) appears to be involved in negative regulation, as the deletion of this region enhances signaling such as tyrosine phosphorylation of the β subunit and Shc (31). A tyrosine phosphatase may bind to this region and negatively regulate the signaling. The best candidate of this negative regulator is PTP-1C (HCP), since it has been shown to bind to the β subunit and is also known to be a negative regulator in Epo signaling (32).

## VI. Signals from the Membrane Proximal Region of the β Subunit

The membrane proximal region is indispensable not only for JAK-2/STAT-5 activation, but also for the induction of DNA synthesis (31,33) (Fig. 2). GM-CSF is able to promote the progression from G1 to S phase and to induce DNA synthesis through the mutant β subunits truncated at either 517 or 544, indicating the signals induced by the membrane proximal region are necessary and sufficient for these functions. However, the mechanism to induce DNA replication by cytokine stimulation needs to be elucidated. In addition, the role of STAT-5 in IL-3/GM-CSF function remains unknown. While STAT-5 was originally identified as a transcription factor for the β-casein gene by PRL, β-casein is usually not produced by IL-3/GM-CSF or other cytokines in hematopoietic cells (34,35). To identify the target genes of STAT-5, we have isolated cytokine-inducible early response genes by using the truncated receptor mutant that activates JAK-2/STAT-5, but not the Ras/Raf/Map kinase cascade (36,37). The involvement of STAT-5 for induction of these genes was further verified by expression of a dominant negative form of STAT-5 which inhibits expression of STAT-5-regulated genes (38). Using these strategies we identified several immediate early response genes induced by IL-3/GM-CSF through STAT-5 in an IL-3-dependent cell line, BaF3. These genes include Cis, Osm, Id, pim-1, and c-fos.

Among these genes, Cis is a novel gene encoding an SH2 domain without any other known motif and binds the tyrosine phosphorylated β subunit. As overexpression of Cis suppresses IL-3-dependent proliferation, Cis may be a negative feedback regulator in cytokine signaling (36) (Fig. 3). Recently, Cis-related molecules were found to negatively regulate various cytokine signaling (39). Thus it seems likely that there is a mechanism to down-regulate cytokine signaling through Cis-like molecules. Oncostatin M (Osm) is a member of the IL-6/LIF cytokine subfamily that utilizes gp130 as a signal transducer. Although Osm is produced by hematopoietic cells by cytokine stimulation, it has no significant effect by itself on hematopoietic cells. Recent results indicate that Osm plays a major role in the initiation of definitive hematopoiesis in the mouse embryo (40). Both Cis and Osm genes contain STAT-5 binding sites in their promoter region and these sites actually serve as a positive element (36,37). In contrast, the promoter regions of pim-1 and Id-1 do not have a typical STAT-5 binding site, but their expression is clearly affected by STAT-5 (38). Id-1 is a helix-loop-helix (HLH) protein that antagonizes function of various transcription factors with HLH (41). It is known to block differentiation of certain cell types such as pro-B cells and erythroid cells. Pim-1 is a serine kinase that was originally found to collaborate with v-myc in lymphomagenesis, but its role

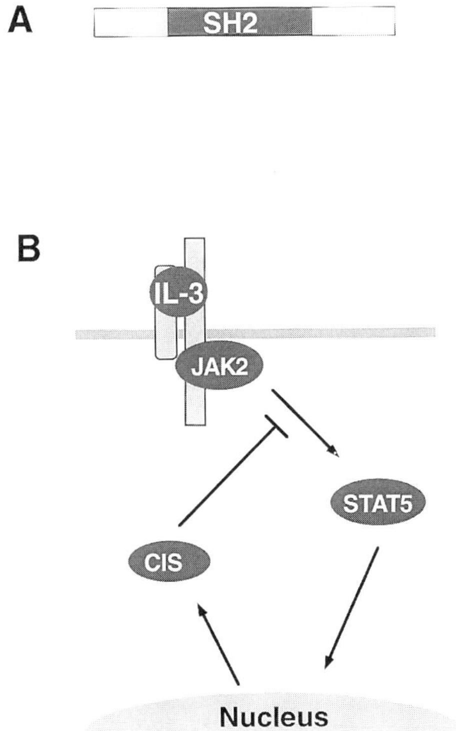


**Figure 3** A feedback mechanism of cytokine signaling. Activation of STAT-5 leads to the induction of Cis, a cytokine-inducible SH2 protein. Cis binds to tyrosine phosphorylated signaling molecules and down-modulates the signaling.

remains unclear (42). As c-fos expression was shown to be controlled by Ras, suppression of c-fos expression by a dominant negative STAT-5 suggests that the optimal induction of c-fos requires multiple signals (38).

Although the membrane proximal domain of the β subunit is also responsible for cytokine-induced c-myc expression, c-myc expression is not affected by a dominant negative STAT-5 (38), indicating that the c-myc expression is independent of STAT-5 and that multiple signaling pathways are activated through the membrane proximal region (Fig. 2). Recently a new adapter molecule, STAM, was found to link JAK and c-myc expression (43). It remains to be tested if STAM also controls STAT-5 activation. Induction of c-myc has been implicated in cell cycle progression. Interestingly, as the net result of the expression of a dominant negative STAT-5 was suppression of DNA synthesis, some of the genes controlled by STAT-5 also contribute to cell cycle progression.

## VII. Role of Ras in IL-3/GM-CSF/IL-5 Function

The membrane distal region of $\beta_c$ is required for the activation of the Ras-Raf-MAPK pathway (Fig. 2). Analysis of signaling molecules activated by the mutant β subunits with a C-terminal truncation, as well as substitution mutants in which tyrosine residues are substituted with phenylalanine within the β cytoplasmic domain, suggest that multiple molecules mediate the Ras activation (23,31): Shc is an adapter molecule that is bound to the tyrosine phosphorylated receptor and recruits SOS, a Ras-guanine nucleotide exchange factor, to membranes where Ras activation takes place. Phosphorylation of Shc by GM-CSF requires the tyrosine residue at 577. A protein tyrosine phosphatase, PTP-1D, is also known to serve as an adapter to recruit SOS, and tyrosine phosphorylation of PTP-1D is mediated through tyrosine 577 as well as other tyrosine residues downstream (23). Thus activation of Ras appears to be mediated by multiple pathways.

Ras activates the Raf kinase cascade that includes Raf, MEK, and MAPK, and also the PI-3 kinase cascade that is supposed to include S6 kinase and c-Akt (27,28). MAPK is believed to be a positive regulator for the induction of gene expression of members of AP-1 transcription factor family including c-fos and c-Jun. Since the activation of the Ras-Raf-MAPK pathway was abolished when the membrane proximal region was deleted, the membrane proximal region is also important for the activation of the Ras pathway. This is also supported by the finding that expression of a dominant negative JAK-2 abrogated the GM-CSF-induced c-fos expression (44). While activation of Ras alone induced c-fos expression, the level of expression was much lower than that of IL-3/GM-CSF stimulation. As described above, expression of a dominant negative STAT-5 also suppressed co-fos induction, and the optimal induction of c-fos appears to be achieved by a combination of two pathways (38).

BaF3 cells expressing the mutant human GM-CSF receptor with truncation at 544, which lacks the ability to activate Ras, follow the cell cycle from G1 to S and induce DNA synthesis in response to GM-CSF (31,33). However, these cells do not proliferate and undergo apoptosis even in the presence of GM-CSF. Expression of an active form of Ras blocks apoptosis and confers on cells the ability to proliferate long term in response to GM-CSF. Thus, by utilizing the mutant receptor, signals for DNA synthesis and suppression of apoptosis are completely segregated (33). The mechanism by which Ras suppresses apoptosis is still unknown. Bcl-2 and Bcl-x are known to be antiapoptotic proteins in various types of apoptosis and are induced by activated Ras (45). However, the suppression of apoptosis by expression of Bcl-2 is much weaker than that by activated Ras, indicating that additional molecules are involved in suppression of apoptosis induced by Ras. The Ras effector mutants with a point mutation in the domain that interacts with the downstream molecules were used to dissect the downstream of Ras (46). For example, the V45E Ras mutant, the substitution mutation of Val at 45 with Glu, abrogates the ability of Ras to interact with the Raf kinase, whereas it retains the ability to activate PI-3 kinase. Interestingly, the V45E Ras mutant as well as an active form of Raf kinase were capable of inducing antiapoptotic function. Thus it seems likely that Ras prevents apoptosis through at least two distinct pathways, the Raf/MAP kinase cascade and the pathway including PI-3 kinase (Fig 2).

The finding that Ras activation results in suppression of apoptosis in hematopoietic cells is consistent with the finding that Ras was constitutively activated in juvenile chronic leukemia due to the lack of functional NF1, a Ras GTPase-activating protein (47). More interestingly, bone marrow cells of NF1-deficient mice were hypersensitive to GM-CSF, suggesting the linkage of Ras activation and leukemogenesis through cytokine signaling pathways.

## VIII. Concluding Remarks

In the past eight years, since the common β subunit was moleculerly identified, much progress has been made in our understanding of the structures and function of the IL-3, IL-5, and GM-CSF receptors. However, there are still many important questions to be addressed. Although receptor expression is the most important for cytokine response, the control mechanism of the receptor expression still remains to be studied. This is particularly important for understanding how cell fate is determined. While huge amounts of information regarding intracellular signaling have been accumulated, these studies were mostly done by using cell lines such as BaF3 cells. Thus it is possible to argue that the cells in the different lineages may use different signaling pathways in the body. In fact, many controversial results have been reported in cytokine signaling even in cell lines. For example, activation of Ras prevents apoptosis in BaF3 cells as described earlier (33), however, it is rather apoptotic in embryonic fibroblasts (46) and is also involved in differentiation of PC12 pheochromocytoma (48). Thus function of a signaling pathway can be variable depending on the cells, and it is therefore important to set up the most physiological cellular system to study cytokine signaling. The results obtained with cell lines need to be reevaluated in more physiological systems such as a primary culture system or mutant animals.

## References

1. Arai K, Lee F, Miyajima A, Miyatake S, Arai N, Yokota T. Cytokines: coordinators of immune and inflammatory responses. Annu Rev Biochem 1990;59:783–836.
2. Miyajima A, Mui ALF, Ogorochi T, Sakamaki K. Receptors for granulocyte-macrophage colony-stimulating factor, interleukin-3, and interleukin-5. Blood 1993;82:1960–1974.
3. Miyajima A, Kitamura T, Harada N, Yokota T, Arai K. Cytokine receptors and signal transduction. Annu Rev Immunol 1992;10:295–331.
4. Sakamaki K, Wang HM, Miyajima I, Kitamura T, Todokoro K, Harada N, Miyajima A. Ligand-dependent activation of chimeric receptors with the cytoplasmic domain of the interleukin-3 receptor β subunit ($\beta_{IL3}$). J Biol Chem 1993;268:15833–15839.
5. Muto A, Watanabe S, Itoh T, Miyajima A, Yokota T, Arai K. Roles of the cytoplasmic domains of the α and β subunits of human granulocyte-macrophage colony-stimulating factor receptor. J Allergy Clin Immunol 1995;96:1100–1114.
6. Eder M, Ernst TJ, Ganser A, Jubinsky PT, Inhorn R, Hoelzer D, Griffin JD. A low affinity chimeric human alpha/beta-granulocyte-macrophage colony-stimulating factor receptor induces ligand-dependent proliferation in a murine cell line. J Biol Chem 1994;269:30173–30180.
7. Hara T, Miyajima A. Two distinct functional high affinity receptors for mouse IL-3. EMBO J 1992;10:1875–1884.
8. Sato N, Caux C, Kitamura T, Watanabe Y, Arai K, Banchereau J, Miyajima A. Expression and factor-dependent modulation of the interleukin-3 receptor subunits on human hematopoietic cells. Blood 1993;82:752–761.
9. Morikawa Y, Tohya K, Hara T, Kitamura T, Miyajima A. Expression of the IL-3 receptor in testis. Biochem Biophys Res Commun 1996;226:107–112.
10. Korpelainen EI, Gamble JR, Smith WB, Goodall GJ, Qiyu S, Woodcock JM, Dottore M, Vadas MA, and Lopez AF. The receptor for interleukin 3 is selectively induced in human endothelial cells by tumor necrosis factor α and potentiates interleukin 8 secretion and neutrophil transmigration. Proc Natl Acad Sci USA 1993;90:11137–11141.
11. Gearing DP, King JA, Gough NM, and Nicola NA. Expression cloning of a receptor for human granulocyte-macrophage colony-stimulating factor. EMBO J 1989;8:3667–3676.
12. Gorman DM, Itoh N, Kitamura T, Schreurs J, Yonehara S, Yahara I, Arai K, and Miyajima A. Cloning and expression of a gene encoding an interleukin 3 receptor-like protein: identification of another member of the cytokine receptor gene family. Proc Natl Acad Sci USA 1990;87:5459–5463.
13. Takatsu K, Takaki S, Hitoshi Y. Interleukin-5 and its receptor: implications in the immune system and inflammation. Adv Immunol 1994;57:145–190.
14. Takagi M, Hara T, Ichihara M, Takatsu K, Miyajima A. Multi-colony stimulating activity of interleukin 5 (IL-5) on hematopoietic progenitors from transgenic mice that express IL-5 receptor α subunit constitutively. J Exp Med 1995;181:889–899.

15. Liboi E, Carroll M, D'Andrea AD, and Mathey-Prevot B. Erythropoietin receptor signals both proliferation and erythroid-specific differentiation. Proc Natl Acad Sci USA 1993;90:11351–11355.
16. Chiba T, Nagata Y, Kishi A, Sakamaki K, Miyajima A, Yamamoto M, Engel JD, Todokoro K. Induction of erythroid-specific gene expression in lymphoid cells. Proc Natl Acad Sci USA 1993;90:11593–11597.
17. Nishijima I, Nakahata T, Hirabayashi Y, Inoue T, Kurata H, Miyajima A, Hayashi N, Iwakura Y, Arai K, Yokota T. A human GM-CSF receptor expressed in transgenic mice stimulates proliferation and differentiation of hemopoietic progenitors to all lineages in response to human GM-CSF. Mol Biol Cell 1995;6:497–508.
18. Wakao H, Chida D, Damen JE, Krystal G, Miyajima A. A possible involvement of Stat5 in erythropoietin-induced hemoblobin synthesis. Biochem Biophys Res Commun 1997; 234:198–205.
19. Dubart A, Feger F, Lacout C, Goncalves F, Vanichenker W, Dumenil D. Murine pluripotent hematopoietic progenitors constitutively expressing a normal erythropoietin receptor proliferate in response to erythropoietin without preferential erythroid cell differentiation. Mol Cell Biol 1994;14:4834–4842.
20. Nishinakamura R, Nakayama N, Hirabayashi Y, Inoue T, Aud D, McNeil T, Azuma S, Yoshida S, Toyoda Y, Arai K, Miyajima A, Murray R. Mice deficient for the IL-3/GM-CSF/IL-5 βc receptor exhibit lung pathology and impaired immune response, while beta IL3 receptor-deficient mice are normal. Immunity 1995;2:211–222.
21. Dranoff G, Crawford AD, Sadelain M, Ream B, Rashid A, Bronson RT, Dickersin GR, Bachurski CJ, Mark EL, Whitsett JA, Mulligan RC. Involvement of granulocyte-macrophage colony-stimulating factor in pulmonary homeostasis. Science 1994;264:713–716.
22. Nishinakamura R, Miyajima A, Mee PJ, Tybulewicz VLJ, Murray R. Hematopoiesis in mice lacking the entire granulocyte macrophage-colony stimulating factor/interleukin-3/interleukin-5 functions. Blood 1996;88:2458–2464.
23. Itoh T, Muto A, Watanabe S, Miyajima A, Yokoa T, Arai K. Granulocyte-macrophage colony-stimulating factor provoles RAS activation and transcription of c-fos through different modes of signaling. J Biol Chem 1996;271:7587–7592.
24. Torigoe T, O'Conner R, Santoli D, Reed JC. Interleukin-3 regulates the activity of the Lyn protein-tyrosine kinase in myeloid-committed leukemic cell lines. Blood 1992;80:617–624.
25. Li T, Tsukada S, Satterthwaite A, Havlik MH, Park H, Takatsu K, Witte ON. Activation of Bruton's tyrosine kinase (BTK) by a point mutation in its pleckstrin homology (PH) domain. Immunity 1995;2:451–460.
26. Ihle JN. Cytokine receptor signalling. Nature 1995;377:591–594.
27. Bollag G, McCormick F. Regulators and effectors of ras proteins. Annu Rev Cell Biol 1991;7:601–632.
28. Rodriguez-Viciana P, Warne PH, Dhand R, Vanhaesebroeck B, Gout I, Fry MJ, Waterfield MD, Downward J. Phosphatidylinositol-3-OH kinase as a direct target of Ras. Nature 1994;52:527–532.
29. Ihle JN. STATs: signal transducers and activators of transcription. Cell 1996;84:331–334.

30. Quelle FW, Sato N, Witthuhn BA, Inhortn RC, Eder M, Miyajima A, Griffin JD, Ihle JN. JAK2 associates with the βc chain of the receptor for granulocyte-macrophage colony stimulating factor, and its activation requires the membrane-proximal region. Mol Cell Biol 1994;14:4335–4341.
31. Sato N, Sakamaki K, Terada N, Arai K, Miyajima A. Signal transduction by the high-affinity GM-CSF receptor: two distinct cytoplasmic regions of the common β subunit responsible for different signaling. EMBO J 1993;12:4181–4189.
32. Yi T, Mui AL, Krystal G, Ihle JN. Hematopoietic cell phosphatase associates with the interleukin-3 (IL-3) receptor β chain and down-regulates IL-3-induced tyrosine phosphorylation and mitogenesis. Mol Cell Biol 1993;13:7577–7586.
33. Kinoshita T, Yokota T, Arai K, Miyajima A. Suppression of apoptotic death in hematopoietic cells by signaling through the IL-3/GM-CSF receptors. EMBO J 1995;14:266–275.
34. Mui AL, Wakao H, O'Farrell AM, Harada N, Miyajima A. Interleukin-3, granulocyte-macrophage colony stimulating factor and interleukin-5 transduce signals through two STAT5 homologs. EMBO J 1995;14:1166–1175.
35. Wakao H, Harada N, Kitamura T, Mui AL, Miyajima A. Interleukin 2 and erythropoietin activate STAT5/MGF via distinct pathways. EMBO J 1995;14:2527–2535.
36. Yoshimura A, Ohkubo T, Kiguchi T, Jenkins NA, Gilbert DJ, Copeland NG, Hara T, Miyajima A. A novel cytokine-inducible gene CIS encodes an SH2-containing protein that binds to tyrosine-phosphorylated interleukin 3 and erythropoietin receptors. EMBO J 1995;14:2816–2826.
37. Yoshimura A, Ichihara M, Kinjyo I, Moriyama M, Copeland NG, Gilbert DJ, Jenkins NA, Hara T, Miyajima A. Mouse oncostatin M: an immediate early gene induced by multiple cytokines through the JAK-STAT5 pathway. EMBO J 1996;15:1055–1063.
38. Mui AL-F, Wakao H, Kinoshita T, Kitamura T, and Miyajima A. Suppression of interleukin-3-induced gene expression by a C-terminal truncated Stat5: role of Stat5 in proliferation. EMBO J 1996;15:2425–2433.
39. Endo T, Masuhara M, M. Y, Suzuki R, Sakamoto H, Mitsui K, Matsumoto A, Tanimura S, Ohtsubo M, Misawa H, Miyazaki T, Leonor N, Taniguchi T, Fujita T, Kanekura Y, Komiya S, Yoshimura A. A new protein containing an SH2 domain that inhibits JAK kinases. Nature 1997; 387:921–924.
40. Mukouyama Y, Hara U Xu M-J, Tamura K, Kim H-J, Kogo H, Tsuji K, Nakahata T, Miyajima A. In vitro expansion of murine multipotential hematopoietic progenitors from embryonic aorta-gonad-mesonephros region. Immunity 1998; 8:105–114.
41. Sun XH. Constitutive expression of the Id1 gene impairs mouse B cell development. Cell 1994;79:893–900.
42. Domen J, Van Der Lugt NM, Laird PW, Saris CJ, Clarke AR, Hooper ML, Berns A. Impaired interleukin-3 response in Pim-1-deficient bone marrow-derived mast cells. Blood 1993;82:1445–1452.
43. Takeshita T, Arita T, Higuchi M, Asao H, Endo K, Kuroda H, Tanaka N, Murata K, Ishii N, Sugamura K. STAM, signal transducing adaptor molecule, is associated with Janus kineases and involved in signaling for cell growth and c-myc induction. Immunity 1997; 6:449–457.

44. Watanabe S, Itoh T, Arai K. JAK2 is essential for activation of c-fos and c-myc promoters and cell proliferation through the human granulocyte-macrophage colony-stimulating factor receptor in BA/F3 cells. J Biol Chem 1996;271:12681–12686.
45. Kinoshita T, Yokota T, Arai K, Miyajima A. Regulation of Bcl-2 expression by oncogenic Ras protein in hematopoietic cells. Oncogene 1995;10:2207–2212.
46. Kinoshita T, Shirouzu M, Kamiya A, Hashimoto K, Yokoyama S, Miyajima A. Raf/MAPK and rapamycin-sensitive pathways mediate the anti-apoptotic function of p21Ras in IL-3-dependent hematopoietic cells. Oncogene 1997;15:619–627.
47. Largaespada DA, Brannan CI, Jenkins NA, Copeland NG. Nf1 deficiency causes Ras-mediated granulocyte/macrophage colony stimulating factor hypersensitivity and chronic myeloid leukaemia. Nat Genet 1996;12:137–143.
48. Serrano M, Lin AW, McCurrach ME, Beach D, Lowe SW. Oncogenic ras provokes permature cell senescence associated with accumulation of p53 and p16$^{INK4a}$. Cell 1997;88:593–602.

# 14

# Interleukin-5 Receptor and Signal Transduction

**KIYOSHI TAKATSU**

University of Tokyo
Tokyo, Japan

## I. Introduction

IL-5 is a dimeric cytokine secreted by several cell types including stimulated helper T (TH) cells, mast cells, and eosinophils (1). While initially identified by its ability to support the growth and differentiation of B cells (2), IL-5 is now known to have pleiotropic effects on the immune system and inflammation (3). Analysis of the three-dimensional structure of crystallized IL-5 revealed that IL-5 possesses a four-$\alpha$-helix bundle motif (4,5) which is conserved among several hematopoietic cytokines. IL-5 exists as a homodimer formed by the interdigitation of two identical monomers (5). Reduction and alkylation of these cysteines, as well as mutation of these cysteines to serines, demonstrated that a native IL-5 monomer lacks all function.

Over the past decade IL-5, IL-3, and GM-CSF with overlapping biological activities have been focused on their role in the pathogenesis of inflammation, allergy, and asthma (6). IL-5, IL-3, and GM-CSF are originally described as hematopoietic growth factors but are now clarified to have pleiotropic activities which include cell activation, proliferation, mobilization, and survival. The gene for IL-5 clusters with the genes for IL-3 and GM-CSF, and their similar exon-intron organization suggests an evolutionary relationship. Among these cytokines, IL-5 is a cytokine more restricted in its properties, regulating the production and function of B cells and eosinophils (3,6).

The IL-5 signal can be transduced through the high-affinity IL-5R that consists of an IL-5-specific subunit, the IL-5 receptor $\alpha$ chain (IL-5R$\alpha$), and a second subunit, IL-5 receptor $\beta$ chain (IL-5R$\beta$) (7–11). Both IL-5R$\alpha$ and IL-5R$\beta$ belong to the cytokine receptor superfamily. IL-5R$\alpha$ specifically binds IL-5 and exists as a transmembrane receptor and as a soluble receptor (7,8). IL-5R$\beta$ is necessary for signal transduction (9,10), which is shared with IL-3R$\alpha$ and GM-CSFR$\alpha$ (12,13) and is called the common beta chain ($\beta_c$) (14). The cytoplasmic domains of both IL-5R$\alpha$ and $\beta_c$ lack domains with known signaling molecules. However, stimulation of cells with IL-5 induces activation of various tyrosine kinases which are essential for IL-5 signaling.

A key question regarding the action of IL-5 in responsive cells has been the molecular mechanism of signal transduction cascade after IL-5 binding to the functional IL-5R which bind IL-5 with high affinity. Here I will overview the structure and function of IL-5 and its receptor system and discuss the current view of IL-5 signaling and its abnormality.

## II. Biological Function of IL-5

### A. Cellular Source of IL-5

Within lymphocyte lineages, the major source of IL-5 is a subset of helper T cells. Among the myeloid lineages, mast cells and eosinophils are the major producers of IL-5. CD4 T cells potentiate the inflammatory and humoral immune responses through the action of Th1 and Th2, respectively, which are distinguished by their patterns of cytokine production (15). Th1 cells produce IFN-$\gamma$, TNF-$\beta$, and IL-2. In contrast, Th2 cells produce IL-4, IL-5, IL-6, IL-10, and IL-13. The most potent factors that influence Th1 and Th2 differentiation are IL-12 (16) and IL-4 (17), respectively. However, the molecular basis of differentiation of these cells from naive T-cell precursors is still unclear. Zheng and Flavell recently reported that GATA-3 is selectively expressed in Th2 cells, but subsides to a minimal level of Th1 (18). Their analyses using antisense GATA-3 and GATA-3 transgenic mice revealed that elevated GATA-3 in CD4 T cells causes Th2 cytokine gene expression.

IL-5 production is regulated in the transcriptional level. Just upstream of the coding sequence of IL-5 is a TATA-like and a CAAT-like transcriptional initiation site. Other positive and negative regulatory elements identified upstream of the IL-5 transcription initiation site include an octamer binding site, a GATA binding site, a CLEO binding site, a CTF binding site, and two GRE binding sites (18–23).

### B. Induction of B-Cell Growth and Differentiation

IL-5 is a synonym of T-cell replacing factor, B-cell growth factor II, IgA enhancing factor, eosinophil differentiation factor, and eosinophil colony-stimulating factor (1). IL-5 induces DNA synthesis of murine chronic leukemic B cells (BCL1) and dextran-sulfate-stimulated splenic B cells. In normal mice, B-cell expression of the IL-5R complex is readily demonstrated on $CD5^+$ B cells which belong to the B-1 lineage that resides largely in the peritoneum (24,25). The B-1 progenitors develop along a stromal cell-dependent IL-5-sensitive pathway, which can bifurcate to $CD5^+$ macrophages under the influence of GM-CSF (reviewed in reference 3). The alternative B-1 pathway leads to B-1a cells which produce natural antibodies that include a spectrum of autoantibodies (26).

B-1 cells from peritoneal washouts respond to IL-5 for polyclonal IgM antibody production. By contrast, the B-2 lineage of B cells is $CD5^-$ and constitute most of the bone marrow and peripheral B cells (27). In mice expressing the IL-5 transgene, B-1 cell population is markedly increased with concomitant hypergammaglobulinemia and autoantibody production (28). Likewise, IL-5-responsive B-1 cells are increased in the spontaneously autoimmune NZB and (NZB $\times$ NZW) $F_1$ mice (29). Resting B cells in spleen do not show proliferative response to IL-5. The potential for conventional B (B-2) cells to express the IL-5R complex and respond to IL-5 can also be demonstrated. IL-5 acts on appropriately activated B cells to induce IgG1 and IgA production (1). Thus evidence has accumulated in murine systems for both an IL-5-sensitive developmental pathway for B-1 cells and a role for IL-5 in the terminal differentiation of mature B-1 cells and appropriately activated B-2 cells. In addition, a role for IL-5 in promoting $C_H$ gene recombination has been demonstrated by synergy with IL-4 which induces recombination in murine B cells activated with anti-IgD dextran (30). Taking all results together, IL-5 is a potent cytokine to induce terminal differentiation of activated mouse B cells and a priming factor to induce accessibility to other cytokines.

In contrast to murine B cells, evidence of a role for IL-5 in human B-cell growth and differentiation has been controversial (31,32). A large collaborative study found no effects on proliferation and Ig production when IL-5 was tested for functional activity on purified human B cells from peripheral blood, tonsils, or spleen using anti-IgM antibodies, phorbolesters, calcium ionophores, *Staphylococcus aureus* Cowan strain I (SAC), or EBV (32). Conversely, several studies subsequently confirmed the potential of human B cells to respond to IL-5. As with mice, IL-5 responsiveness of human B cells depends on the activation signal used. Detection of message for IL-5R$\alpha$ in resting B cells upon the stimulation of B cells with the novel bacteria B-cell mitogen *Moraxella catarrhalis* and Ig synthesis of B cells stimulated with the mitogen in response to IL-5 have provided direct evidence that human B cells are able to respond to IL-5 (31).

### C. Activation of Eosinophil Precursor and Mature Eosinophil

In humans, the biological effects of IL-5 are best characterized for eosinophils. IL-5 induces proliferation and differentiation of eosinophilic precursors in bone marrow. In addition to inducing terminal maturation of eosinophils, IL-5 prolongs eosinophil survival by delaying apoptotic death, possesses eosinophil chemotactic activity, increases eosinophil adhesion to endothelial cells, and enhances eosinophil effector function (6,32–35). In several pathophysiological conditions, an increase in serum and tissue levels of IL-5 and eosinophil numbers have also been described.

Of clinical relevance is a role for IL-5 in hypereosinophilic syndromes, late-phase allergic reaction such as bronchial asthma, and solid organ allograft rejection. The IL-5 mRNA expression has been detected both in bronchial mucosal biopsies and bronchoalveolar lavage T cells of mild atopic asthmatic subjects (36). Selective priming of eosinophil but not neutrophil locomotion by IL-5 suggests that IL-5 plays a significant role in the preferential accumulation of eosinophils at the site of allergic inflammation.

Emerging concepts in understanding the role of IL-5 in asthma have been discussed through the integration of results from animal studies and analyses of clinical disorders. Such an approach could be inhibition of IL-5. Several animal models have been developed to study pulmonary inflammation with characteristic manifestations of airway eosinophilia. Administration of a neutralizing mAb to IL-5 before antigen inhalation suppresses the airway hyperreactivity of mouse, guinea pig, and monkey models (37–39) and appears to be applicable to inhibit the development of allergen-provoked airway eosinophilia and hyperreactivity.

### D. IL-5R-Deficient Mice

IL-5 transgenic (IL-5-Tg) mice expressing the murine IL-5 gene exhibit elevated serum levels of IgM, IgA, and IgE, an increase in number of B-1 cells, autoantibody production, and persistent eosinophilia (28). IL-5-Tg mice also show massive eosinophilia in peripheral blood and infiltration of eosinophils into various tissues. These prominent features of IL-5-Tg mice are waved by passive administration of anti-IL-5 or anti-IL-5Rα mAb. These results imply that IL-5 is deeply involved in the development and activation of B cells and eosinophils in vivo. This was further confirmed by generating IL-5 and IL-5R-deficient mice.

We generated the IL-5Rα-deficient (IL-5R$\alpha^{-/-}$) mice by means of gene targeting in embryonic stem cells (40). We constructed targeting vector to in-activate four cysteine residues in the extracellular domain. Our IL-5Rα$^{-/-}$ mice lack the expression of not only the mRNA expression but also the surface expression of IL-5Rα (40,41). The IL-5Rα$^{-/-}$ mice were born and grew up normally. Total nucleated cell number of spleen, thymus, and lymph node are unaltered in the IL-5Rα$^{-/-}$ mice as compared with these in age-matched wild-type littermates. They are healthy and show normal development of T and B cells. Expression levels of CD4 and CD8 on peripheral T cells and of IgM, B220, CD44, BP-1, CD23, IL-7R, CD43, and CD38 on B cells in spleen are not changed between wild-type and the IL-5Rα$^{-/-}$ mice. Thus knocking out of IL-5R is not lethal, and the IL-5 and IL-5Rα system is not essential for early development of lymphoid systems.

Interestingly, total cell number of the peritoneal cavity of the IL-5Rα$^{-/-}$ mice is significantly lower (one-third) than in wild-type littermates. Furthermore, the IL-5Rα$^{-/-}$ mice show the decreased number of B-1 cells and peripheral eosinophils concomitant with low serum concentration of IgM and IgG3 (41). B cells and eosinophil precursors of the IL-5Rα$^{-/-}$ mice show no IL-5 response for proliferation and differentiation. Thus the IL-5/IL-5Rα system is required to regulate development of B-1 cells, production of natural antibody, and eosinophilopoiesis. Impaired eosinophilopoiesis in IL-5Rα$^{-/-}$ mice enhances the survival of intracranial worms of *Angiostrongylus cantonensis*, while intracranial worms in IL-5 transgenic mice are expelled (40,41). These results clearly indicate that IL-5-induced eosinophils serve as a potent effector cell in the killing of the intracranial worms in mice.

IL-5-deficient (IL-5$^{-/-}$) mice were also generated (42). The phenotype of the IL-5$^{-/-}$ mice is essentially identical to that of IL-5Rα$^{-/-}$ mice.

## III. Structure of IL-5 Receptor

### A. Molecular Constitution of IL-5 Receptor

IL-5 binds to a specific cell surface receptor (IL-5R) that consists of two distinct membrane proteins, IL-5Rα and $\beta_c$.

#### *IL-5Rα*

The gene for IL-5Rα maps to the long arm of human and mouse chromosome 3 (43) and chromosome 6 (44), respectively, although its human gene map is not complete. The murine IL-5Rα gene is known to consist of 11 exons (44). The 5′ regulatory elements of the murine gene include binding sites for AP-1, Sp1, NF-κB, NF-IL-6, and GATA-1 (44,45). The IL-5Rα cDNA encodes a 420 amino acid protein consisting of a leader sequence, an extracellular domain, a transmembrane domain, and a cytoplasmic domain (8). In addition, a soluble form of IL-5Rα (sIL-5Rα) is expressed (46,47). A human sIL-5Rα is derived from alternatively spliced mRNA which excludes the last three exons that encode the transmembrane and cytoplasmic domains (9,46).

The extracellular portion of IL-5Rα is composed of three fibronectin type-III-like modules (7,8). The two membrane proximal modules contain the conserved superfamily structures; four conserved cysteines in the middle domain and the tryptophan-serine-X-tryptophan-serine or WSXWS (where X is any amino acid) motif (48) in the membrane proximal domain. The cytoplasmic domain of IL-5Rα has no homology with signaling molecules such as kinases, phosphatases, nucleotide binding proteins, and src homology domains, but it has regions rich in proline (Pro-Pro-X-Pro) following the transmembrane domain (7) that is well conserved between IL-5Rα as well as among receptors for IL-3, GM-CSF, prolactin, and growth hormone. This region shows homology with a part of the actin-binding domain of β-spectrin (49).

Recombinant mouse IL-5Rα with a molecular mass of 60 kDa binds IL-5 with low affinity and is not capable of transducing a signal. The native IL-5 dimer binds IL-5Rα in a 1:1 stoichiometry (46). Alone, human IL-5Rα can bind either human or murine IL-5 with a dissociation constant of approximately 1 nM (50,51). This is in contrast to murine IL-5Rα, which binds murine IL-5 with much greater affinity than it binds human IL-5 despite the 70% homology for IL-5 between these two species (52,53). Although deglycosylated IL-5 is functional, only glycosylated IL-5Rα is capable of binding IL-5 (8,51). Alone IL-5Rα is not capable of transducing a signal (11).

A region involved in IL-5 binding in the N-terminal module of IL-5Rα was first targeted by covalent modification using isothiazolones (54). Derivatization of Cys66 on its free sulfhydryl group disrupted IL-5 binding. However, a cysteine to serine mutant at this position still bound IL-5. Asp55, Asp56, Tyr57, and Glu58 within N-terminal module as crucial for binding IL-5 are identified by alanine scanning mutagenesis. This cluster of negatively charged amino acids may interact with the cluster of positively charged amino acids in the β-strand region of IL-5 that has been identified as important for IL-5Rα binding. Five putative binding determinants including Arg188, Cys249, and Cys296 of the third module are targeted for site-directed mutagenesis to be important for binding IL-5.

The sIL-5Rα binds IL-5 with an affinity similar to membrane bound IL-5Rα, suggesting that the transmembrane and cytoplasmic domains of IL-5Rα contribute little energetically to IL-5 binding (8,9,51). The biological role of sIL-5Rα is unknown but is hypothesized to act as an IL-5 carrier in vivo and thereby prolong the cytokines' half-life. Conversely, the ability of sIL-5Rα to neutralize IL-5 ($IC_{50}$ = 12 nM) suggests a role in down-regulating IL-5-mediated immune responses (51).

The dimeric configuration of IL-5 suggests the possibility of receptor bivalency. However, several complementary techniques, including analytical ultracentrifugation, titration microcalorimetry, analysis of gel filtration, and plasmon resonance have exhaustively demonstrated that the native IL-5 dimer binds IL-5Rα in a 1:1 stoichiometry (51,55). Based on titration microcalorimetry and plasmon resonance results, it is also speculated that a possible conformation change occurs upon IL-5 engagement of IL-5Rα although the mechanism is entirely unknown.

### $\beta_c$

The gene for $\beta_c$ is on human chromosome 22, but details of its structure are limited. The murine gene is on chromosome 15 and contains 14 exons spanning 28 kb (56). In the 5′ flanking sequence, potential recognition sequences for the hematopoietic transcription factors GATA-1 and PU.1 are present, in addition to a TATA-like transcriptional initiation sequence. Expression of $\beta_c$ is induced with LPS or IL-1 stimulation (57–59). The translated $\beta_c$ protein consists of a 16 amino acid leader sequence, a 422 amino acid extracellular domain, a 28 amino acid transmembrane domain, and a 432 amino acid cytoplasmic domain (15). The extracellular domains consist of a double repeat of the classic two module superfamily domain. Each domain includes two fibronectin type-III-like modules with the more N terminal containing the four conserved cysteines and the more C terminal including the WSXWS motif. The proline-rich region of the cytoplasmic domain of the $\beta_c$ contains a Pro-X-Pro sequence that exists in the membrane proximal, box-1, region of other members of the cytokine receptor family (14). The $\beta_c$ has a relatively large cytoplasmic domain (~440 amino acid residues) and its cytoplasmic domain has no homology with signaling molecules such as kinases, phosphatases, nucleotide binding proteins and src homology domains. Studies using a series of cytoplasmic deletion mutants of the human $\beta_c$ have revealed that there are at least two distinct regions in the cytoplasmic domain of $\beta_c$ required for growth signal transduction (60,61).

The $\beta_c$ subunit does not bind IL-5 alone, but in the human system $\beta_c$ associates with IL-5Rα to enhance the affinity for IL-5 by a few-fold, resulting in a high-affinity dissociation constant on the order of 300 pM. This enhancement of affinity is accounted for by a reduction in the off rate of IL-5, as the on rate is unchanged from that of IL-5Rα alone (62). The $\beta_c$ subunit also enhances the efficiency of IL-5 internalization, which explains the reduction in surface expression of high-affinity IL-5R following IL-5 stimulation (62). The $\beta_c$ is absolutely necessary for signal transduction. There is no significant association between $\beta_c$ and sIL-5Rα, which explains the ability of sIL-5Rα to neutralize IL-5 activity. This is in contrast to the related IL-6 receptor system in which sIL-6R is capable of binding to gp130 and IL-6 to transduce a signal

(63,64). The binding stoichiometry between IL-5 and $\beta_c$ in the high-affinity complex is suggested by indirect cross-linking studies to be 1:1 like that for IL-5R$\alpha$ (55).

## IV. IL-5 Signal Transduction

The molecular mechanism by which IL-5 binding to its receptor elicits diverse responses by subsets of leukocytes remains an enigma. Accumulating evidence suggests that phosphatidyl inositol turnover, calcium mobilization, and activation of protein kinase A are not essential for IL-5-induced differentiation signals (65). Although tyrosine phosphorylation is usually one of the earliest biochemical events in the signal transduction cascade induced by growth factors whose receptors possess endogenous enzymatic activity (66), the cytoplasmic domains of IL-5R$\alpha$ and $\beta_c$, like other cytokine receptors, have no homology with signaling molecules such as kinases, phosphatases, nucleotide binding proteins, and src homology domains. Nevertheless, IL-5 does induce rapid tyrosine phosphorylation of cellular proteins (67,68) and enhances the transcription of nuclear proto-oncogenes (69). The suppression of IL-5-induced proliferation with a tyrosine kinase inhibitor (70) indicates that activation of tyrosine kinases is indispensable in IL-5 signal transduction. At least three different signaling pathways can be activated by IL-5 stimulation.

### A. Activation of the Ras Pathway and Proto-Oncogenes

One of the earliest events that occurs after IL-5 binds to its receptor is the rapid tyrosine phosphorylation of $\beta_c$ and several cellular substrates including Shc and Vav. The tyrosine phosphorylated Shc can initiate the Ras pathway by binding to an adapter protein called Grb2 through its SH2 domain (71,72). Grb2 also binds through its SH3 domain to a proline-rich motif of Sos, a nucleotide exchange protein. Sos then activates Ras, which is a GTP binding protein that works downstream of tyrosine kinases in the growth signaling pathway (73–75). Downstream of Ras is a serine/threonine kinase called Raf which activates the unique bifunctional kinase MEK that can phosphorylate both tyrosine and serine/threonine. The only known substrate for MEK is the serine/threonine kinase MAPK. Once activated, MAPK triggers nuclear transcription factors that lead to the induction of several gene products including proto-oncogenes. Activation of the Ras cascade is dependent on both the cytoplasmic region of IL-5R$\alpha$ and the region between Leu626 and Ser763 of $\beta_c$ (56).

It is well established that induction of tyrosine phosphorylation and nuclear proto-oncogene expression are critical for cytokine signal transduction (69). Expression of *c-fos*, *c-jun*, and *c-myc* proto-oncogene mRNA is rapidly induced upon stimulation with IL-5 (76). This proto-oncogene expression is not induced in cells transfected with IL-5Rα mutants that lack either the proline-rich motif or a sequence just downstream of the proline-rich region in the cytoplasmic domain (76). The region between Leu626 and Ser763 of $\beta_c$ is also necessary for induction of *c-fos* and *c-jun* expression, while the region between Arg455 and Glu517 is responsible for induction of c-myc expression and pim-1, a proto-oncogene which encodes a serine/threonine kinase that cooperates with *c-myc* and plays a role in the cell proliferation (60).

### B. Activation of JAK Kinases and STAT Proteins

A family of cytoplasmic protein tyrosine kinases called Janus kinases (alternatively referred to as just another kinase family) has been described and includes JAK-1, JAK-2, JAK-3, and TYK-2 has been described (reviewed in reference 77). These proteins contain a kinase domain and a kinase-like domain, but lack SH2, SH3, and membrane-spanning domains. Recent studies revealed that the JAK family of kinases couples ligand binding to cytokine receptors with tyrosine phosphorylation of cellular proteins (77). JAK kinases associate with a proline-rich segment of a cytokine receptors cytoplasmic domain called the box-1 region. Upon ligand engagement of the receipt, activated JAK kinases phosphorylate tyrosines on cytoplasmic proteins which function as signal transducers and activators of transcription (STAT) (77,78). These phosphorylated STAT proteins dimerize, translocate to the nucleus, and bind to DNA response elements (79,80).

JAK-2 is rapidly tyrosine phosphorylated in response to IL-5 (69,76,81). A significant but lesser extent of tyrosine phosphorylation of JAK-1 is also observed in response to IL-5 (81). However, JAK-3 is not tyrosine phosphorylated. The membrane proximal proline-rich sequence of the cytoplasmic domain of IL-5Rα, which is conserved among the α chains of IL-3R, IL-5R, and GM-CSFR, is essential for tyrosine phosphorylation of JAK-2 (76,82). The six amino acids downstream from the proline-rich region is also important, though not essential. A role for the box-1 region of $\beta_c$ in JAK-2 activation is also demonstrated (83).

Treatment of human peripheral blood monocytes or basophils with IL-3, IL-5, IL-10, or GM-CSF activates DNA binding proteins which are tyrosine phosphorylated (84). An IL-3 and GM-CSF responsive STAT protein has been identified as STAT-5 (85), which is one of the substrates for JAK-2 kinase. IL-5 also induces STAT-5 activity (81,85,86), which is mediated by both JAK-2 and to a lesser extent JAK-1. Activation of JAK-2 and STAT-1 has been shown in eosinophils in response to IL-5 (86–91). These results suggest different JAK-STAT signaling pathways for B cells and eosinophils.

The activation of STAT-5 in response to IL-3, IL-5, and GM-CSF suggests a common signaling pathway through IL-3R, IL-5R, and GM-CSFR, all of which share $\beta_c$. Transfection of the dominant negative form of STAT-5 into a GM-CSF responsive cell line inhibits GM-CSF-induced cell proliferation (92), indicating the involvement of STAT-5 activation in signaling through the $\beta_c$. As IL-3, GM-CSF, and IL-5 exert different functions in some cell types, more subtle modulation of STAT-5 or other signaling molecules may result in a cytokine-specific response. Although the specificity of IL-5 is mainly due to the restricted expression of IL-5R$\alpha$ (93,94), efforts are continuing to determine whether IL-5R$\alpha$-specific cytoplasmic residues also contribute to IL-5-specific signaling pathways. The genes activated by STAT-5 have been examined and found that STAT-5 can induce the gene expression of Oncostatin M and a cytokine-inducible SH2 protein Cis (95,96).

### C. The Activation of Bruton and Src-Family Tyrosine Kinases

Nonreceptor protein tyrosine kinases are key regulators of the development and function of lymphocytes. The structures of these kinases are characterized by the src homology domains which serve as protein-protein interaction sites. The Bruton tyrosine kinase (Btk) belongs to a new subfamily of nonreceptor tyrosine kinases, which includes TecI, TecII, Itk, and DSrc28C (97). Btk, a B-cell-specific tyrosine kinase, contains SH2 and SH3 domains and is the defective gene in human X-linked agammaglobulinemia (XLA) (98,99) and murine X-linked immunodeficiency (XID). In XLA patients, various point mutations and insertions of nucleotide in the *btk* gene are found and in XID mouse a single conserved amino acid residue within the pleckstrin homology (PH) domain of mouse Btk is mutated (100,101). XLA patients have less than 1% of the normal levels of mature B cells in the peripheral blood and dramatically reduced immunoglobulin levels. In XID mice, B-cell numbers are reduced to around 50% of normal and levels of IgM and IgG3 are greatly decreased. B cells from XID mice are unresponsiveness to IL-10, CD38, and CD40 stimulation (102–104). This indicates that Btk is critical for multiple pathways important in B-cell function and Btk dependence of human B cells appears to be more potent than that of mouse B cells.

The number of IL-5 responsive B cells and their capacity to respond to IL-5 is greatly reduced in XID mice because of impaired IL-5 signaling (105,106). However, eosinophil progenitors and mature eosinophils in XID mice respond to IL-5 to an extent similar to normal mice (105). We obtained essentially the same results as above by using B cells from $Btk^{-/-}$ mice (Uehara et al., unpublished data). These results indicate that low responsiveness to IL-5 in XID mice is lineage restricted and that IL-5-mediated signaling cascades in eosinophils are somehow different from those in B cells.

The kinase activity of Btk in IL-5-stimulated early B-cell line Y16 was examined by an immune complex kinase assay. Significantly enhanced Btk activity was detected in anti-Btk immunoprecipitates following 5 to 20 min of IL-5 stimulation (70). No enhanced Btk activity was detected in IL-5-stimulated cells which lacked the cytoplasmic domain of IL-5Rα. Btk contains SH2 and SH3 domains, which are important for signal transduction in many nonreceptor tyrosine kinases. Recently, signaling through IL-5R, which ordinarily provides a costimulus with other mitogenic factors, was completely blocked in fynTnull B cells, while an IL-5-inducible increase in Btk kinase activity was observed from both wild-type and fynTnull animals (107). B cells from $Lyn^{-/-}$ mice are unable to respond to CD38 ligation for proliferation by virtue of the inability of Btk activation (108). Furthermore, B cells from either $Fyn^{-/-}$ and $Lyn^{-/-}$ mice showed the impaired proliferative response to IL-5 (Yasue et al. unpublished data). Interaction of Btk with Fyn and Lyn has been shown in various experimental systems in vitro (109). If Btk, Lyn, and Fyn are all part of the same signaling cascade, the above observations suggest that Btk is the more IL-5R proximal element than Fyn and Lyn is upstream of Btk.

A critical role of Btk in IL-5 signaling was further supported by isolation of a gain-of-function Btk mutant, Btk*, which drives growth of NIH3T3 cells in soft agar (110). Btk* results from a single-point mutation in the PH domain, where a glutamic acid is mutated to a lysine at position 41. Expression of Btk* also relieves IL-5 dependence of a B-lineage cell line. This transforming activity required kinase activity, a putative autophosphorylation site, and a functional PH domain. These results show that Btk may play a critical role in B-cell development and activation by stimuli such as IL-5 and CD38.

## V. Mechanism of IL-5 Receptor Activation

### A. Recruitment of $\beta_c$ to IL-5Rα is an IL-5-Dependent Process

Functional complexes of many cytokine receptors are composed of two distinct subunits and undergo ligand-induced dimerization or multimerization (80). For example, IL-6R is composed of two subunits, IL-6Rα and gp130, whose functional form is a heterotetramer composed of two molecules each of two subunits, and homodimerization of gp130 was displayed to be involved n activation of IL-6R (111). The functional receptors for IL-3, GM-CSF, and IL-5 are composed of two subunits, ligand-specific α chain and $\beta_c$. The $\beta_c$ has been reported to form a homodimer in hGM-CSFR and hIL-5R systems irrespective of ligand stimulation and be tyrosine phosphorylated after association with their α chain in response to relevant ligand (80,112,113). The precise stoichiometry of each subunit of hIL-5R remains to be elucidated for better understanding of hIL-5 signal transduction.

To address this issue cellular extract of nonstimulated IL-5-responsive human cell line TF-h5Rα was immunoprecipitated with anti-IL-5Rα mAb.

Western blot analyses using anti-IL-5Rα or anti-$\beta_c$ mAb revealed that in the absence of IL-5, anti-IL-5Rα mAb did not coimmunoprecipitate $\beta_c$ (90). Coimmunoprecipitation of $\beta_c$ with hIL-5Rα was observed only when stimulated with IL-5. We did not find a homodimer of $\beta_c$ in the immune complexes. Anti-βc mAb was also able to immunoprecipitate hIL-5Rα together with tyrosine phoshorylated $\beta_c$ only when cells were stimulated with IL-5. Although tyrosine phosphorylation of $\beta_c$ was also observed in cellular extracts of GM-CSF-stimulated TF-h5Rα, no association with hIL-5Rα was observed. Taken collectively, our results imply that hIL-5Rα and $\beta_c$ do not preform heterodimer in the absence of hIL-5. The hIL-5Rα recruits $\beta_c$ in the presence of IL-5 resulting in formation of a heterodimer and activate IL-5 signaling pathway.

To test whether multimerization of $\beta_c$ is able to transduce IL-5 signal, chimeric IL-5R possessed the extracellular domain of IL-5Rα and the transmembrane and cytoplasmic domains of $\beta_c$ are constructed (76). Transfectants expressing the chimeric IL-5R together with a native $\beta_c$ proliferative in response to IL-5, although they require 100-fold as much as IL-5 compared with transfectants expressing wild-type IL-5Rα. Furthermore, JAK-1/STAT-5 activation is observed and JAK-2 activation is hardly detectable (76,82). These results imply that dimerization of the cytoplasmic domain of $\beta_c$ confers the ability, in part, to transduce a growth signal through JAK-1/STAT-5 pathway in the absence of the cytoplasmic domain of IL-5Rα. Therefore we conclude that an IL-5 signal appears to be mainly transduced through an IL-5Rα/$\beta_c$ heterodimer via JAK-2/STAT-5 pathway and through cytoplasmic dimerization of $\beta_c$ in part via JAK-1/STAT-5 pathway.

### B. Association of JAK-2 and JAK-1 with hIL-5Rα and $\beta_c$, Respectively

Although IL-5-induced tyrosine phosphorylation of cellular proteins are essential for biological activities, both IL-5Rα and $\beta_c$ subunits do not contain intrinsic kinases involved in signaling, suggesting that the receptor closely associates with kinases, of which most suspected candidates are JAK-1 and JAK-2. In the hGM-CSFR system, JAK-2 has been shown to be associated constitutively with $\beta_c$ (112,113). Lyn kinase was also reported to be associated with $\beta_c$ and activated by IL-5. However, there has been no report about kinases associated with hIL-5Rα. We evaluated physical association of JAK-1 and JAK-2 with each component of hIL-5R complex.

Cellular extracts of TF-h5Rα were immunoprecipitated with anti-hIL-5Rα mAb followed by western blotting with anti-JAK-2 and anti-JAK-1 mAbs. Results revealed that JAK-2 was coimmunoprecipitated with hIL-5Rα regardless of IL-5 stimulation (90). On the other hand, JAK-1 was not found in the immunoprecipitates with anti-hIL-5Rα mAb in the absence of IL-5, but was coprecipitated in the presence of IL-5. JAK-1 was coimmunoprecipitated with

$\beta_c$ by anti-$\beta_c$ mAb regardless of IL-5 stimulation. Furthermore, JAK-2 as well as JAK-1 were tyrosine phosphorylated only when cells were stimulated with hIL-5. These results indicate that JAK-2 and JAK-1 are constitutively associated with hIL-5R$\alpha$ and $\beta_c$, respectively, and are activated by IL-5 stimulation.

To determine the region necessary for binding of JAK-2 to hIL-5R$\alpha$, we generated several glutathion S-transferase (GST) fusion proteins that contained the complete cytoplasmic domain or C-terminal truncated cytoplasmic domain of hIL-5R$\alpha$. The GST fusion protein of the cytoplasmic region of $\beta_c$ was also prepared. Cellular extracts were incubated with beads coupled with GST fusion proteins and proteins bound to the beads were analyzed by western blotting. GST fusion proteins containing the complete cytoplasmic domain of hIL-5R$\alpha$ is able to bind to JAK-2 (90). Using five different GST fusion proteins of the truncated cytoplasmic domain of hIL-5R$\alpha$, we found that hIL-5R$\alpha$ lacks at least the C-terminal membrane distal region bound to JAK-2. In contrast, GST fusion proteins with the cytoplasmic region of $\beta_c$ were comprised of box-1- and box-2-bound JAK-1. Taking all results together, JAK-2 and JAK-1 constitutively associate with IL-5R$\alpha$ and $\beta_c$, respectively, and both JAK-1 and JAK-2 are activated in response to IL-5. It is not clear at this moment whether JAK-2 is associated with $\beta_c$.

### C. Role of Proline-Rich Region in the Cytoplasmic Domain of the IL-5R$\alpha$ Chain in Signal Transduction

Transfectants expressing $\beta_c$ and IL-5R$\alpha$ which lacks an entire cytoplasmic region can bind IL-5 with high affinity, but cannot respond to IL-5 (11). The results indicate the critical role of the cytoplasmic domain of IL-5R$\alpha$ together with $\beta_c$ in IL-5 signal transduction. To identify region(s) critical for the IL-5-mediated signal transduction, four different mutant cDNAs of IL-5R$\alpha$ have been created, each of which has a deletion of six amino acid residues in its cytoplasmic domain (76). Regardless of the cytoplasmic deletions, all four different transfectants express similar levels of high-affinity IL-5R on their cell surface with $K_d$ values equivalent to those of transfectants and expressing the wild-type IL-5R$\alpha$. Mutated IL-5R$\alpha$ proteins are processed properly with the correct size, indicating that mutations induced in the cytoplasmic domain of IL-5R$\alpha$ do not affect the interactions of IL-5R$\alpha$ with IL-5 or $\beta_c$, thereby facilitating reconstitution of the high-affinity IL-5R.

Transfectants expressing mutant IL-5R$\alpha$, having deletions in the carboxy-terminal region that is unique to IL-5R$\alpha$, respond to IL-5 for proliferation, JAK-2 activation, and proto-oncogene expression. In contrast, transfectants expressing the mutant IL-5R$\alpha$ have a deletion in the region rich in proline residues (Pro-Pro-X-Pro) and do not respond to IL-5. The proximal region, downstream from the proline-rich area, has been shown to be important, though not essential. Deletion of the membrane proximal cytoplasmic domain of IL-5Rα containing the sequence $Pro^{352}$-$Pro^{353}$-X-$Pro^{355}$ (ppvp motif) disrupts all IL-5-mediated signal transduction including tyrosine phosphorylation of cellular proteins, the JAK-2/STAT-5 activation, and induction of nuclear proto-oncogene expression (76,81). Essentially identical results were reported in the human IL-5R system (82). These results indicate that the region rich in proline residues is essential for IL-5-mediated growth signal transduction.

To better characterize the functional residues within the proline-rich domain, analysis of a panel of IL-5Rα alanine replacement mutants was generated. JAK-1 and JAK-2 are phosphorylated following IL-5 stimulation of cells expressing the mIL-5Rα mutant pAvA, AAvp, or to a much lesser extent ApvA (where A represents an alanine substitution), while cells expressing the AAvA mutant are not. Similar effects on proliferation and proto-oncogene induction are also demonstrated (76). These results indicate that the existence of at least one of three proline residues in the Pro-Pro-x-Pro motif, which is conserved among the α chains of IL-3R, IL-5R, and GM-CSFR, is indispensable for signal transduction and that $Pro^{352}$ and $Pro^{355}$ are more critical than $Pro^{353}$.

The proline-rich region ($Pro^{352}$-$Pro^{353}$-$Val^{354}$-$Pro^{355}$-$Ala^{356}$-$Pro^{357}$) in the cytoplasmic domain of mouse IL-5Rα appears to belong to the Pro1-X-A1-Pro2-X-Pro3 (where A1 is any aliphatic residue) motif of the PRM1 family (113). Recently, another proline-rich motif, Pro-X-Pro, important for signaling of other cytokines, has been elucidated. Results with IL-5Rα mutants showed that neither of the proline residues of the Pro-X-Pro sequence in the Pro-Pro-X-Pro motif is critical for IL-5R-induced JAK-2-STAT-5 activation or for cell growth. However, $Pro^{357}$ of IL-5Rα, which is not conserved in IL-3Rα or GM-CSFRα, may play a role in IL-5 signaling. It is possible that $Pro^{357}$ of IL-5Rα plus one of the N-terminal prolines in the Pro-Pro-X-Pro motif is sufficient for IL-5 signal transduction (114). Our analysis using alanine substitution mutants of $Pro^{357}$ suggest that $Pro^{357}$ is not a critical residue for IL-5 signaling (Kouro et al., unpublished).

### D. Role of Proline-Rich Region in the Cytoplasmic Regions of $\beta_c$ in Signaling

Deletion mutants of $\beta_c$ revealed that a region between Leu626 and Ser763 is also important for tyrosine phosphorylation of Shc and PI-3K, while the region between Val578 and Leu626 is associated with the tyrosine phosphorylation of other cellular proteins (115). Alanine substitutions of $\beta_c$ revealed that Tyr365, His367, and Ile368 influence the binding affinity of the receptor heterodimer for IL-5. These residues are also important to GM-CSF, but not to IL-3. These data provide evidence that high-affinity binding of IL-5 can be dissociated from that of the other cytokines which share the $\beta_c$. Taking all results together, IL-5Rα binds to a region near the junction of loop 3 with helix D and the N-terminal end of helix D, while the $\beta_c$ chain binding localizes to a portion of helix A centered around Glu13.

## VI. Closing Remarks

### A. Functional Properties of IL-5

IL-5 has pleiotropic activities on various target cells, as like other cytokines. It is quite important to clarify what is a major role of IL-5 in growth and differentiation of hematopoietic cells. One of the issues we are currently interested in is the role of IL-5 in Ig-isotype switching and apoptosis of B cells. IL-5 appears to sustain survival of TGF-β/LPS-stimulated B cells in vitro culture. Concerning role of IL-5 in Ig-isotype switching, we need a good model to evaluate molecular mechanisms of isotype selection. We and others have evidence that IL-5 partially rescues anti-IgM-induced apoptosis of WEHI-231 cells and in vitro apoptosis of eosinophils, but its molecular mechanism is totally unknown.

In this review I do not focus on role of IL-5 in eosinophilopoiesis and activation of eosinophils. There is considerable evidence supporting the notion that IL-5 plays a critical role in pathogenesis of asthmatic diseases. Mice disrupted IL-5 or IL-5Rα genes may provide us useful tools for clarifying the exact role of IL-5 in eosinophil development and triggering.

### B. IL-5R-Mediated Signaling Pathways

IL-3, IL-5, and GM-CSF make up a subfamily of cytokines displaying a variety of overlapping actions during hematopoiesis. These three hematopoietic factors bind to distinct specificity-determining α receptor components, but share $\beta_c$ as a common signal transducer; the unique distributions of the individual α subunits determine which hematopoietic cells are capable of responding to each of the factors. The signals generated by IL-5, IL-3, and GM-CSF appears to be equivalent, and different functions of these cytokines are due to the stage of development of cells expressing the receptors. Alternatively, different signal-transducing molecules which generate a specific signal for each cytokine, may be associated with respective ligand-binding α subunits of each receptor. These possibilities are not mutually exclusive. Analyses of molecular mechanisms of IL-5Rα gene expression will be a quite important step for understanding IL-5 biology.

Each α subunit of IL-5R, IL-3R, and GM-CSFR has a conserved region underneath of the transmembrane domain. This region is important to interact with the cytoplasmic domain of $\beta_c$. The cytoplasmic domain, particularly the membrane proximal proline-rich sequences and the adjacent downstream proline-rich region, of the IL-5Rα is essential and important, respectively, for IL-5-mediated signal transduction in transduction of the IL-5 growth signal. These two regions are well conserved among IL-5Rα, IL-3Rα, and GM-CSFRα, prolactin, and growth hormone receptors and are able to speculate a critical role in transducing common growth signals. The carboxy-terminal regions of the α chains of IL-5R, IL-3R, and GM-CSFR are different from each other. The latter regions may contribute to the transduction of ligand-specific signals or important to induce differentiation of cells.

We have been particularly interested in the tyrosine phosphorylation of Shc and HS1 proteins and in the activation of Btk kinase in IL-5 signaling. Btk is activated by IL-5 stimulation. The Btk protein has potential to interact in a novel way with proteins involved in an IL-5R-mediated signaling pathway. Search for cellular molecules that can interact with IL-5Rα and Btk through its amino-terminal unique region should shed light on the complexed signaling requirements of B-cell differentiation in response to cytokines including IL-5.

It is also important to clarify differences of signal transduction pathways between B cells and eosinophils. Eosinophils from XID mice respond to IL-5 for prolonged survival, while B cells from XID mice do not respond IL-5. These results strongly suggest that there are at least two different signaling pathways for IL-5; one is operated in B cells and the other is operated in eosinophils. If we can find specific inhibitors for IL-5R-mediated signaling in eosinophils, such inhibitors may be good candidates for antiasthmatic drugs.

## References


1. Takatsu K, Takaki S, Hitoshi Y. Interleukin-5 and its receptor system in the immune system and inflammation. Adv Immunol 1994;54:145–190.
2. Kinashi T, Harada N, Severinson E, Tanabe T, Sideras P, Konishi M, Azuma C, Tominaga A, Bergstedt-Lindqvist S, Takahashi M, Matsuda F, Yaoita Y, Takatsu K, Honjo T. Cloning of complementary DNA encoding T-cell replacing factor and identity with B-cell growth factor II. Nature 1986;324:70–73.
3. Takatsu K. Interleukin-5 and Its Receptor System: From Genes to Disease. Austin, TX: R. G. Landes, 1995:1-167.
4. Rozwarski DA, Gronenborn AM, Clore GM, Bazan JF, Bohm A, Wlodawer A, Hatada M, Karplus PA. Structural comparison among the short-chain helical cytokines. Structure 1994;2:159–173.
5. Milburn MV, Hassell AM, Lambert MH, Jordan SR, Proudfoot AE, Graber P, Wells TN. A novel dimer configuration revealed by the crystal structure at 2.4 Å resolution of human interleukin-5. Nature 1993;363:172–116.
6. Sanderson CJ. Interleukin-5, eosinophils, and disease. Blood 1992;79:3101–3109.
7. Takaki S, Tominaga A, Hitoshi Y, Mita S, Sonoda E, Yamaguchi N, Takatsu K. Molecular cloning and expression of the murine interleukin-5 receptor. EMBO J 1990;9:4367–4374.
8. Murata Y, Takaki S, Migita M, Kikuchi Y, Tominaga A, Takatsu K. Molecular

cloning and expression of the human interleukin 5 receptor. J Exp Med 1992;175:341-351.
9. Tavernier J, Devos R, Cornelis S, Tuypens T, Van der Heyden J, Fiers W, Plaetinck G. A human high affinity interleukin-5 receptor (IL5R) is composed of an IL5-specific alpha chain and a beta chain shared with the receptor for GM-CSF. Cell 1991;66:1175–1184.
10. Takaki S, Mita S, Kitamura T, Yonehara S, Tominaga A, Yamaguchi N, Miyajima A, Takatsu K. Identification of the second subunit of the murine interleukin-5 receptor: interleukin-3 receptor-like protein, AIC2B is a component of the high affinity interleukin-5 receptor. EMBO J 1991;10:2833–2838.
11. Takaki S, Murata Y, Kitamura T, Miyajima A, Tominaga A, Takatsu K. Reconstitution of the functional receptors for murine and human interleukin 5. J Exp Med 1993;177:1523–1529.
12. Kitamura T, Sato N, Arai K, Miyajima A. Expression cloning of the human IL-3 receptor cDNA reveals a shared β subunit for the human IL-3 and GM-CSF receptors. Cell 1991;66:1165–1174.
13. Hayashida K, Kitamura T, Gorman DM, Arai K, Yokota T, Miyajima A. Molecular cloning of a second subunit of the receptor for human granulocyte-macrophage colony-stimulating factor (GM-CSF): reconstitution of a high-affinity GM-CSF receptor. Proc Natl Acad Sci USA 1990;87:9655–9659.
14. Miyajima A, Mui AL, Ogorochi T, Sakamaki K. Receptor for granulocyte-macrophage colony-stimulating factor, interleukin-3, and interleukin-5. Blood 1993;82:1960–1974.
15. Mosmann TR, Coffman RL. TH1 and TH2 cells: different patterns of lymphokine secretion lead to different functional properties. Annu Rev Immunol 1989;7:145–173.
16. Trinchieri G. Biology of human natural killer cells. Adv Immunol 1989;47:187–376.
17. Hsieh CS, Macatonia SE, Tripp CS, O'Garra A, Murphy KM. Development of Th1 CD4+ T cells through IL-12 produced by listeria-induced macrophages. Science 1993;260:547–549.
18. Zheng W-P, Flavell RA. The transcription factor GATA-3 is necessary and sufficient for Th2 cytokine gene expression in CD4 T cells. Cell 1997;89:587–596.
19. Le Beau MM, Lemons RS, Espinosa R 3d, Larson RA, Arai N, Rowley JD. Interleukin-4 and interleukin-5 map to human chromosome 5 in a region encoding growth factors and receptors and are deleted in myeloid leukemias with a del(5q). Blood 1989;73:647–650.
20. Wang Y, Campbell HD, Young IG. Sex hormones and dexamethasone modulate interleukin-5 gene expression in T lymphocytes. J Steroid Biochem Mol Biol 1993;44:203–210.
21. Bousquet J, Chanez P, Lacoste JY, Barneon G, Ghavanian N, Enander I, Venge P, Ahlstedt S, Simony-Lafontaine J, Godard P, Michel FB. Eosinophilic inflammation in asthma. N Engl J Med 1990;23:1033–1039.
22. Gruart-Gouilleux V, Engels P, Sullivan M. Characterization of the human

interleukin-5 gene promoter: involvement of octamer binding sites in the gene promoter activity. Eur J Immunol 1995;25:1431–1435.

23. Yamagata T, Nishida J, Sakai R, Tanaka T, Honda H, Hirano N, Mano H, Yazaki Y, Hirai H. Of the GATA-binding proteins, only GATA-4 selectively regulates the human interleukin-5 gene promoter in interleukin-5-producing cells which express multiple GATA-binding proteins. Mol Cell Biol 1995;15:3830–3839.
24. Hitoshi Y, Yamaguchi N, Mita S, Sonoda E, Takaki S, Tominaga A, Takatsu K. Distribution of IL-5 receptor-positive B cells. Expression of IL-5 receptor on Ly-1(CD5)+ B cells. J Immunol 1990;144:4218–4225.
25. Rolink AG, Thalmann P, Kikuchi Y, Erdei A. Characterization of the interleukin 5-reactive splenic B cell population. Eur J Immunol 1990;20:1949–1956.
26. Shirai T, Hirose S, Okada T, Nishimura N. CD5$^+$ B cells in autoimmune disease and lymphoid malignancy. Clin Immunol Immunopathol 1991;59:173–186.
27. Hayakawa K, Hardy RR, Herzenberg LA. Progenitors for Ly-1 B cells are distinct from progenitors for other B cells. J Exp Med 1995;161:1554–1568.
28. Tominaga A, Takaki S, Koyama N, Katoh S, Matsumoto R, Migita M, Hitoshi Y, Hosoya Y, Yamauchi S, Kanai Y, Miyazaki J-I, Usuku G, Yamamura KI, Takatsu K. Transgenic mice expressing a B cell growth and differentiation factor gene (interleukin 5) develop eosinophilia and autoantibody production. J Exp Med 1991;173:429–437.
29. Herron LR, Coffman RL, Bond MW, Kotzin BL. Increased autoantibody production by NZB/NZW B cells in response to IL-5. J Immunol 1988;141:842–848.
30. Mandler R, Chu CC, Paul WE, Max EE, Snapper CM. Interleukin 5 induces S mu-S gamma 1 DNA rearrangement in B cells activated with dextran-anti-IgD antibodies and interleukin 4: a three component model for Ig class switching. J Exp Med 1993;178:1577–1586.
31. Huston MM, Moore JP, Mettes H, Tavana G, Huston DP. Human B cells express IL-5 receptor messenger ribonucleic acid and respond to IL-5 with enhanced IgM production after mitogenic stimulation with *Moraxella catarrhalis*. J Immunol 1996;156:1392–1401.
32. Clutterbuck E, Shields JG, Gordon J, Smith SH, Boyd A, Callard RE, Campbell HD, Young IG, Sanderson CJ. Recombinant human interleukin 5 is an eosinophil differentiation factor but has no activity in standard human B cell growth factor assays. Eur J Immunol 1987;17:1743–1750.
33. Yamaguchi Y, Hayashi Y, Sugama Y, Miura Y, Kasahara T, Kitamura S, Torisu M, Mita S, Tominaga A, Takatsu K. Highly purified murine interleukin 5 (IL-5) stimulates eosinophil function and prolongs in vitro survival. IL-5 as an eosinophil chemotactic factor. J Exp Med 1988;67:1737–1742.
34. Yamaguchi Y, Suda T, Ohta S, Tominaga K, Miura Y, Kasahara T. Analysis of the survival of mature human eosinophils: interleukin-5 prevents apoptosis in mature human eosinophils. Blood 1991;78:2542–2547.
35. Takatsu K, Dickason RA, Huston D. Interleukin-5. In: Leroith D, Bondy C, eds. Growth Factors and Cytokines in Health and Disease London: JAI Press, 1997:143–200.

36. Hamid Q, Azzawi M, Ying S, Moqbel R, Wardlaw AJ, Corrigan CJ, Bradley B, Durham SR, Collins JV, Jeffery PK. Expression of mRNA for interleukin-5 in mucosal bronchial biopsies from asthma. J Clin Invest 1991;87:1541–1546.
37. Akutsu I, Kojima K, Kariyone A, Makino S, Takatsu K. Passive administration of anti-IL-5 antibody into chronically ovalbumin-sensitized guinea pigs induces suppression of eosinophilia and bronchial hyperreactivity. Immunol Lett 1995;45:109–116.
38. Kung TT, Stelts DM, Zurcher JA, Adams GK, Egan RW, Kreutner W, Watnick AS, Jones H, Chapman RW. Involvement of IL-5 in a murine model of allergic pulmonary inflammation: prophylactic and therapeutic effect of an anti-IL-5 antibody. Am J Respir Cell Mol Biol 1995;13:360–365.
39. Mauser PJ, Pitman AM, Fernandez X, Foran SK, Adams GK III, Kreutner W, Egan RW, Chapman RW. Effects of an antibody to IL-5 in a monkey model of asthma. Am J Respir Crit Care Med 1995;152:467–472.
40. Yoshida T, Ikuta I, Sugaya H, Maki K, Takagi M, Kanazawa H, Sunaga S, Kinashi T, Yoshimura K, Miyazaki J, Takaki S, Takatsu K. Defective B-1 cell development and impaired immunity against *Angiostrongylus cantonensis* in IL-5Rα deficient mice. Immunity 1996;4:483–494.
41. Yoshida T. Targeted disruption of murine IL-5 receptor a gene: defective B-1 cell development and impaired immunity against *Angiostrongylus cantonensis*. Ph.D. dissertation. Tokyo University, Tokyo, Japan, 1997.
42. Kopf M, Bronbacher F, Hodgkin PD, Ramsey AJ, Mibourne EA, Dai WJ, Ovington KS, Behm CA, Kohler G, Young IG, Matthaei KI. IL-5 deficient mice have a developmental defect in CD5+ B-1 cells and lack eosinophilia but have normal antibody and cytotoxic T cell responses. Immunity 1996;4:15–24.
43. Isobe M, Kumura Y, Murata Y, Takaki S, Tominaga A, Takatsu K, Ogita Z. Localization of the gene encoding the alpha subunit of human interleukin-5 receptor (IL5Rα) to chromosome region 3p24-3p26. Genomics 1992;14:755–758.
44. Imamura F, Takaki S, Akagi K, Miyazaki J-I, Yamamura K-I, Takatsu K, Tominaga A. The murine interleukin-5 receptor alpha-subunit gene: characterization of the gene structure and chromosome mapping. DNA Cell Biol 1994;13:283–292.
45. Sun Z, Yergeau DA, Tuypens T, Tavernier J, Paul CC, Baumann MA, Tenen DG, Ackerman SJ. Identification and characterization of a functional promoter region in the human eosinophil IL-5 receptor a subunit gene. J Biol Chem 1995;270:1462–1471.
46. Tavernier J, Tuypens T, Plaetinck G, Verhee A, Fiers W, Devos R. Molecular basis of the membrane-anchored and two soluble isoforms of the human interleukin 5 receptor alpha subunit. Proc Natl Acad Sci USA 1992;89:7041–7045.
47. Kikuchi Y, Migita M, Takaki S, Tominaga A, Takatsu K. Biochemical and functional characterization of soluble form of IL-5 receptor α (sIL-5Rα): development of ELISA system for detection of sIL-5Rα. J Immunol Meth 1994;167:289–298.
48. Bazan JF. Structural design and molecular evolution of a cytokine receptor superfamily. Proc Natl Acad Sci USA 1990;87:6934–6938.

49. Yamaguchi N, Hitoshi Y, Takaki S, Murata Y, Migita M, Kamiya T, Minowada J, Tominaga A, Takatsu K. Murine interleukin 5 receptor isolated by immunoaffinity chromatography: comparison of determined N-terminal sequence and deduced primary sequence from cDNA and implication of a role of the intracytoplasmic domain. Int Immunol 1991;3:889–898.
50. Morton TA, Bennett DB, Appelbaum ER, Cusimano DM, Johanson KO, Matico RE, Young PR, Doyle M, Chaiken IM. Analysis of the interaction between human interleukin-5 and the soluble domain of its receptor using a surface plasmon resonance biosensor. J Mol Recognit 1994;7:47–55.
51. Johanson K, Appelbaum E, Doyle M, Hensley P, Zhao B, Abdel-Meguid SS, Young P, Cook R, Carr S, Matico R, Cusimano D, Dul E, Angelichio M, Brooks I, Winborne E, McDonnell P, Morton T, Bennett D, Sokoloski T, McNulty D, Rosenberg M, Chaiken I. Binding interactions of human interleukin 5 with its receptor alpha subunit. J Biol Chem 1995;270:9459–9471.
52. Tsuruoka N, Yamashiro K, Tsujimoto M. Purification of soluble murine interleukin 5 (IL-5) receptor alpha expressed in Chinese hamster ovary cells and its action as an IL-5 antagonist. Arch Biochem Biophys 1993;307:133–137.
53. Cornelis S, Plaetinck G, Devos R, Van der Heyden J, Tavernier J, Sanderson CJ, Guisez Y, Fiers W. Detailed analysis of the IL-5-IL-5R alpha interaction characterization of crucial residues on the ligand and the receptor. EMBO J 1995;14:3395–3402.
54. Devos R, Guisez Y, Plaetinck G, Cornelis S, Tavernier J, Van Der Heyden J, Foley LH, Scheffler JE. Covalent modification of the interleukin-5 receptor by isothiazolones leads to inhibition of the binding of interleukin-5. Eur J Biochem 1994;225:635–640.
55. Devos R, Guisez Y, Cornelis S, Verhee A, Heyden JVD, Manneberg M, Lahm W, Fiers W, Tavernier J, Plaetinck G. Recombinant soluble human interleukin-5 (hIL-5) receptor molecules. Cross-linking and stoichiometry of binding to IL-5. J Biol Chem 1993;268:6581–6587.
56. Gorman DM, Itoh N, Jenkins NA, Gilbert DJ, Copeland NG, Miyajima A. Chromosomal localization and organization of the murine genes encoding the beta subunits (AIC2A and AIC2B) of the interleukin 3, granulocyte/macrophage colony-stimulating factor, and interleukin 5 receptors. J Biol Chem 1992;267:15842–15848.
57. Mita S, Tominaga A, Hitoshi Y, Sakamoto K, Honjo T, Akagi M, Kikuchi Y, Yamaguchi N, Takatsu K. Characterization of high-affinity receptors for interleukin 5 on interleukin 5-dependent cell lines. Proc Natl Acad Sci USA 1989;86:2311–2315.
58. Kitamura T, Takaku F, Miyajima A. IL-1 up-regulates the expression of cytokine receptors on a factor-dependent human hemopoietic cell line, TF-1. Int Immunol 1991;3:571–577.
59. Watanabe Y, Kitamura T, Hayashida K, Miyajima A. Monoclonal antibody against the common beta subunit (beta c) of the human interleukin-3 (IL-3), IL-5, and

granulocyte-macrophage colony-stimulating factor receptors shows upregulation of beta c by IL-1 and tumor necrosis factor-alpha. Blood 1992;80:2215–2220.
60. Sato N, Sakamaki S, Terada N, Arai K-I, Miyajima A. Signal transduction by the high-affinity GM-CSF receptor: two distinct cytoplasmic regions of the common β subunit responsible for different signaling. EMBO J 1993;12:4181–4189.
61. Sakamaki K, Miyajima I, Kitamura T, Miyajima A. Critical cytoplasmic domains of the common b subunit of the human GM-CSF, IL-3 and IL-5 receptor for growth signal transduction and tyrosine phosphorylation. EMBO J 1993;11:3541–3549.
62. Mita S, Takaki S, Tominage A, Takatsu K. Comparative analysis of kinetics of binding and internalization of IL-5 murine IL-5 receptor of high and low affinity. J Immunol 1993;151:6924–6932.
63. Taga T, Hibi M, Hirata Y, Yamasaki K, Yasukawa K, Matsuda T, Hirano T, Kishimoto T. Interleukin-6 triggers the association of its receptor with a possible signal transducer, gp130. Cell 1989;58:573–581.
64. Hibi M, Murakami M, Sito M, Hirano T, Taga T, Kishimoto T. Molecular cloning and expression of an IL-6 signal transduction, gp130. Cell 1990;63:1149–1161.
65. Yamaguchi N, Takahashi T, Harada N, Takatsu K. Mechanisms of the interleukin 5-induced differentiation of B cells. J Biochem (Tokyo) 1989;106:837–843.
66. Ullrich A, Schlessinger J. Signal transduction by receptors with tyrosine kinase activity. Cell 1990;61:203–211.
67. Morla AO, Schreurs J, Miyajima A, Wang JY. Hematopoietic growth factors activate the tyrosine phosphorylation of distinct sets of proteins in interleukin-3-dependent murine cell lines. Mol Cell Biol 1988;8:2214–2218.
68. Murata Y, Yamaguchi N, Hitoshi Y, Tominaga A, Takatsu K. Interleukin 5 and interleukin 3 induce serine and tyrosine phosphorylations of several cellular proteins in an interleukin 5-dependent cell line. Biochem Biophys Res Commun 1990;173:1102–1108.
69. Conscience JF, Verrier B, Martin G. Interleukin-3-dependent expression of the c-myc and c-fos proto-oncogenes in hematopoietic cell lines. EMBO J 1986;5:317–323.
70. Sato S, Katagiri T, Takaki S, Kikuchi Y, Hitoshi Y, Yonehara S, Tsukada S, Kitamura D, Watanabe T, Witte ON, Takatsu K. IL-5 receptor-mediated tyrosine phosphorylation of SH2/SH3-containing proteins and activation of Bruton's tyrosine and Janus 2 kinases. J Exp Med 1994;180:2101–2111.
71. Pelicci G, Lanfrancone L, Grignani F, McGlade J, Cavallo F, Forni G, Nicoletti I, Grignani F, Pawson T, Pellicci PG. A novel transforming protein (SHC) with an SH2 domain is implicated in mitogenic signal transduction. Cell 1992;70:93–104.
72. Egan SE, Giddings BW, Brooks MW, Buday L, Sizeland AM, Weinberg RA. Association of Sos Ras exchange protein with Grb2 is implicated in tyrosine kinase signal transduction and transformation. Nature 1993;363:45–51.
73. Smith MR, DeGudicubus SJ, Stacey DW. Requirement for c-ras proteins during viral oncogene transformation. Nature 1986;320:540–543.

74. Satoh T, Nakafuku M, Miyajima A, Kaziro Y. Involvement of p21ras protein in signal-transduction pathways from interleukin 2, interleukin 3 and granulocyte/macrophage colony-stimulating factor, but not from interleukin 4. Proc Natl Acad Sci USA 1991;88:3314–3318.
75. Duronio V, Welham MJ, Abraham S, Dryden P, Schrader JW, Welham MJ, Abraham S. p21ras activation via hemopoietic receptors and c-kit requires tyrosine kinase activity but not tyrosine phosphorylation of p21ras GTPase-activating protein. Proc Natl Acad Sci USA 1992;89:1587–1591.
76. Takaki S, Kanazawa H, Shiiba M, Takatsu K. A critical cytoplasmic domain of the interleukin-5 (IL-5) receptor alpha chain and its function in IL-5-mediated growth signal transduction. Mol Cell Biol 1994;14:7404–7413.
77. Ihle JN. Cytokine receptor signaling. Nature 1995;377:591–594.
78. Darnell JE Jr, Kerr IM, Stark GR. Jak-STAT pathways and transcriptional activation in response to IFNs and other extracellular signaling transduction. Science 1994;264:1415–1418.
79. Akira S, Nishio Y, Inoue M, Wang XJ, Wei S, Matsusaka T, Yoshida K, Sudo T, Naruto M, Kishimoto T. Molecular cloning of APRF, a novel IFN-stimulated gene factor 3 p91-related transcription factor involved in the gp130-mediated signaling pathway. Cell 1994;77:63–71.
80. Kishimoto T, Taga T, Akira S. Cytokine signal transduction. Cell 1994;76:253–262.
81. Kouro T, Kikuchi Y, Kanazawa H, Hirokawa K, Harada N, Shiiba M, Wakao H, Takaki S, Takatsu K. Critical proline residues of the cytoplasmic domain of the IL-5 receptor alpha chain and its function in IL-5 mediated activation of JAK kinase and STAT5. Int Immunol 1996;8:237–246.
82. Cornelis S, Fache I, Van der Heyden J, Guisez Y, Tavernier J, Devos R, Fiers W, Plaetinck G. Characterization of critical residues in the cytoplasmic domain of the human interleukin-5 receptor alpha chain required for growth signal transduction. Eur J Immunol 1995;25:1857–1864.
83. Weiss M, Yokoyama C, Shikama Y, Naugle C, Druker B, Sieff CA. Human granulocyte-macrophage colony-stimulating factor receptor signal transduction requires the proximal cytoplasmic domain of the alpha and beta subunits. Blood 1993;82:3298–3303.
84. Larner AC, David M, Feldman GM, Igarashi H, Hackett RH, Webb DS, Sweitzer SM, Petricoin EF, Finbloom DS. Tyrosine phosphorylation of DNA binding proteins by multiple cytokines. Science 1993;261:1730–1733.
85. Mui AL-F, Wakao H, O'Farrell A-M, Harada N, Miyajima A. Interleukin-3, granulocyte-macrophage colony-stimulating factor and interleukin-5 transduce signals through two STAT5 homologues. EMBO J 1995;14:1166–1172.
86. Ogata N, Kikuchi Y, Kouro T, Takatsu K. Activation of JAK2/STAT5 pathway is commonly involved in signaling through the human interleukin-5 receptor. Int Arch Allergy Immunol 1997; 114(suppl 1):24–27.
87. Van der Brugger T. Caldenhover E. Kanters D. Coffer P. Raaijimakers JA. Lammers JW. Koenderman L. IL-5 signaling in human eosinophils involves JAK2 tyrosine kinase and Stat1a. Blood 1995;85:1442–1448.

88. Pazdrak K, Justement L, Alam R. Mechanism of inhibition of eosinophils activation by transforming growth factor-β. Inhibition of Lyn, MAP, Jak2 kinases and STAT1 nuclear factor J Immunol 1995;155:4454.
89. Bates ME, Bertcs PJ, Busse WW. IL-5 activates a 45-kilodalton mitogen-activated protein (MAP) kinase and Jak-2 tyrosine kinase in human eosinophils. J Immunol 1996;156:711-.
90. Ogata N, Kouro T, Yamada A, Koike M, Hanai M, Ishikawa T, Takatsu K. The association of the IL-5 receptor a chain with the b chain depends on the IL-5 stimulation. Blood 1998;
91. Pazdrak K, Stafford S, Alam R. The activation of the Jak-STAT1 signaling pathway by IL-5 in eosinophils. J Immunol 1995;155:397–402.
92. Mui AL, Wakao H, Kinoshita T, Kitamura T, Miyajima A. Suppreession of interleukin-3-induced gene expression by a C-terminal truncated Stat5: role of Stat5 in proliferation. EMBO J 1996;15:2425-2433.
93. Takagi M, Hara T, Ichihara M, Hara T, Ichihara M, Takatsu K, Miyajima A. Multi-colony stimulating activity of interleukin-5 (IL-5) on hematopoietic progenitors from transgenic mice that express IL-5 receptor alpha subunit constitutively. J Exp Med 1995;181:889–899.
94. Shiiba M, Takaki S, Takatsu K. Interleukin-3 (IL-3) and granulocyte-macrophage colony-stimulating factor (GM-CSF) can induce differentiation of chronic B cell leukemia expressing the a subunit of IL-3 and GM-CSF receptor. Int Arch Allergy Immunol 1996;111(suppl):11–14.
95. Yoshimura A, Ichihara M, Kinjo I, Moriyama M, Copeland NG, et al. Mouse oncostatin M: an immediate early response gen induced by multiple cytokine through the JAK/STAT5 pathway. EMBO J 1996;15:1055–1063.
96. Matsumoto A, Masuhara M, Mitsui K, Yokouchi M, Ohtsubo M, Misawa H, Miyajima A, Yoshimura A. CIS, a cytokine inducible S2 protein, is a target of the JAK-STAT5 pathway and modulates STAT5 activation. Blood 1997; 89:3148–3154.
97. Tsukada S, Rawlings DJ, Witte ON. Role of Bruton's tyrosine kinase in human and murine B cell immunodeficiency. Curr Opin Immunol 1994;6:623–630.
98. Tsukada S, Saffran DC, Rawlings DJ, Parolini O, Allen RC, Klisak I, Sparkes RS, Kubagawa H, Mohandas T, Quan S, Belmont JW, Cooper MD, Conley ME, Witte ON. Deficient expression of a B cell cytoplasmic tyrosine kinase in human X-linked agammaglobulinemia. Cell 1993;72:279–290.
99. Vetrie D, Vorechovsky I, Sideras P, Holland J, Davies A, Flinter F, Hammarstrom L, Kinnon C, Levinsky R, Bobrow M. The gene involved in X-linked agammaglobulinaemia is a member of the src family of protein-tyrosine kinases. Nature 1993;361:226–233.
100. Rawlings D, Saffran DC, Tsukada S, Largaespada DA, Grimaldi JC, Cohen L, Mohr RN, Bazan JF, Howard M, Copeland NG, Jenkins NA, Witte ON. Mutation of unique region of Bruton's tyrosine kinase in immunodeficient Xid mice. Science 1993;261:358–360.
101. Thomas JD, Sideras P, Smith CIE, Vorechovsky I, Chapman V, Paul WE. Colocalization of X-linked agamma-globulinemia and X-linked immunodeficiency genes. Science 1993;261:355–361.

102. Go NF, Castle BE, Barrett R, Kastelein R, Dang W, Mosmann TR, Moore KW, Howard M. Interleukin 10, novel B cell stimulatory factor: unresponsiveness of X chromosome-linked immunodeficiency B cells. J Exp Med 1990;172:1625–1631.
103. Hasbold J, Klaus GGB. B cells from CBA/N mice do not proliferate following ligation of CD40. Eur J Immunol 1994;24:152–157.
104. Kikuchi Y, Yasue T, Miyake K, Kimoto M, Takatsu K. Cross-linking of CD38 induces tyrosine phosphorylation of Bruton's tyrosine kinase and expression of IL-5 receptor: synergistic effect with IL-5. Proc Natl Acad Sci USA 1995;92:10879–10883.
105. Hitoshi Y, Sonoda E, Kikuchi Y, Yonehara S, Nakauchi H, Takatsu K. Interleukin-5 receptor positive B cells, but not eosinophils are functionally and numerically influenced in the mice carried with Xlinked immunodeficiency. Int Immunol 1993;9:1183–1190.
106. Koike M, Kikuchi Y, Tominaga A, Takaki S, Akagi K, Miyazaki J-I, Yamamura K-I, Takatsu K. Defect of IL-5-receptor-mediated signaling in B cells of X-linked immunodeficient (XID) mice. Int Immunol 1995;7:21–30.
107. Appleby MW, Kerner JD, Chien S, Maliszewski CR, Bondadaa S, Perlmutter RM. Involvement of p59fynT in IL-5 receptor signaling. J Exp Med 1995;182:811–820.
108. Yasue T, Kikuchi Y, Nishizumi M, Yamamoto T, Takatsu K. Lyn kinase is involved in B cell triggering by CD38 ligation and IL-5 for IgG1 production. Proc Natl Acad Sci USA 1997; 94:10307–10312.
109. Cheng G, Ye ZS, Baltimore D. Binding of Bruton's tyrosine kinase to Fyn, Lyn, or Hck through a Src homology domain-mediated interaction. Proc Natl Acad Sci USA 1994;91:8152–8155.
110. Li T, Tsukada S, Satterthwaite A, Havlik MH, Park H, Takatsu K, Witte OH. Activation of Bruton's tyrosine kinase (BTK) by a point mutation in its pleckstrin homology (PH) domain. Immunity 1995;2:451–460.
111. Murakami M, Hibi M, Nakagawa N, Nakagawa T, Yasukawa K, Yamanishi K, Taga T, Kishimoto T. IL-6-induced homodimerization of gp130 and associated activation of a tyrosine kinase. Science 1993;260:1808–1810.
112. Quelle FW, Sato N, Witthuhn BA, Inhorn RC, Eder M, Miyajima A, Griffin JD, Ihle J. JAK2 associates with the βc chain of the receptor for granulocyte-macrophage colony-stimulating factor, and its activation requires the membrane-proximal region. Mol Cell Biol 1994;14:4335–4341.
113. Muto A, Watanabe S, Miyajima A, Yokota T, Arai K. The β subunit of human granulocyte-macrophage colony-stimulating factorreceptor forms a homodimer and is activated via association with the α subunit. J Exp Med 1996;183:1911–1916.
113. O'Neal KD, Yu-Lee L. The proline-rich motif (PRM): a novel feature of the cytokine/hematopoietin receptor superfamily, lymphokine. Cytokine Res 1993;12:309–312.
114. O'Neal KD, Shearer WT. Letter to the Editor. Clarification of the role of Pro-X-Pro sequence in IL-5 receptor signal transduction. Mol Cell Biol 1995;15:4657–4658.

115. Woodcock JM, Zacharakis B, Plaetinck G, Bagley CJ, Qiyu S, Hercus TR, Tavernier J, Lopez AF. Three residues in the common beta chain of the human GM-CSF, IL-3 and IL-5 receptors are essential for GM-CSF and IL-5 but not IL-3 high affinity binding and interact with Glu21 of GM-CSF. EMBO J 1994;13:5176–5185.

# 15

# Regulation of Interleukin-5 Gene Expression

**COLIN J. SANDERSON, MONICA L. DE BOER, MONICA SENNA SALERNO, GRETCHEN T. F. SCHWENGER, MARC THOMAS, and VIATCHESLAV A. MORDVINOV**

TVW Telethon Institute for Child Health Research
West Perth, Western Australia

**STÉPHANE KARLEN**

University of Berne
Inselspital, Switzerland

## I. Introduction

The expression of IL-5 is synonymous with the production of eosinophils. These blood and tissue leukocytes are produced in a very limited range of disease types, indicating a unique control of the production of IL-5 in the T-cell response to antigen. Clearly this control is regulated at the level of gene expression. Considering the tight control of IL-5 expression, as well as the similarity in the development of eosinophilia in different species, it might be expected that the specific regulatory elements would by highly conserved. However, it is surprising that the flanking region of the human and mouse genes has very limited homology. The region -80 to -20 is highly conserved, but upstream and 3′ regions give little indication of common elements that might be involved in the specific regulation of the gene. This conserved proximal region is important for expression, but as discussed below, other elements outside this region are required for overall regulation.

## II. Cell Systems for Analysis of Regulation

A feature in reviewing published work on the regulation of IL-5 transcription is the lack of agreement between different groups. This probably derives from four technical issues: (1) the use of limited promoter fragments which may not express correctly; (2) the use of cell lines which express IL-5 in an abnormal fashion; (3) the use of human gene constructs in mouse cell lines; and (4) the use of different cell activation stimuli.

One of the main factors limiting studies on IL-5 expression has been the limited number of cell lines available which express IL-5 in an inducible fashion. Studies with primary T cells is limiting because of the low efficiency of transfection and the difficulty in obtaining undegraded nuclear extracts The mouse EL4-23 cell line was used in the original characterization of IL-5 and has been widely used to study gene regulation. Not all sublines of EL4 produce IL-5. In our original studies induction with phorbol ester (PMA) was found to stimulate IL-5 production, but subsequent work demonstrated that dibutyryl cyclic AMP (cAMP) markedly enhanced IL-5 expression (1). The mouse T-cell line D10.G4.1 (D10) was derived as an antigen responsive T-cell clone (2). It produces a number of cytokines including IL-5 and has the advantage that it can be achieved via the T-cell receptor, either by antigen (conalbumin), concanavalin A (ConA), or anti-CD3, as well as by PMA. A T-cell hybrid (NIMP-TH1) was developed by fusing spleen cells from a parasitized mouse with the mouse lymphoma BW5147 and then selecting for IL-5 production following stimulation with PMA (3). This cell line has the interesting property of producing IL-5 but apparently no other cytokine. This observation again points to a different mechanism in IL-5 gene activation. This cell line is readily transfected but so far has found little application in gene regulation studies.

Human Jurkat cells have been used for the study of IL-4 regulation, but none of the clones that we tested produced IL-5 under any conditions of stimulation. Surprisingly they do express luciferase under the control of 500 bp of the IL-5 promoter when stimulated with PMA and the calcium ionophore A23187. This compares with a significant constitutive expression of an IL-4 promoter-luciferase construct, and this is increased less than twofold when stimulated with A23187 (see Fig. 1). These results indicate that Jurkat cells are not a useful model for IL-5 expression. The human HSB-2 cell line provides a model for inducible IL-5 gene regulation, but in our hands produces only very low amounts of IL-5 (C. J. Sanderson, unpublished data). However, IL-5 expression is inducible with PMA, and ionomycin and mRNA can be monitored by nuclear run-on using PCR (4). The human T-cell leukemia cell line ATL-16T constitutively expresses IL-5, but the mechanism behind this abnormal activation of the IL-5 gene is not known. More recently we have worked with a human T-cell line, PER-117 (5) which inducibly expresses IL-5 as well as other

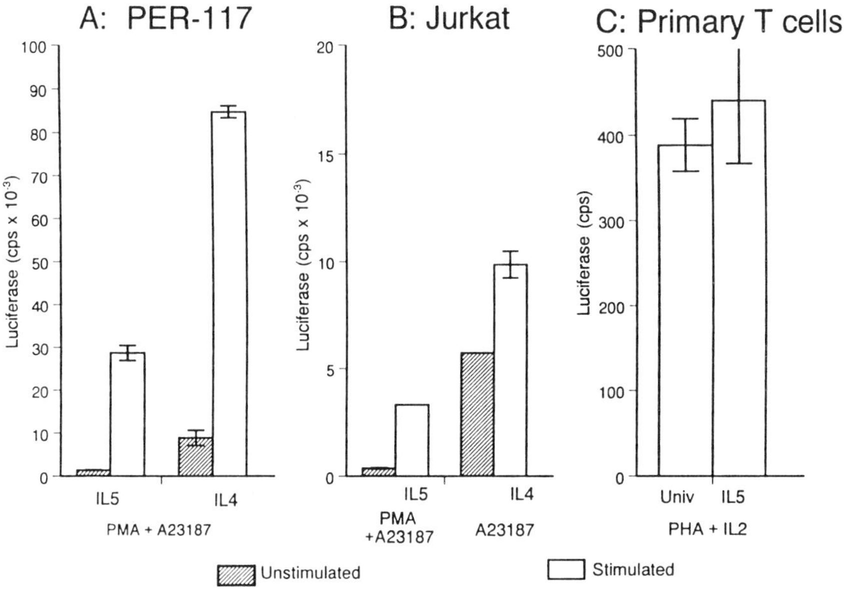


**Figure 1** Transient expression of reporter constructs in human T cells. The conditions of stimulation are shown for each case. (A): PER-117 cell line. (B): Jurkat cell line. (C): Peripheral blood mononuclear cells, comparing a universal promoter with the IL-5 promoter. Note the different scales on the Y axis.

cytokines, including IL-2 and IL-4. There is no detectable constitutive expression of IL-5 but it can be induced with PMA (Fig. 1) and further enhanced by cAMP and ionomycin. IL-5 production is inhibited by dexamethasone and cyclosporin A, depending on the method of stimulation, and so the gene appears to be functioning normally. This cell line has the disadvantage that it does not express the T-cell receptor and so cannot be activated by ConA or anti-CD3. All these tumor lines have disadvantages, and while they can be used as a first approach to IL-5 regulation, it will be important to follow up with primary T cells. Although this has been regarded as technically difficult, recent results have been more encouraging. By optimizing conditions we have successfully measured luciferase reporter activity in both primary mouse and human T cells. For successful transfection of primary T cells, the cells have to be prestimulated prior to transfection. Under these conditions an IL-5 reporter construct containing 507 bp of the IL-5 promoter can be successfully introduced and expressed in primary human T cells (Fig. 1). Mori et al. (6) successfully used human T-cell clones to study IL-5 regulation by dexamethasone, indicating that primary T cells can be used as well.

## III. Deletion Analysis

It is surprising that for a gene product that is highly conserved both structurally and in its biological activity, alignment of gene sequences from different species gives few clues to the control of gene expression. The exception is the region between −20 and −80, which is highly conserved and which is critical for expression. However, as illustrated in Figure 2, while there are well-defined elements upstream of this conserved region, they are different between mouse and man. This raises the possibility that these elements, which are common to many other genes, may not be the elements crucial to the specific regulation of IL-5.

Several groups have carried out deletion analysis, but there is considerable difference between the results reported. This is exemplified when the results of different deletion experiments are represented graphically (Fig. 3). This

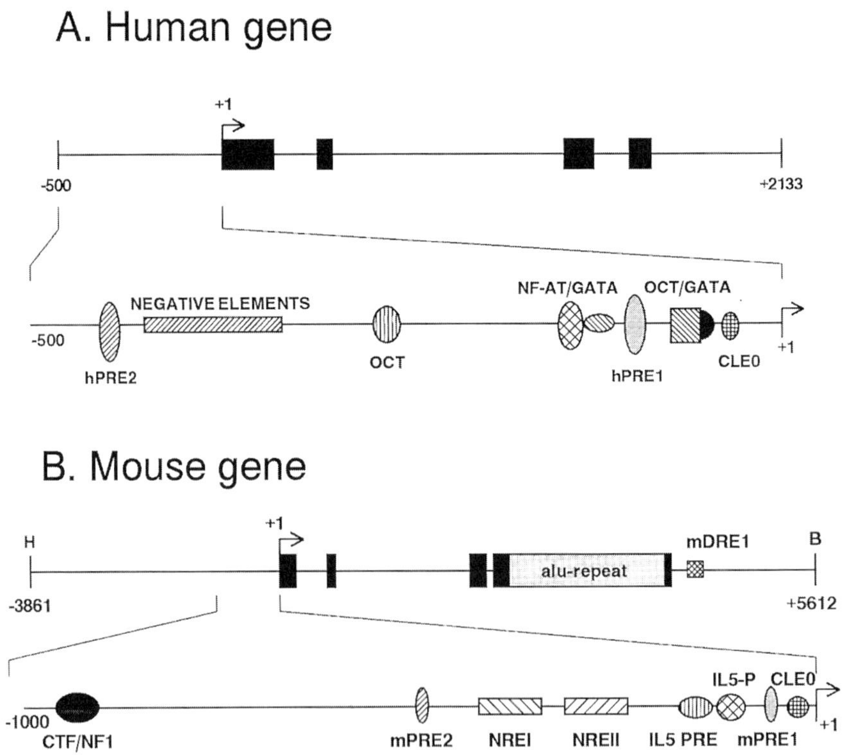


**Figure 2** Maps of the human (A) and mouse (B) IL-5 genes with details of regulatory elements in the promoter region. See text for details.

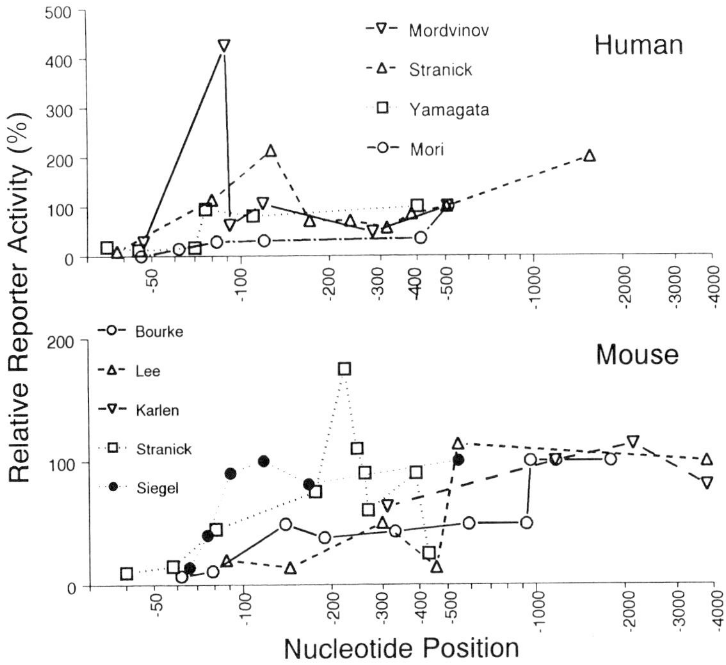


**Figure 3** Graphical representation of the results from deletions of the 5′ region of the IL-5 gene. Nucleotides numbered from the initiation of transcription. Analysis of the human gene is expressed relative to the expression of a 511 bp construct (100%) or 417 bp fragment in the results reported by Stranick et al. (13). See also, V. A. Mordvinov et al., unpublished data and references 10 and 14. Analyses of the mouse gene are expressed relative to a 1147 bp construct, or where this was not included, the longest fragment tested (9,11,14,17, and S. Karlen et al., unpublished data).

illustrates that while there is a consensus that distal regions have little effect and the proximal region is of major importance, there is little agreement about the intervening sequences.

A key question in gene regulation is understanding the spacial limits of regulatory elements. It is well known that distal elements in both the upstream and downstream flanking sequences can be important. Transgenic mice generated with a 10 kb fragment containing the IL-5 gene as well as the human CD2 locus control region (LCR) give some clues that this fragment might contain all the key regulatory elements. This construct provides IL-5 expression under the control of its own promoter, and the CD2 LCR provides a low-level constitutive expression which induces constitutive eosinophilia (7). When infected with the cestode *Mesocestoides corti* these mice develop very high levels of IL-

5, consistent with the normal activation of the transgenes. Furthermore, activation of spleen cells in vitro with ConA leads to much higher levels of IL-5 production than from normal spleen cells. The magnitude of this response is approximately proportional to the number of transgenes (8).

We have therefore used this 10 kb fragment as the starting point for reporter studies in EL4 cells. This fragment consists of –3361 to +5612 relative to the cap site. The luciferase gene was inserted at the cap site without deleting any sequences. It gave high-level inducible expression. A deletion analysis reveals three important facts. First, deleting to –1170 had little effect on expression, so the region from –3361 to –1170 is unlikely to contain any critical elements. Second, deleting to –313 increased the constitutive expression and decreased the level of inducible expression, indicating that the region between –1170 and –313 does contain important elements.

### A. Proximal Promoter Activators

For the purposes of this discussion, the proximal region is defined as the conserved region from –80 to –20, which contains a number of regulatory motifs as well as the TATA box (Fig. 2). The most studied is the conserved lymphokine element 0 (CLE0). This element was first identified because of its high homology between human and mouse genomic sequences, as well as its conservation in the GM-CSF gene. Related sequences also exist in other cytokine genes.

Deletion and linker scanner analysis in EL4 cells showed that the CLE0 element was crucial for IL-5 expression. Mutations in this element almost completely abolished expression in response to PMA and PMA + cAMP (9). Similarly the importance of this element was demonstrated by the establishment of stable transfectants in EL4 and D10 cells. Mutation of CLE0 markedly reduced expression of the gene in D10 cells induced by antigen (10) and in EL4 cells when induced by PMA (11). In all these studies, as well as work from this laboratory using EL4 cells (12), proteins binding to the CLE0 element were inducible, with little if any protein detected in unstimulated cells. Proteins of similar mobility were noted in an EL4 subline which did not produce IL-5, as well as in the human Jurkat cell line which also does not produce IL-5. Thus induction of the protein complexes appears to be essential for expression but is not specifically related to the expression of the IL-5 gene. Mori et al. (69) found that successive deletions decreased the ratio of induced to uninduced expression, but it is not clear from the results presented whether this results from a decrease in induced expression or an increase in constitutive expression. Mutation of the CLE0 element largely abrogated reporter expression. However, the role of the CLE0 element is not universally accepted. In one study, deletion to –80 increased the constitutive expression and removed inducibility in mouse D10 cells (13). This led the authors to the conclusion that CLE0, which is left intact, is not responsible for inducible expression. This cannot be reconciled with results from other groups, as discussed above.

Surprisingly, in other studies with the D10 T-cell line (14) it was reported that all the protein complexes were expressed constitutively. In fact, examination of Figure 5 in that article shows a protein band which appears to be induced, but this was not discussed by the authors. Furthermore, mutations in the CLE0 element had little effect on reporter expression, which lead the authors to conclude that the CLE0 element was of little importance to the expression of the gene. There are two possible explanations for this difference with the studies discussed above. First, this latter study was done in the context of only a 431 bp promoter fragment, which may give incomplete or misleading reporter expression. Second, results are expressed as a fraction of expression of the reporter under control of an SV40 promoter. This is itself an inducible system, making interpretation of data difficult.

The CLE0 consists of an overlapping AP-1 and an inverted NFAT-like sequence. The major inducible band in EL4 cells in inhibited by an AP-1 consensus sequence, and is supershifted by antisera to the AP-1 family members c-fos and JunB. Two minor bands which are present in unstimulated EL4 cells and not increased by stimulation were partially inhibited by consensus NFAT sequences. Mutation of the AP-1 moiety destroyed the ability to compete for binding to CLE0, whereas mutation of the NFAT-like sequence had little effect. This suggests that, at least in EL4 cells, the AP-1 sequence is critical to the binding of all the complexes to CLE0. Taking all these reports together we conclude that the binding of c-fos and JunB to the CLE0 element is critical to the expression of IL-5 (12).

The CLE0 element is thought to work in concert with other activation elements in the proximal region of the promoter. However, again it is difficult to reconcile results from different laboratories. First we will discuss studies on the human promoter. Yamagata et al. (15) demonstrated that deletion to base −76 had little effect on reporter expression compared to a fragment to −400, when tested in ATL-16T cell line which expresses IL-5 constitutively. However, deletion of a further 6 bases (to −70) markedly inhibited expression. This effect was attributed to a GATA element, and it was demonstrated that GATA-4 protein bound to this site. On the other hand, Gruart-Gouilleux et al. (16) working with the human promoter in mouse EL4 cells, found that deleting down to −80 had little effect on expression. Deletion to −67, which would delete the GATA site, had no additional effect. In EMSA experiments with an oligo corresponding to −67 to −30, which includes the CLE0 element, binding of Oct factors was demonstrated, suggesting a role for this group of transcription factors in the activation of IL-5. In our own studies using the human promoter in the human PER-117 cell line, deletion from −507 to −92 had little effect upon stimulation with PMA and cAMP. Deleting an additional 3 bases caused an enhancement of expression which is discussed in the next section. Further deletion to -47, which deletes most of CLE0, markedly decreased expression.

A study of the mouse gene in mouse EL4 cells indicated that activation via the combination of the adjacent GATA and CLE0 elements in response to elevated levels of cAMP results in selective expression of IL-5 (17). In this case GATA-3 was demonstrated to bind to the GATA element. The question of which GATA protein was important was addressed by Zhang et al. (18), who produced convincing evidence that GATA-3 was critical to the Th2-specific expression of IL-5. These authors argued that the observation that GATA-4 was important (15) (discussed above) may have been due to aberrant expression of this protein by the cell line used in the study.

### B. Distal Promoter Elements

As mentioned above, deleting from -3361 to -1174 of the mouse gene has no effect when compared to a 10 kb fragment encompassing the whole gene, but further deletions altered the pattern of expression. This is consistent with results obtained with stable transfectants in D10 cells, where an enhancer element between -940 to -928 was identified. Mutation of a CTF/NF1 site in this region converted the stable transfectants to constitutive expression (11), although it is important to note that induction was done with PMA which produces only a fraction of the activation compared with PMA plus cAMP. In other experiments, deleting to -932 decreased transient expression by about 50% when the cells are induced with PMA and cAMP, with no apparent effect on constitutive expression (9). This is an important element but its precise role in gene regulation requires further work.

Deletion and mutation analysis revealed an NFAT-related element (IL-5P) between -117 and -92 which is important in the activation of the gene (9). A functionally analogous (but not homologous nor spatially related) regulator was identified in the human gene between -123 and -92 (IL-5-REII) when tested in mouse D10 cells. This region contained sequences with homology to NFAT, NF-Y, and AP-1 binding sites. Proteins binding to the region reacted with antibodies to NFAT (13).

In a study with the human promoter expressed in mouse EL4 cells an octamer (Oct) element was located at -244 to -237 and formed complexes with factors antigenically related to members of the Oct group. Mutation of this element reduced IL-5 expression by 90%. In contrast, a deletion analysis of the human gene tested in mouse D10 cells failed to identify activity in this region. No effect was reported when deleting from -1547 to -172, but a negative regulatory element was identified between -172 and -127. This region showed weak binding to nuclear proteins from a human T-cell clone (SP-B13), but binding was not effected by cell activation (13). One must assume that because the footprinting was done with a human cell line but the transfections with a mouse cell line, the human cells could not be transfected. The lack of correlation between protein binding and expression following activation, as well as the species differences, suggests more work is required to confirm the relevence of these findings.

## IV. Upstream Repressor Elements

Deletion analysis of the human promoter revealed a promoter element between –404 and –312 when expressed in mouse EL4 cells. The nature of the repressor was not investigated further (16).

We have identified two novel related regulatory elements in the IL-5 promoter. The first of these elements consists of a 5 bp inverted repeat and a 7 bp core sequence and is called the human palindromic element (hPRE1). The hPRE1 is located between the positive regulatory complexes CLE0/Oct/GATA and NF-AT/GATA at positions –78 to –94 of the promoter. This site covers the sequence *ATGCC*attatta*GGCAT* which is unique to IL-5. The hPRE1 element was identified as an IL-5 repressor with deletion of the element resulting in a increase in human IL-5 promoter activity (V. A. Mordvinov, unpublished data). By EMSA, binding of a specific complex to the hPRE1 sequence was observed using nuclear extracts prepared from different T-cell and non-T-cell lines. However, treatment of cells with PMA and cAMP greatly reduced hPRE1 protein binding only in PER-117 T cells. This observation suggests that in T cells exhibiting inducible IL-5 expression the hPRE1 sequence may act as a constitutive repressor. The element appears only in IL-5 gene sequences and thus may be a specific regulator of IL-5.

Expression of several cytokines has been shown to be partly regulated by repressor elements. Negative regulatory element (NRE) has been identified in the human IL-4 promoter. It has been shown that the IL-4 promoter activity is normally down-regulated by NRE via repression of the enhancer-positive regulatory element (19). The CK1/CK2 region of the IL-3 and GM-CSF genes acts as a repressor of basal-level expression (20,21). In resting T lymphocytes, the IL-2 gene is silenced by a repressor biding to the Pud element present in the promoter region. Upon T-cell activation, this silencer is displaced by a positive transcription factor and the gene is derepressed and transcribed (22).

Interestingly the hPRE1 sequence is located amidst the positive regulatory elements of the hIL-5 proximal promoter. By virtue of its location, hPRE1 binding proteins could be involved in direct contact with GATA transcription factors (Fig. 2). The GATA element as well as CLE0 and Oct are an integral part of the positive regulatory domain which is critical for inducible expression of the gene. The second palindromic element present in the human IL-5 gene is the hPRE2 element which has inverted repeats similar to hPRE1 but a dissimilar core sequence. This element is located between nucleotides –452 and –462 and also forms four DNA-protein complexes with PER-117 cells. These proteins can be competed out by the hPRE1 sequence and vice versa, indicating similarity in the binding of the two elements. It is proposed that there exists negative regulatory proteins common to both the hPRE1 and hPRE2 sequences. Thus it is possible that common regulatory proteins allow the hPRE1 and hPRE2 to interact with each other, and could be involved in interactions with positive elements to fine tune the regulation of expression.

Two related palindromic elements (mPRE1 and mPRE2) have also been identified in the mouse IL-5 promoter. The mPRE1 sequence is located at positions –79 to –90 of the promoter. This element has high homology to hPRE1 and consists of a 3 bp inverted repeat and a 5 bp core sequence. However, in contrast to the human element, mPRE1 has been shown to be involved in positive induction of the mouse IL-5 gene. We have no explanation for this surprising result. A second element, mPRE2, similar to hPRE2 is located at a distal site upstream in the promoter (–459 to –470). This element has identical inverted repeats but a dissimilar core sequence and is also involved in positive induction of the gene. These elements bind proteins of identical electrophoretic mobility from nuclear extracts of the mouse T-cell line EL4-23 and murine primary T cells and can cross-compete for DNA-protein complex formation. A model for interaction of these two elements resulting in formation of a higher-order nucleoprotein complex has been proposed due to the additive effect observed upon IL-5 promoter activity when these elements are mutated in parallel (G. T. F. Schwenger, unpublished data).

Interestingly, the PRE1 and PRE2 elements are present in all known IL-5 genes (mouse, rat, human, and ovine) but not in any other gene on the database. This suggests the possibility of a role for these elements in the specific regulation of the IL-5 gene.

## V. Downstream Repressor Elements

A 3 kb fragment of the 3′ region of the murine gene cloned upstream or downstream of luciferase reduced expression to 10 to 15%. Further analysis of this region (M. Senna Salerno, unpublished data) was carried out by cloning the fragment downstream of the luciferase reporter in the pGL3-promoter vector (Promega, Madison, Wisconsin). This caused a decrease in expression compared to the vector in both stimulated and unstimulated conditions. A series of deletions made in this construct identified a 258 bp fragment downstream of the poly(A) attachment site which showed a strong repressor activity. Upon stimulation with PMA and cAMP the repressor activity was diminished but not completely abolished. To locate potential regulatory elements in vitro footprinting was carried out with both strands of the 258-bp fragment using nuclear extracts of EL4-23 cells. A protected site was observed on both the DNA strands with nuclear extracts from unstimulated cells. Protection was not observed in activated cells. This protected site indicated the presence of constitutively expressed protein complexes and was named mouse downstream regulatory element 1 (mDRE1). This element is remarkable both for the length of sequence protected (47 bp) and for the sequence which consists of four repeats of ATGAATGA, all in the same orientation. The first and last pairs of repeats are separated by four nonrelated nucleotides, so the whole mDRE1 structure is symmetrical, apart from the final seven protected nucleotides.

EMSA using an oligonucleotide corresponding to the protected area indicated that two protein complexes show specific binding. Interestingly nuclear extracts of activated EL4 cells gave weaker binding than the nonactivated cell extracts, supporting the footprinting results and indicating that binding decreases upon cell stimulation. Competition experiments with smaller and mutated oligonucleotides indicated that a sequence containing two of the repeats are the main motif involved in protein binding (underlined on the sequence). Up to four nucleotides could be inserted between the two repeats without disrupting binding. This suggests that the motif binds multiple copies of the same proteins.

## VI. Pathways Leading to the Activation of the IL-5 Gene

Activation of T cells requires the interaction of the TCR complex with antigen in association with the major histocompatibility complex, which leads to an increase in intracellular calcium concentration and activation of protein kinase C (PKC) (23). In vitro activation of T cells can be achieved by stimulating the TCR with anti-CD3 mAb or by treating the cells with PHA or PMA in combination with ionomycin. The TCR-CD3 pathway is sensitive to CsA and FK506. Stimulation of the TCR alone, however, is insufficient to fully activate most T cells and a second signal provided by antigen presenting cells (APC) is also required (24). This costimulatory signal can be generated through the CD28 signaling pathway (25). Interestingly CD28 signal transduction is resistant to CsA but is sensitive to rapamycin (26).

Efficient production of IL-5 requires the activation of both the TCR and a second signaling pathway. Anti-CD28 mAb, in combination with PMA, was shown to be necessary for optimal induction of IL-5 synthesis (27–29). This CD28-mediated induction was insensitive to CsA (27). However, several studies demonstrated that IL-5 secretion can be inhibited by CsA (30–32). This suggests that an alternative, CsA-sensitive, costimulatory pathway can be used for the induction of the gene. Indeed, synergy between PMA and cAMP has been reported for the activation of IL-5 (1,16). Recent pharmacological studies have shown that cAMP signaling involves the $Ca^{2+}$-dependent phosphate calcineurin whose activity is suppressed by CsA (33). We recently demonstrated that cAMP-induced transcription of the IL-5 gene is CsA sensitive (12). It is important to note that while cAMP markedly enhances the expression of IL-5, it has an inhibitory effect on Il-2, IL-3, IL-10, and GM-CSF (1,34,35) and has no effect on IL-4 (36). Histamine has been shown to increase the production of IL-5 in activated T cells, whereas the production of IL-4 was not affected (37). The induction by histamine was mediated via $H_2$ receptors which are known to activate the cAMP-dependent protein kinase A (PKA) signaling pathway.

Such observations are of importance, since they provide us with a model to understand the specific control mechanisms regulating the expression of the IL-5 gene. Upon stimulation with an allergen (or antigen), the TCR/CD3 complex is activated and delivers signals toward the nucleus through the PKC and the $Ca^{2+}$-dependent signaling pathways. This results in the activation of a broad range of transcription factors including AP-1 and NF-AT. Through interaction of CD28 with its ligands B7 and B7-2 on the surface of APC, a costimulatory signal is delivered that fully activates transcription. As a consequence, expression of most cytokine genes is achieved. Eosinophils are eventually activated by IL-3, GM-CSF, and IL-5, whereas IL-4-stimulated B-cells start to produce IgE. In certain circumstances, however, it is believed that allergen can provoke the direct release of histamine by mast cells (38). By interacting with $H_2$ receptors, histamine generates cAMP-mediated signals which simultaneously activate the IL-5 gene (through stimulation of AP-1 binding by PKA) (39) and suppresses the synthesis of the other pro-inflammatory cytokines (via inhibition of NF-κB binding) (34). In that particular case, IL-5 is the only mediator of eosinophil activation produced and the inflammatory symptoms characteristic of asthma are independent of the presence or the absence of IgE.

This is of course an oversimplified view of gene regulation by T cells. The model, for example, does not take into account additional accessory receptor molecules which could modulate T-cell activation. Adhesion molecules such as LFA-1, VLA-4, CD2, and CD44 have been reported to mediate transmembrane signaling events (40). The binding of certain cytokines to their receptors can also dramatically affect the magnitude and pattern of T-cell lymphokine expression. Studies indicate that IL-2 increases IL-5 production by T lymphocytes (29,41). Signaling through IL-2 receptors was recently shown to involve at least three distinct pathways (42). Finally, the use of alternative signaling pathways can also lead to the activation of regulatory factors which cross-compete for control of the T-cell response. A good candidate for such differential activation would be the AP-1 transcription factor. AP-1 binding is mainly controlled by PKC. However, in response to cAMP induction, PKA promotes the formation of active AP-1 complexes containing JunB (43). In similar conditions, JunB is also a potent inhibitor of c-Jun and JunD (44,45). Therefore one can imagine that through activation of the PKC pathway expression of a broad range of genes responding to AP-1 would be induced, whereas in cAMP-treated cells only those under the control of particular JunB/AP-1 complexes would be activated. This hypothesis could be considered for the regulation of IL-5, as we recently demonstrated that induction of IL-5 expression in cAMP-stimulated mouse T cells is mainly regulated via a JunB-containing AP-1 complex (12).

## VII. Posttranscriptional Effects

Posttranscriptional regulation plays an important role in the regulation of several cytokine genes. The control of mRNA stability is seen in several cytokines (e.g., IL-1, IL-2, IL-3, IL-6, GM-CSF, and G-CSF) (46–50). Modulation of translational efficiency is also an important posttranscriptional regulatory event in eukaryotic gene expression and is seen in such cytokines as TNF-α and IFN-β (51,52). In both these instances, regulation is commonly mediated by way of its 3′-UTR. To investigate the role of the 3′-UTR in regulating mIL-5 gene expression, two IL-5 cDNA expressing clones were used (53). The first corresponded to the full-length mRNA (IL-5cFL) of 1534 nt in length. The second encoded a truncated version in which most of the 3′-UTR was missing (IL-5cTR). To compare the mRNA levels between the two, both constructs were electroporated into COS7 cells and the RNA extracted at various time points following transfection. A northern blot analysis revealed very similar kinetics of IL-5 mRNA accumulation between the two, suggesting that the 3′-UTR has a minimal effect on IL-5 RNA stability. Analysis of the translational efficiency between the two transcripts was also performed. The two cDNA plasmids were cloned into a vector with the SP6 promoter and translation levels were assayed by $^{35}$S-labeled methionine incorporation into IL-5 using the reticulocyte lysate expression system. No significant difference in translation was observed between the two clones, suggesting little involvement of the 3′-UTR in mIL-5 regulation. These results suggest that posttranscriptional control may not be a major factor in controlling IL-5 production.

## VIII. Drug Effects on IL-5 Production

### A. Glucocorticoids

Glucocorticoids are the most effective treatment for asthma available today (54). Their clinical efficacy is believed to arise from their ability to inhibit cytokine-mediated leukocyte recruitment into the airways (55). One such important cytokine involved in this process is IL-5. IL-5 is believed to play a pivotal role in the activation and specific migration of eosinophils from the bloodstream into various tissues. Granule proteins released from activated eosinophils damage the respiratory epithelium in vitro and induce bronchial hyperresponsiveness. A role for IL-5 and eosinophils in bronchial hyperreactivity and allergic airway disease has been shown recently in vivo (56). Inhibiting the production of IL-5 may represent a useful approach in the treatment of asthma.

Glucocorticoids have been shown to inhibit IL-5 production. Corticosteroid treatment in patients with moderate asthma revealed a decrease in bronchial responsiveness, bronchial eosiniphilia, and the number of BAL (bronchalveolar lavage) cells expressing mRNA for IL-5 (57,58). In another study, corticosteroid treatment was found to significantly decrease peripheral blood eosinophil counts and serum IL-5 (59). Using the Th2 clone D10.G4.1, corticosteroids were shown to inhibit α-CD3-induced IL-5 production in a dose-dependent manner (60). Dexamethasone, a synthetic glucocorticoid, was also shown to inhibit IL-5 production from Th-0, Th-1, and Th2-like T-cell clones derived from BAL fluid, blood, and from randomly cloned and allergen-specific T-cell clones (61,62).

The ability of dexamethasone to inhibit IL-5 gene expression has been found to be dependent on the type of stimulation. Rolfe et al. (63) reported that dexamethasone could inhibit IL-5 gene expression in PBMC after treatment with PHA, PMA, and rIL-2, but not ionomycin. In our own studies using PER-117 cells, we have observed that dexamethasone exhibits a reduced ability to stimulate IL-5 production when cells are stimulated with PMA + A23187 as compared to PMA or PMA + cAMP (M. L. De Boer, V. A. Mordvinov, and S. E. Peroni, unpublished data). Taken together, this suggests that dexamethasone interferes with a pathway requiring PKC, but not one involving an increase in intracellular calcium (63). However, a conflicting report has shown that dexamethasone used at similar concentrations as in the two latter studies could completely inhibit IL-5 production from PBMC when stimulated with PMA and ionomycin (31). The reason for this discrepancy is not immediately clear, but may be due in part to the level of sensitivity of the various assays used to measure IL-5.

Mori et al. (6) have recently shown that glucocorticoids can inhibit IL-5 at the level of protein production, IL-5 mRNA induction, and at the level of transcriptional activity in T-cell clones stimulated with α-CD3 or rIL-2. It was found that dexamethasone can suppress the transcriptional activity mediated by a 500 bp IL-5 reporter construct, indicating that this region is responsible for regulation by glucocorticoids. In agreement, we have found that an IL-5 reporter construct containing 2 kb of the IL-5 promoter is not more susceptible to the inhibitory effects of dexamethasone than a 500 bp IL-5 reporter construct when transiently transfected into PER-117 cells (M. L. De Boer, unpublished data). Using consensus oligonucleotides for various transcription factors as probes in EMSA, it was shown that altogether α-CD3 could induce NFAT, NF-κB, or

AP1, only NF-κB and AP1 were sensitive to dexamethasone (6). IL-2R stimulation in contrast, did not induce NFAT, NF-κB, or AP-1, even though IL-5 gene expression was abolished by treatment with dexamethasone. This suggests that NF-κB and AP-1 may be important for IL-5 synthesis after TCR stimulation, but they are not necessary upon stimulation with IL-2. Whether glucocorticoids act on these transcription factors in the context of bona fide human IL-5 sequences remains to be determined.

### B. Other Drugs

Other drugs have been used in the treatment of asthma include CsA (cyclosporin A), FK506, and rapamycin. Although all have been shown to inhibit IL-5 production (31,32,64,65), their mode of action is not yet known. CsA and FK506, complexed to immunophilins, can inhibit calcineurin, a $Ca^{2+}$-dependent phosphatase that is believed to play a role in $Ca^{2+}$-dependent T-cell activation (66). Calcineurin dephosphorylates NFAT (67), allowing it to translocate to the nucleus and bind to the regulatory regions of various genes (68). CsA and FK506 have been shown to inhibit the phosphorylation and nuclear translocation of NFAT (66–68). Recently, it has been shown that a region of the human IL-5 promoter located between −123 and −92 (REII) is critical for inducible IL-5 promoter activity in the murine Th2 cell clone D10.G4.1 (13). As mentioned previously, proteins that bind to this region react with antibodies to NFAT. This region was also found to be a specific target of CsA inhibition (13). In addition, FK506 was found to inhibit protein binding to CLE0 upon activation of T-cell clones with α-CD3 (69). CLE0 contains consensus sites for AP-1 and NFAT transcription factors. Whether a potential mechanism of IL-5 suppression results from the ability of CsA and FK506 to inhibit NFAT binding to these regions in the human IL-5 promoter remains to be determined. In contrast to CsA and FK506, rapamycin inhibits T-cell activation by interfering with $Ca^{2+}$-independent signaling pathway (66,70,71). Recently it has been shown that CsA and FK506 do not inhibit IL-5 expression by effecting IL-5 mRNA stability (64).

As observed with dexamethasone, the mode of stimulation also appears to play a role in the ability of these drugs to effect T-cell function. CsA and FK506 strongly inhibit IL-5 mRNA expression in response to PHA, PMA, and/or ionomycin (64,65), whereas rIL-2-induced IL-5 expression is resistant to CsA and rapamycin (65). This again illustrates that different signaling pathways are involved in IL-5 expression depending on whether cells are stimulated via the IL-2R or TCR. These observations underscore the usefulness of these drugs in dissecting out the various signaling pathways involved in IL-5 expression. The mechanisms that mediate inhibition of T-cell function by CsA and dexamethasone also appear to be different (72), and as a result, CsA has been shown to be clinically effective in the treatment of glucocorticoid-resistant asthma (73,74).

Interestingly a new agent, OM-01, has been found to suppress IL-5 protein production, mRNA expression, and transcriptional activity in PBMC with no effect observed on IL-2 or IL-4 (75). Additionally, it was reported that this agent could inhibit late-phase eosinophil infiltration when used in a murine experimental asthma model. Further studies are clearly warranted to determine if this agent will be useful in treating eosinophilic disorders.

## IX. Conclusions

Although our understanding of the regulation of IL-5 production is far from complete, a clearer picture is emerging. There is a major role for the highly conserved proximal promoter region, where the CLE0 and GATA elements are critical to expression. More distal upstream and downstream elements are also involved and may fine-tune the levels of expression in individual cells. The species differences in these more distal regions is an enigma, as the regulation of eosinophilia is highly conserved in mammalia. Presumably different species have found slightly different ways to fine-tune the production of IL-5 to give a similar overall effect.

It is frequently asserted that the expression of IL-4 and IL-5 is coordinately controlled, implying a common mechanism of gene expression. This is largely based on the frequent association of IgE and eosinophilia, and the coexpression in long-term T-cell clones. There is no good evidence for this at the gene level. Although the two cytokines are frequently coexpressed in certain diseases such as atopic allergy, a more likely process would be that they are induced by essentially different molecular mechanisms. This allows the differential expression of the two genes at both the population and the single-cell level. This provides an explanation for the differential expression of IgE and eosinophilia, as seen in intrinsic asthma, without ruling out the coexpression of the two genes when a disease process provokes them simultaneously.

## References

1. Lee HJ, Koyano-Nakagawa N, Naito Y, Nishida J, Arai N, Arai K-I, Yokota T. cAMP activates the IL-5 promoter synergistically with phorbol ester through the signaling pathway involving protein kinase A in mouse thymoma line EL-4. J Immunol 1993;151:6135–6142.
2. Kaye J, Porcelli S, Tite J, Jones B, Janeway CA, Jr. Both a monoclonal antibody and antisera specific for determinants unique to individual cloned helper T cell lines can substitute for antigen and antigen-presenting cells in the activation of T cells. J Exp Med 1983;158:836–856.
3. Warren DJ, Sanderson CJ. Production of a T-cell hybrid producing a lymphokine stimulating eosinophil differentiation. Immunology 1985;54:615–623.

4. Rolfe FG, Sewell WA. Analysis of human interleukin-5 gene transcription by a novel nuclear run on method based on the polymerase chain reaction. J Immunol Meth 1997;202:143–151.
5. Kees UR, Peroni SE, Ranford PR, Ford J. A new human cell line for the molecular dissertation of the requirement for interleukin-1 in the production of interleukin-2 by immature T cells. J Immunol Meth 1994;168:1–8.
6. Mori A, Kaminuma O, Suko M, Inoue S, Ohmura T, Hoshino A, Asakura Y, Miyazawa K, Yokota T, Okumura Y, Ito K, Okudaira H. Two distinct pathways of interleukin-5 synthesis in allergen-specific human T-cell clones are suppressed by glucocorticoids. Blood 1997;89:2891–2900.
7. Dent LA, Strath M, Mellor AL, Sanderson CJ. Eosinophilia in transgenic mice expressing interleukin 5. J Exp Med 1990;172:1425–1431.
8. Strath M, Dent L, Sanderson C. Infection of IL5 transgenic mice with *Mesocestoides corti* induces very high levels of IL5 but depressed production of eosinophils. Exp Hematol 1992;20:229–234.
9. Lee HJ, Masuda ES, Arai N, Arai K, Yokota T. Definition of cis-regulatory elements of the mouse interleukin-5 gene promoter. Involvement of nuclear factor of activated T cells-related factors in interleukin-5 expression. J Biol Chem 1995;270:17541–17550.
10. Naora H, Young IG. Comparison of the mechanisms regulating IL-5, IL-4, and three other lymphokine genes in the Th2 clone D10.G4.1. Exp Hematol 1995;23:597–602.
11. Bourke PF, Van Leeuwen BH, Campbell HD, Young IG. Localization of the inducible enhancer in the mouse interleukin-5 gene that is responsive to T-cell receptor stimulation. Blood 1995;85:2069–2077.
12. Karlen S, D'Ercole M, Sanderson CJ. Two pathways can activate the interleukin-5 gene and induce binding to the conserved lymphokine element 0. Blood 1996;88:211–221.
13. Stranick KS, Zambas DN, Uss AS, Egan RW, Billah MM, Umland SP. Identification of transcription factor binding sites important in the regulation of the human interleukin-5 gene. J Biol Chem 1997;272:16453–16465.
14. Stranick KS, Payvandi F, Zambas DN, Umland SP, Egan RW, Billah MM. Transcription of the murine interleukin 5 gene is regulated by multiple promoter elements. J Biol Chem 1995;270:20575–20582.
15. Yamagata T, Nishida J, Sakai R, Tanaka T, Honda H, Hirano N, Mano H, Yazaki Y, Hirai H. Of the GATA-binding proteins, only GATA-4 selectively regulates the human interleukin-5 gene promoter in interleukin-5-producing cells which express multiple GATA-binding proteins. Mol Cell Biol 1995;15:3830–3839.
16. Gruart-Gouilleux V, Engels P, Sullivan M. Characterization of the human interleukin-5 gene promoter: involvement of octamer binding sites in the gene promoter activity. Eur J Immunol 1995;25:1431–1435.
17. Siegel MD, Zhang DH, Ray P, Ray A. Activation of the interleukin-5 promoter by cAMP in murine EL-4 cells requires the GATA-3 and CLE0 elements. J Biol Chem 1995;270:24548–24555.
18. Zhang DH, Cohn L, Ray P, Bottomly K, Ray A. Transcription factor GATA-3 is

differentially expressed murine Th1 and Th2 cells and controls Th2-specific expression of the interleukin-5 gene. J Biol Chem 1997;272:21597-21603.
19. Li-Weber M, Krafft H, Krammer PH. A novel enhancer element in the human IL-4 promoter is suppressed by a position-independent silencer. J Immunol 1993;151:1371-1382.
20. Ryan GR, Vadas MA, Shannon MF. T-cell functional regions of the human IL-3 proximal promoter. Mol Reprod Dev 1994;39:200–207.
21. Coles LS, Occhiodoro F, Vadas MA, Shannon MF. A sequence-specific single-strand DNA binding protein that contacts repressor sequences in the human GM-CSF promoter. Nucleic Acids Res 1994;22:4276–4283.
22. Mouzaki A, Dai Y, Weil R, Rungger D. Cyclosporin A and FK506 prevent the derepression of the IL-2 gene in mitogen-induced primary T lymphocytes. Cytokine 1992;4:151-160.
23. Perlmutter RM, Levin SD, Appleby MW, Anderson SJ, Alberola-Ila J. Regulation of lymphocyte function by protein phosphorylation. Annu Rev Immunol 1993;11:451–499.
24. Rincon M, Flavell RA. AP-1 transcriptional activity requires both T-cell receptor-mediated and co-stimulatory signals in primary T lymphocytes. EMBO J 1994;13:4370–4381.
25. Jenkins MK, Johnson JG. Molecules involved in T-cell costimulation. Curr Opin Immunol 1993;5:361-367.
26. Lai JH, Tan TH. CD28 signaling causes a sustained down-regulation of I kappa B alpha which can be prevented by the immunosuppressant rapamycin. J Biol Chem 1994;269:30077-30080.
27. Schandene L, Alonso-Vega C, Willems F, Gerard C, Delvaux A, Velu T, Devos R, De Boer M, Goldman M. B7/CD28-dependent IL-5 production by human resting T cells is inhibited by IL-10. J Immunol 1994;152:4368–4374.
28. Wierenga EA, Snoek M, Jansen HM, Bos JD, van Lier RAW, Kapsenberg ML. Human atopen-specific types 1 and 2 T helper cell clones. J Immunol 1991;147:2942-2949.
29. Kuiper HM, de Jong R, Brouwer M, Lammers K, Wijdenes J, van Lier RAW. Influence of CD28 co-stimulation on cytokine production is mainly regulated via interleukin-2. Immunology 1994;83:38–44.
30. Okudaira H, Mori A, Suko M, Etoh T, Nakagawa H, Ito K. Enhanced production and gene expression of interleukin-5 in patients with bronchial asthma: possible management of atopic diseases by down-regulation of interleukin-5 gene transcription. Int Arch Allergy Immunol 1995;107:255–258.
31. Mori A, Suto M, Nishizaki Y, Kaminuma O, Matsuzaki G, Ito K, Etoh T, Nakagawa H, Tsuruoka N, Okudaira H. Regulation of interleukin-5 production by peripheral blood mononuclear cells from atopic patients with FK506, cyclosporin A and glucocorticoid. Int Arch Allergy Immunol 1994;104(suppl 1):32–35.
32. Andersson J, Nagy S, Groth C-J, Andersson U. Effects of FK506 and cyclosporin A on cytokine production studied in vitro at a single-cell level. Immunology 1992;75:136–142.
33. Schwaninger M, Blume R, Kruger M, Lux G, Oetjen E, Knepel W. Involvement

of the Ca(2+)-dependent phosphatase calcineurin in gene transcription that is stimulated by cAMP through cAMP response elements. J Biol Chem 1995;270:8860–8866.
34. Chen D, Rothenberg EV. Interleukin-2 transcription factors as molecular targets of cAMP inhibition: delayed inhibition kinetics and combinatorial transcription roles. J Exp Med 1994;179:931–942.
35. Derig HG, Burgess GS, Klinberg D, Dahreine TS, Mochizuki DY, Williams DE, Boswell HS. Role for cyclic AMP in the postreceptor control of cytokine stimulated stromal cell growth factor production. Leukemia 1990;4:471–479.
36. Novak TJ, Rothenberg EV. cAMP inhibits induction of interleukin-2 but not of interleukin-4 in T-cells. Proc Natl Acad Sci USA 1990;87:9353–9357.
37. Schmidt J, Fleissner S, Heimann-Weitschat I, Lindstaedt R, Szelenyi I. Histamine increases anti-CD3 induced IL-5 production of T-type T cells via histamine H2-receptors. Agents Actions 1994;42:81–85.
38. Corrigan CJ, Kay AB. T cells and eosinophils in the pathogenesis of asthma. Immunol Today 1992;13:501–505.
39. de Groot RP, Auwerx J, Karperien M, Staels B, Kruijer W. Activation of junB by PKC and PKA signal transduction through a novel cis-acting element. Nucleic Acids Res 1991;19:775–781.
40. Fraser JD, Straus D, Weiss A. Signal transduction events leading to T-cell lymphokine gene expression. Immunol Today 1993;14:357–362.
41. Bohjanen PJ, Okajima M, Hodes RJ. Differential regulation of interleukin 4 and interleukin 5 gene expression: a comparison of T-cell gene induction by anti-CD3 antibody or by exogenous lymphokines. Proc Natl Acad Sci USA 1990;87:5283–5287.
42. Miyazaki T, Liu Z-J, Kawahara A, Minami Y, Yamada K, Tsujimoto Y, Barsoumian EL, Perlmutter RM, Taniguchi T. Three distinct IL-2 signaling pathways mediated by bcl-2, c-myc, and lck cooperate in hematopoietic cell proliferation. Cell 1995;81:223–231.
43. Hsu J-C, Cressman DE, Raub R. Promoter-specific trans-activation and inhibition mediated by JunB. Cancer Res 1993;53:3789–3794.
44. Chiu R, Angel P, Karin M. Jun-B differs in its biological properties from, and is a negative regulator of c-Jun. Cell 1989;59:979–986.
45. Kobierski LA, Chu H-M, Tan Y, Comb MJ. cAMP-dependent regulation of proenkephalin by JunD and JunB: positive and negative effects of AP-1 proteins. Proc Natl Acad Sci USA 1991;88:10222–10226.
46. Lindsten T, June CH, Ledbetter JA, Stella G, Thompson CB. Regulation of lymphokine messenger RNA stability by a surface-mediated T cell activation pathway. Science 1989;244:339–343.
47. Guba SC, Stella G, Turka LA, June CH, Thompson CB, Emerson SG. Regulation of interleukin 3 gene induction in normal human T cells J Clin Invest 1989;84:1701–1706.
48. Elias JA, Lentz V. IL-1 and tumor necrosis factor synergistically stimulate fibroblast IL-6 production and stabilize IL-6 messenger RNA. J Immunol 1990;145:161–166.

49. Koeffler HP, Gasson J, Tobler A. Transcriptional and posttranscriptional modulation of myeloid colony-stimulating factor expression by tumor necrosis factor and other agents. Mol Cell Biol 1988;8:3432–3438.
50. Shaw G, Kamen R. A conserved AU sequence from the 3′ untranslated region of GM-CSF mRNA mediates selective mRNA deregulation. Cell 1986;46:659–667.
51. Kruys V, Wathelet M, Poupart P, Contreras R, Fiers W, Contnet J, Huez G. The 3′ untranslated region of the human interferon-beta mRNA has an inhibitory effect on translation. Proc Natl Acad Sci USA 1987;84:6030–6034.
52. Kruys V, Huez G. Translational control of cytokine expression by 3′ UA-rich sequences. Biochimie 1994;76:862–866.
53. Campbell HD, Sanderson CJ, Wang Y, Hort Y, Martinson ME, Tucker WQ, Stellwagen A, Strath M, Young IG. Isolation, structure and expression of cDNA and genomic clones for murine eosinophil differentiation factor. Comparison with other eosinophilopoietic lymphokines and identity with interleukin-5. Eur J Biochem 1988;174:345–352.
54. Barnes PJ. Inhaled glucocorticoids for asthma [review]. N Engl J Med 1995;332:868–875.
55. Schwiebert LM, Beck LA, Stellato C, Bickel CA, Bochner BS, Schleimer RP, Schwiebert LA. Glucocorticosteroid inhibition of cytokine production: relevance to antiallergic actions [published erratum appears in J Allergy Clin Immunol 1996;98(3):718 [review]. J Allergy Clin Immunol 1996;97:143–152.
56. Hogan S, Koskinen A, Foster P. Interleukin-5 and eosinophils induce airway damage and bronchial hyperreactivity during allergic airway inflammation in BALB/c mice. Immunol Cell Biol 1997;75:284–288.
57. Robinson D, Hamid Q, Ying S, Bentley A, Assoufi B, Durham S, Kay AB. Prednisolone treatment in asthma is associated with modulation of bronchoalveolar lavage cells interleukin-4, interleukin-5, and interferon-gamma cytokine gene expression. Am Rev Respir Dis 1993;148:401–406.
58. Leung DY, Martin RJ, Szefler SJ, Sher ER, Ying S, Kay AB, Hamid Q. Dysregulation of interleukin 4, interleukin 5, and interferon gamma gene expression in steroid-resistant asthma. J Exp Med 1995;181:33–40.
59. Corrigan CJ, Haczku A, Gemou-Engesaeth V, Doi S, Kikuchi Y, Takatsu K, Durham SR, Kay AB. DC4 T-lymphocyte activation in asthma is accompanied by increased serum concentrations of interleukin-5. Effect of glucocorticoid therapy. Am Rev Respir Dis 1993;147:540–547.
60. Schmidt J, Fleissner S, Heimann-Weitschat I, Lindstaedt R, Szelenyi I. The effect of different corticosteroids and cyclosporin A on interleukin-4 and interleukin-5 release from murine Th2-type T cells. Eur J Pharmacol 1994;260:247–250.
61. Krouwels FH, van der Heijden JF, Lutter R, van Neerven RJ, Jansen HM, Out TA. Glucocorticosteroids affect functions of airway- and blood-derived human T-cell clones, favoring the Th1 profile through two mechanisms. Am J Respir Cell Mol Biol 1996;14:388–397.
62. Braun C, Huang S, Bashian G, Kagey-Sobotka A, Lichtenstein L, Essayan D. Corticosteroid modulation of human, antigen-specific Th1 and Th2 responses. Clin Immunol 1997;100:400–407.

63. Rolfe FG, Hughes JM, Armour CL, Sewell WA. Inhibition of interleukin-5 gene expression by dexamethasone. Immunol 1992;77:494–499.
64. Rolfe F, Valentine J, Sewell W. Cyclosporin A and FK506 reduce interleukin-5 mRNA abundance by inhibiting gene transcription. Am J Respir Cell Mol Biol 1997;17:243–250.
65. Valentine J, Sewell W. Induction of IL-5 expression by IL-2 is resistant to the immunosuppressive agents cyclosporin A and rapamycin. Int Immunol 1997;9:975–982.
66. Fruman DA, Klee CB, Bierer BE, Burakoff SJ. Calcineurin phosphatase activity in T lymphocytes is inhibited by FK 506 and cyclosporin A. Proc Natl Acad Sci USA 1992;89:3686–3690.
67. Luo C, Burgeon E, Carew JA, McCaffrey PG, Badalian TM, Lane WS, Hogan PG, Rao A. Recombinant NFAT1 (NFATp) is regulated by calcineurin in T cells and mediates transcription of several cytokine genes. Mol Cell Biol 1996;16:3955–3966.
68. Shaw KT, Ho AM, Raghavan A, Kim J, Jain J, Park J, Sharma S, Rao A, Hogan PG. Immunosuppressive drugs prevent a rapid dephosphorylation of transcription factor NFAT1 in stimulated immune cells. Proc Natl Acad Sci USA 1995;92:11205–11209.
69. Mori A, Kaminuma O, Mikami T, Hoshino A, Ohmura T, Miyazawa K, Suko M, Okudaira H. Dissection of human IL-5 promoter—essential role of CLE0 element in human IL-5 gene transcription. Int Arch Allergy Immunol 1997;113:272–274.
70. Dumont FJ, Staruch MJ, Koprak SL, Melino MR, Sigal NH. Distinct mechanisms of suppression of murine T cell activation by the related macrolides FK-506 and rapamycin. J Immunol 1990;144:251–258.
71. Bierer BE, Mattila PS, Standaert RF, Herzenberg LA, Burakoff SJ, Crabtree G, Schreiber SL. Two distinct signal transmission pathways in T lymphocytes are inhibited by complexes formed between an immunophilin and either FK506 or rapamycin. Proc Natl Acad Sci USA 1990;87:9231–9235.
72. Corrigan CJ, Brown PH, Barnes NC, Tsai JJ, Frew AJ, Kay AB. Glucocorticoid resistance in chronic asthma. Peripheral blood T lymphocyte activation and comparison of the T lymphocyte inhibitory effects of glucocorticoids and cyclosporin A. Am Rev Respir Dis 1991;144:1026–1032.
73. Alexander AG, Barnes NC, Kay AB. Trial of cyclosporin in corticosteroid-dependent chronic severe asthma [see comments]. Lancet 1992;339:324–328.
74. Lock SH, Kay AB, Barnes NC. Double-blind, placebo-controlled study of cyclosporin A as a corticosteroid-sparing agent in corticosteroid-dependent asthma [see comments]. Am J Respir Crit Care Med 1996;153:509–514.
75. Okudaira H, Mori A, Mikami T, Kaminuma O, Ohmura T, Hoshino A, Suko M. Selective suppression of IL-5 synthesis by OM-01—pinpoint treatment of atopic diseases by IL-5 gene transcription inhibitor. Int Arch Allergy Immunol 1997;113:331–334.

# 16

# Regulation of Interleukin-5 Expression in T Lymphocytes: Repression by Dexamethasone

**IAN G. YOUNG, CHIOK L. TAN, JULIET A. FISHER, BARBARA H. VAN LEEUWEN, and KLAUS I. MATTHAEI**

Australian National University
Canberra, Australia

## I. Introduction

IL-5 is an unusually specific cytokine and one of its best established activities is to promote the growth, differentiation, and activation of eosinophils (1–4). The production of IL-5 by T lymphocytes is believed to generate the eosinophilia which occurs during immune responses to helminth parasites and in allergic diseases such as asthma. Evidence supporting an obligatory role in IL-5 in the regulation of eosinophilia has been obtained recently in studies with IL-5-deficient mice (5,6). Additionally IL-5 and eosinophils were shown to play a central role in aeroallergen-induced lung damage and airway hyperresponsiveness in a mouse model of asthma (7–10). IL-5 and eosinophils also appear to contribute to host defense against some parasites (reviewed in reference 11). Recent studies have also shown that IL-5 synergises with eotaxin in the homing of eosinophils (12).

The cytokines produced by activated T lymphocytes play a central regulatory role in the coordination of immune and inflammatory responses. Helper T cells vary in the cytokine genes expressed after T-cell activation and mouse T-cell clones have been classified into two main classes (Th1 and Th2) on the basis of the cytokines they express. Their cytokine expression phenotypes correlate with the proposed roles of Th2 cells in regulating B-cell effector functions and of Th1 cells in controlling delayed-type hypersensitivity and cytotoxic responses (13). IL-5 is coordinately expressed by the Th2 class of mouse helper T cells with a variety of other lymphokines including IL-3, IL-4, IL-6, IL-10, and GM-CSF following antigenic stimulation. T-cell activation is a complex process that involves cell surface-mediated activation of multiple intracellular signaling pathways and results in the activation of protein kinase C (PKC) and an elevation in intracellular $Ca^{2+}$ (14).

In recent years we have been interested in defining the mechanisms that regulate the expression of IL-5 in Th2 lymphocytes and this article summarizes our work on IL-5 regulation in the Th2 T-cell clone D10.G4.1, studies with transgenic animals, and some recent work on the mechanism of repression by dexamethasone.

## II. Signaling Pathways Involved in IL-5 Regulation

In order to establish whether IL-5 is regulated by mechanisms shared with other coordinately expressed cytokines in Th2 cells, the effect of a variety of activators and inhibitors of known signaling pathways on the expression of IL-5 and five other cytokines was studied in the Th2 clone D10.G4.1 (15,16). Using northern blot analysis it was shown that, whereas none of the six cytokine mRNAs could be detected in unstimulated D10.G4.1 cells, the lectin ConA was effective in inducing all of the cytokine genes. This agent is believed to stimulate a number of glycosylated cell surface molecules including the TCR-CD3 complex which triggers activation of two parallel second messenger pathways involving PKC activation and $Ca^{2+}$ mobilization. The $Ca^{2+}$ signal appears to be largely mediated via a cyclosporin A (CsA)-sensitive pathway in D10.G4.1 cells and this pathway was shown to be essential for TCR-CD3-induced expression of the IL-3, IL-4, and GM-CSF genes. The $Ca^{2+}$ signal was optimally induced by the $Ca^{2+}$ ionophore A23187 which produces sustained elevation of intracellular $Ca^{2+}$ levels. In contrast, the TCR-CD3-stimulated expression of the IL-5, IL-6, and IL-10 genes was relatively resistant to CsA. Furthermore, these three genes were induced by PMA stimulation alone, suggesting that the PKC signaling pathway may independently regulate these genes. The IL-5, IL-6, and IL-10 genes were also selectively induced by stimulation of the IL-1 receptor and by forskolin. Studies by other workers with a subline of D10.G4.1 (17) have indicated that stimulation of the IL-1 receptor induces PKC activation and increased intracellular cAMP flux. Since forskolin activates adenylate cyclase it would appear that the IL-5, IL-6, and IL-10 genes can be induced by PKC- and cAMP-dependent pathways in D10.G4.1 cells.

Although the six different cytokine genes could be subdivided into the two broad groups outlined above, each gene behaved differently in terms of induction by combinations of activators, the requirement for protein synthesis during induction, and the relative importance of transcriptional and posttranscriptional mechanisms in their expression. This indicated that there were unique mechanisms involved in the regulation of the six genes in D10.G4.1 cells. It therefore follows that there may be circumstances in which they are differentially expressed depending on the nature of the immune response and the signals received by the T cells during antigen presentation. An example of differential expression of IL-5 and IL-4 is in intrinsic asthma where eosinophilia occurs without elevated IgE levels, in contrast to atopic asthma where the two cytokines appear to be coordinately expressed (18).

In the studies described above, IL-5 expression was shown to be regulated predominantly at the transcriptional level, to require protein synthesis for induction irrespective of the stimulus used, and to be induced in response to activation of PKC and adenylate cyclase (15,16). These results are supported by studies with other Th2 clones (17,19) and the murine T lymphoma EL4.23 (20).

## III. Localization of the Enhancer Responsive to TCR Stimulation

In order to investigate the transcription factors and transcriptional mechanisms regulating IL-5 expression in T lymphocytes we developed a stable transfection assay using the Th2 clone D10.G4.1 and the lymphoma EL4.23 (21). The use of stable transfection was designed to allow the study of promoter constructs in a normal chromatin environment. Since stable transfection involves random integration of reporter genes into the chromosomes of individual transfectants, a polyclonal population of transfectants was used to minimize any possible position effects.

We were able to demonstrate that the expression characteristics of a chloramphenicol acetyltransferase (CAT) reporter construct carrying 3859 bp of upstream sequence from the mouse IL-5 gene were the same as those of the endogenous chromosomal IL-5 gene (21). These properties included inducibility by ConA, PMA, or TCR-CD3 stimulation, repression by dexamethasone, and inefficient repression by CsA. Subsequent studies indicated that 1170 bp of upstream sequence was sufficient for optimal inducibility and retention of dexamethasone repression (21,22).

In keeping with the signaling studies described above, the strongest induction of the −1170 mIL-5 CAT reporter construct when stably transfected into D10.G4.1 cells was achieved with a combination of PMA and dibutyryl cAMP

(23). Uninduced signals were close to background and expression was regularly induced 100-fold by synergistic stimulation with these two agents. Many separate stable transfection experiments have been carried out with the –1170 mIL-5 CAT reporter construct. The consistently low uninduced levels obtained together with a reproducible pattern of synergistic stimulation by PMA and dibutyryl cAMP indicate that our results are not being distorted by variable position effects arising, for example, from the influence of enhancers in neighboring genes.

In contrast to the high levels of inducibility of the –1170 mIL-5 CAT construct in the Th2 clone D10.G4.1, expression of this construct was reduced to close to background levels in the Th1 clone H66 (23). This indicated that the region of the promoter to –1170 may carry all of the information necessary for tissue-specific regulation of IL-5 gene expression, namely inducible expression in Th2 but not Th1 T lymphocytes.

To test the ability of the region of the promoter to –1170 to direct inducible expression in T lymphocytes in vivo, transgenic mice carrying the –1170 mIL-5 CAT reporter gene were prepared (24). In case other elements in and around the IL-5 gene were involved, a second reporter construct was also used which carried a 10 kb fragment covering the IL-5 gene and which included 3859 bp of upstream sequence. Using RT-PCR it was shown that both reporter constructs were inducibly expressed in splenic T lymphocytes prepared from these mice after stimulation with anti-CD3 monoclonal antibodies. These results provide further evidence supporting the in vitro findings that the upstream region to –1170 is sufficient to give the characteristic expression pattern of the IL-5 gene.

## IV. Positive Regulatory Elements in the Promoter

Truncation of the upstream region in the –1170 mIL-5 CAT reporter construct to –88 resulted in retention of high levels of inducibility (over 100-fold) but loss of repression by dexamethasone (see below). Analysis of the proximal promoter region identified two regions of transcription factor binding designated mIL-5A (–41 to –61) and mIL-5B (–62 to –76) (22,23,25). The mIL-5A region (also designated CLE0 by Lee et al.; 26) encompasses an AP1-like binding site (–ve strand, –48 to –54) adjacent to a site with similarities to binding sites for the NFAT and Ets families (–ve strand, –41 to –47). The mIL-5B region carries a consensus GATA site (–ve strand, –67 to –72). Mutagenesis of either the TCATTT region of the mIL-5A site or the GATA region of the mIL-5B site in the context of the –1170 mIL-5 CAT reporter construct reduced expression dramatically to less than 5% of that obtained with the complete –1170 mIL-5 CAT (22,23). Deletion of segments between –920 and –88 and deletion of the region –980 to –940 gave no indication of any other positive control elements in these regions having significant effects on IL-5 expression in D10.G4.1 cells (23). A functional CTF/NF-1 binding site at –928 to –940 was identified (see below). CTF/NF-1 in this case appears to be acting as a negative regulator.

In nuclear extracts from the D10.G4.1 cells transcription factor binding to the mIL-5A and mIL-5B regions was shown to be inducible but not present in similar extracts from Th1 cells (22,25). This suggests that the proximal region of the promoter may be involved in the tissue-specific regulation of the IL-5 gene.

Although there is not complete agreement on the positive control elements involved in regulating the IL-5 gene, several other studies have supported a critical role for the mIL-5A (CLE0) and mIL-5B (GATA) regions (26–29). A role for NFAT and Oct binding to sites further upstream of the proximal promoter region has also been reported (26,30).

## V. Repression by Dexamethasone

As described above, the –88 mIL-5 CAT construct was highly inducible after stable transfection into D10.G4.1 cells, but was not repressed by dexamethasone. Indeed, an approximately twofold stimulation of CAT activity occurred (31). Inspection of the sequence in the region to –88 showed the presence of a consensus binding site (TGTCCT) for the glucocorticoid receptor immediately upstream of the GATA site at –67 to –72 which may be involved in this stimulation. In contrast, the –1170 mIL-5 CAT reporter construct was strongly repressed (about 90%) by dexamethasone (31). The repression of the reporter construct by dexamethasone indicates that the action of dexamethasone is occurring at the level of transcription. In these experiments dexamethasone was added at the time of stimulation.

Attempts were made to locate elements involved in repression by dexamethasone. Deletion of segments covering collectively –88 to –920 did not significantly block dexamethasone repression (31). We had previously identified a binding site for CTF/NF-1 located between –928 to –940 and have recently confirmed the constitutive presence of CTF/NF-1 in nuclear extracts of D10.G4.1 cells using antibody supershift experiments. CTF/NF-1 binding could be abolished by mutation of the binding site (31). Inactivation of the CTF binding site in the context of the –1170 mIL-5 CAT reporter construct resulted in a slight elevation of unstimulated levels of CAT activity, but the CTF mutant construct was highly inducible (average of 100-fold). To date three separate transfection experiments have indicated that mutation of the CTF site reduces the dexamethasone repression of the –1170 mIL-5 CAT reporter from tenfold to about twofold. This suggests that CTF/NF-1 plays a significant role in the repression of the IL-5 gene by dexamethasone in D10.G4.1 cells (31).

CTF/NF-1 has been reported to act as both a positive and a negative transcriptional regulator (32), although how it activates transcription is still uncertain (33). We hypothesize that in the case of the IL-5 gene, CTF is acting as a repressor and that repression by CTF is normally reversed by activation with PMA/dibutyryl cAMP. With the CTF mutant construct, absolute levels of CAT activity are significantly elevated (two- to fivefold) supporting the concept that the wild-type –1170 mIL-5 CAT construct is repressed by CTF/NF-1 (31). According to the above model, the action of dexamethasone would be to interfere with the release of CTF repression and to prevent efficient induction of gene expression. Mutation of the CTF site would interfere with the CTF repression and therefore the –1170 mIL-5 CAT reporter construct would be able to be induced efficiently in the presence of dexamethasone.

Glucocorticoids are clinically important because they are effective in controlling inflammation. Both positive and negative effects on gene regulation appear to be involved, although the mechanisms are not well understood (reviewed in reference 34). Glucocorticoids bind to a cytoplasmic receptor protein, the glucocorticoid receptor (GR), which translocates to the nucleus and positively or negatively regulates gene expression. Many of the genes that are regulated as part of the anti-inflammatory actions of glucocorticoids do not have a classical GR binding site but have binding sites for transcription factors such as AP-1 or NF-κB.

It appears that negative effects of the GR may predominate in the anti-inflammatory effects of glucocorticoids (34). Several negative actions of the GR on gene expression have been studied in detail and so far the mechanisms involve either overlapping binding sites or protein-protein interactions. In the former case, the GR competes with positive-acting transcription factors for binding to a common site in the promoter of a gene. Examples include the human osteocalcin and bovine prolactin genes (reviewed in reference 34). Where protein-protein interactions are involved, the GR binds to a transcription factor and reduces its transactivation potential with or without effects on DNA binding. Interactions between the GR and two transcription factors centrally involved in inflammation, AP-1 and NF-κB have been reported (reviewed in reference 34). AP-1 and NF-ATp are involved in the glucocorticoid repression of the human IL-2 gene (35–38) and NF-κB is involved in repression of the human IL-8 gene (39). With NF-κB, an indirect mechanism of glucocorticoid repression involving enhanced expression of its inhibitor (I-κBα) has also recently been identified (40,41).

Although further work is required on the role of CTF/NF-1 in dexamethasone repression of the IL-5 gene, on the basis of the findings described above, the negative regulation of the IL-5 gene by the GR appears to involve a different mechanism to those previously reported. Whether the GR directly interacts with CTF/NF-1, reducing its ability to be activated, or affects this process indirectly awaits further studies.

## References


1. Campbell HD, Tucker WQ, Hort Y, Martinson ME, Mayo G, Clutterbuck EJ, Sanderson CJ, Young IG. Molecular cloning, nucleotide sequence, and expression of the gene encoding human eosinophil differentiation factor (interleukin-5). Proc Natl Acad Sci USA 1987;84:6629–6633.
2. Lopez AF, Sanderson CJ, Gamble JR, Campbell HD, Young IG, Vadas MA. Recombinant human interleukin-5 is a selective activator of human eosinophil function. J Exp Med 1988;167:219–224.
3. Sanderson CJ, Campbell HD, Young IG. Molecular and cellular biology of eosinophil differentiation factor (interleukin-5) and its effects on human and mouse B cells. Immunol Rev 1988;102:29–50.
4. Yamaguchi Y, Hayashi Y, Sugama Y, Miura Y, Kasahara T, Kitamura S, Torisu M, Mita S, Tominaga A, Takatsu K. Highly purified murine interleukin-5 (IL-5) stimulates eosinophil function and prolongs in vitro survival. IL-5 as an eosinophil chemotactic factor. J Exp Med 1988;167:1737–1742.
5. Kopf M, Brombacher F, Hodgkin PD, Ramsay AJ, Milbourne EA, Dai WJ, Ovington KS, Behm CA, Kohler G, Young IG, Matthaei KI. IL-5-deficient mice have a developmental defect in CD5+ B-1 cells and lack eosinophilia but have normal antibody and cytotoxic T cell responses. Immunity 1996;4:15–24.
6. Takamoto M, Ovington KS, Behm CA, Sugane K, Young IG, Matthaei KI. Eosinophilia, parasite burden and lung damage in *Toxocara canis* infections in C57BL/6 mice genetically deficient in IL-5. Immunology 1997;90:511–517.
7. Foster PS, Hogan SP, Ramsay AJ, Matthaei KI, Young IG. Interleukin-5 deficiency abolishes eosinophilia, airways hyperreactivity, and lung damage in a mouse asthma model [see comments]. J Exp Med 1996;183:195–201.
8. Hogan SP, Mould AM, Kikutani H, Ramsay AJ, Foster PS. Aeroallergen-induced eosinophilic inflammation, lung damage and airways hyperreactivity in mice can occur independently of IL-4 and allergen-specific immunoglobulins. J Clin Invest 1997;99:1329–1339.
9. Hogan SP, Koskinen A, Matthaei KI, Young IG, Foster PS. Il-5 producing $CD^{4+}$ T-cells plays a pivotal role in the induction of eosinophilia and allergic airways disease in mice. Am Rev Respir Dis 1998;157:210–218.
10. Hogan SP, Koskinen A, Foster PS. Interleukin-5 and eosinophils induce airways damage and bronchial hyperreactivity during allergic airways inflammation in BALB/c mice. Immunol Cell Biol 1997;75:284–288.
11. Matthaei KI, Foster PS, Young IG. The role of IL-5 in vivo: studies with IL-5 deficient mice. Mem Instit Oswaldo Cruz 1997;92:63–68.
12. Mould AW, Matthaei KI, Young IG, Foster PS. Relationship between interleukin-5 and eotaxin in regulating blood and tissue eosinophilia in mice. J Clin Invest 1997;99:1064–1071.

13. Mosmann TR, Coffman RL. $TH_1$ and $TH_2$ cells: different patterns of lymphokine secretion lead to different functional properties. Annu Rev Immunol 1989;7:145–173.
14. Fraser JD, Straus D, Weiss A. Signal transduction events leading to T-cell lymphokine gene expression. Immunol Today 1993;14:357–362.
15. Naora H, Altin JG, Young IG. TCR-dependent and -independent signaling mechanisms differentially regulate lymphokine gene expression in the murine T helper clone D10.G4.1. J Immunol 1994;152:5691–5702.
16. Naora H, Young IG. Comparison of the mechanisms regulating IL-5, IL-4, and three other lymphokine genes in the $Th_2$ clone D10.G4.1. Exp Hematol 1995;23:597–602.
17. Munoz E, Beutner U, Zubiaga A, Huber BT. IL-1 activates two separate signal transduction pathways in T helper type II cells. J Immunol 1990;144:964–969.
18. Walker C, Bode E, Boer L, Hansel TT, Blaser K, Virchow JC Jr. Allergic and nonallergic asthmatics have distinct patterns of T-cell activation and cytokine production in peripheral blood and bronchoalveolar lavage. Am Rev Respir Dis 1992;146:109–115.
19. O'Neill LA, Bird TA, Saklatvala J. How does interleukin-1 activate cells? Interleukin 1 signal transduction [comment] [see comments]. Immunol Today 1990;11:392–394.
20. Naora H, Young IG. Mechanisms regulating the mRNA levels of interleukin-5 and two other coordinately expressed lymphokines in the murine T lymphoma EL4.23. Blood 1994;83:3620–3628.
21. Bourke PF, van Leeuwen BH, Campbell HD, Young IG. Localization of the inducible enhancer in the mouse interleukin-5 gene that is responsive to T-cell receptor stimulation. Blood 1995;85:2069–2077.
22. Naora H, van Leeuwen BH, Bourke PF, Young IG. Functional role and signal-induced modulation of proteins recognizing the conserved TCATTT-containing promoter elements in the murine IL-5 and GM-CSF genes in T lymphocytes. J Immunol 1994;153:3466–3475.
23. Tan CL, van Leeuwen BH, Young IG. Promoter elements controlling IL-5 transcription in the $TH_2$ clone D10.G4.1. In preparation.
24. Fisher JA, Tan CL, Matthaei KI, Young IG. Localisation of an IL-5 gene enhancer responsive to T-cell activation using transgenic mice. In preparation.
25. Naora H. Regulation of lymphokine gene expression in activated murine T-lymphocytes. Ph.D. dissertation. Australian National University, 1993.
26. Lee HJ, Masuda ES, Arai N, Arai K, Yokota T. Definition of cis-regulatory elements of the mouse interleukin-5 gene promoter. Involvement of nuclear factor of activated T cell-related factors in interleukin-5 expression. J Biol Chem 1995;270:17541–17550.
27. Siegel MD, Zhang DH, Ray P, Ray A. Activation of the interleukin-5 promoter by cAMP in murine EL-4 cells requires the GATA-3 and CLE0 elements. J Biol Chem 1995;270:24548–24555.
28. Yamagata T, Nishida J, Sakai R, Tanaka T, Honda H, Hirano N, Mano H, Yazaki Y, Hirai H. Of the GATA-binding proteins, only GATA-4 selectively regulates the

human interleukin-5 gene promoter in interleukin-5-producing cells which express multiple GAT-binding proteins. Mol Cell Biol 1995;15:3830–3839.

29. Karlen S, D'Ercole M, Sanderson CJ. Two pathways can activate the interleukin-5 gene and induce binding to the conserved lymphokine element 0. Blood 1996;88:211–221.
30. Gruart-Gouilleux V, Engels P, Sullivan M. Characterization of the human interleukin-5 gene promoter: involvement of octamer binding sites in the gene promoter activity. Eur J Immunol 1995;25:1431–1435.
31. Tan CL, van Leeuwen BH, Young IG. Role of CTF/NF-1 in dexamethasone repression of the IL-5 gene. In preparation.
32. Jones KA, Kadonaga JT, Rosenfeld PJ, Kelly TJ, Tjian R. A cellular DNA-binding protein that activates eukaryotic transcription and DNA replication. Cell 1987;48:79–89.
33. Alevizopoulos A, Dusserre Y, Tsai-Pflugfelder M, von der Weid T, Wahli W, Mermod N. A proline-rich TGF-beta-responsive transcriptional activator interacts with histone H3. Gene Dev 1995;9:3051–3066.
34. Cato AC, Wade E. Molecular mechanisms of anti-inflammatory action of glucocorticoids. Bioessays 1996;18:371–378.
35. Vacca A, Felli MP, Farina AR, Martinotti S, Maroder M, Screpanti L. Meco D, Petrangeli E, Frati L, Gulino A. Glucocorticoid receptor-mediated suppression of the interleukin-2 gene expression through impairment of the cooperativity between nuclear factor of activated T cells and AP-1 enhancer elements. J Exp Med 1992;175:637–646.
36. Jain J, McCaffrey PG, Miner Z, Kerppola TK, Lambert JN, Verdine GL, Curran T, Rao A. The T-cell transcription factor NF-ATp is a substrate for calcineurin and interacts with Fos and Jun. Nature 1993;365:352–355.
37. Paliogianni F, Raptis A, Ahuja SS, Najjar SM, Boumpas DT. Negative transcriptional regulation of human interleukin-2 (IL-2) gene by glucocorticoids through interference with nuclear transcription factors AP-1 and NF-AT. J Clin Invest 1993;91:1481–1489.
38. Rao A. NF-ATp: a transcription factor required for the co-ordinate induction of several cytokine genes. Immunol Today 1994;15:274–281.
39. Mukaida N, Morita M, Ishikawa Y, Rice N, Okamoto S, Kasahara T, Matsushima K. Novel mechanism of glucocorticoid-mediated gene repression. Nuclear factor-kappa B is target for glucocorticoid-mediated interleukin-8 gene repression. J Biol Chem 1994;269:13289–13295.
40. Auphan N, DiDonato JA, Rosette C, Helmberg A, Karin M. Immunosuppression by glucocorticoids: inhibition of NF-kappa B activity through induction of I kappa B synthesis [see comments]. Science 1995;270:286–290.
41. Scheinman RI, Cogswell PC, Lofquist AK, Baldwin AS Jr. Role of transcriptional activation of I kappa B alpha in mediation of immunosuppression by glucocorticoids [see comments]. Science 1995;270:283–286.

# 17

# Interleukin-5 and the Interleukin-5 Receptor: Targets for Drug Discovery in Asthma

**MURRAY McKINNON, MARTYN BANKS, ROBERTO SOLARI, and GRAEME ROBERTSON**

Glaxo Wellcome Research and Development
Stevenage, Hertfordshire, United Kingdom

## I. Introduction

The eosinophil is a terminally differentiated leukocyte that appears to play an important protective role in the host defense response to parasitic infections (1). Elimination of parasites is primarily mediated through the targeted release of toxic cationic proteins, such as major basic protein (MBP), from eosinophil granules (2). The generation of toxic oxygen radicals catalyzed by the eosinophil NADPH oxidase complex may also contribute to an efficient killing process (3). However, in contrast to its protective role, the eosinophil has also been implicated in the pathophysiology of allergic diseases such as bronchial asthma, atopic dermatitis, and allergic rhinitis (4–6). In bronchial asthma, for example, eosinophil accumulation in the lung is a consistent finding and there is a good correlation between eosinophil number and the severity of the late-phase asthmatic response (7,8). Furthermore, histologic studies have demonstrated that eosinophil-derived mediators such as MBP are found in the lungs of asthmatics around sites of epithelial damage (7,9). Significantly it has been demonstrated that MBP induces damage to human bronchial epithelium resulting in desquamation and ciliated cell destruction (10), and there is a good relationship between these eosinophil-derived mediators and bronchial hyperreactivity (11,12).

This data would suggest that the eosinophil is a key effector cell in asthma which is capable of inducing damage to respiratory epithelium and thus contributing to the overall lung inflammation. This cell type therefore represents an attractive target for the identification of novel anti-inflammatory drugs for the treatment of asthma.

Eosinophil development is under the control of a family of related T-cell-derived cytokines: interleukin-5 (IL-5), interleukin-3 (IL-3), and granulocyte-macrophage colony stimulating factor (GM-CSF) (13). While the latter two cytokines exhibit biological activities on other hematopoietic lineages, the effects of IL-5 are restricted, at least in humans, to cells of the eosinophil and basophil lineage (4,14). In the decade since its identification IL-5 has emerged as perhaps the key regulator of eosinophil production and function. IL-5, which is produced predominantly by T cells but also by mast cells (15) and eosinophils (16), induces the differentiation and expansion of eosinophil precursors in the bone marrow (13) and plays a key role in regulating many of the specialized functions of mature terminally differentiated eosinophils. These include induction of adhesion to vascular endothelium (17), a prerequisite for diapedesis into tissues, and priming of both degranulation and chemotaxis (18,19). Furthermore, IL-5 is a potent antiapoptotic cytokine and thus prolongs eosinophil survival (20). The biological properties of this cytokine, allied with its specificity for eosinophils, suggest that IL-5 may represent an important molecular target for the development of anti-eosinophil therapeutics. Furthermore the validity of IL-5 as a target has been demonstrated in a variety of animal models of allergic asthma, where administration of neutralizing anti-IL-5 monoclonal antibodies in mouse, guinea pig, or primate models of allergic asthma inhibit the development of both airway eosinophilia and bronchial hyperreactivity (21–25). In addition, mice rendered IL-5 deficient, through deletion of the IL-5 gene, fail to produce either blood or lung eosinophilia, nor do they develop airway hyperreactivity in response to aeroallergen challenge (26).

Clearly there is now good clinical data, albeit circumstantial, supported by experimental evidence in animal models of allergic asthma, to suggest that blocking the actions of IL-5 may prevent not only eosinophil production but their accumulation and activation at sites of lung inflammation thereby potentially producing significant clinical benefit in the treatment of asthma. A clearer definition of the role of both IL-5 and eosinophils in the pathogenesis of bronchial asthma awaits the evaluation of specific IL-5 inhibitors in the clinic.

## II. General Strategies for Inhibiting IL-5 Action

In considering general strategies for inhibiting IL-5 action the paracrine/autocrine nature of cytokine action affords opportunities for intervention at multiple cel-

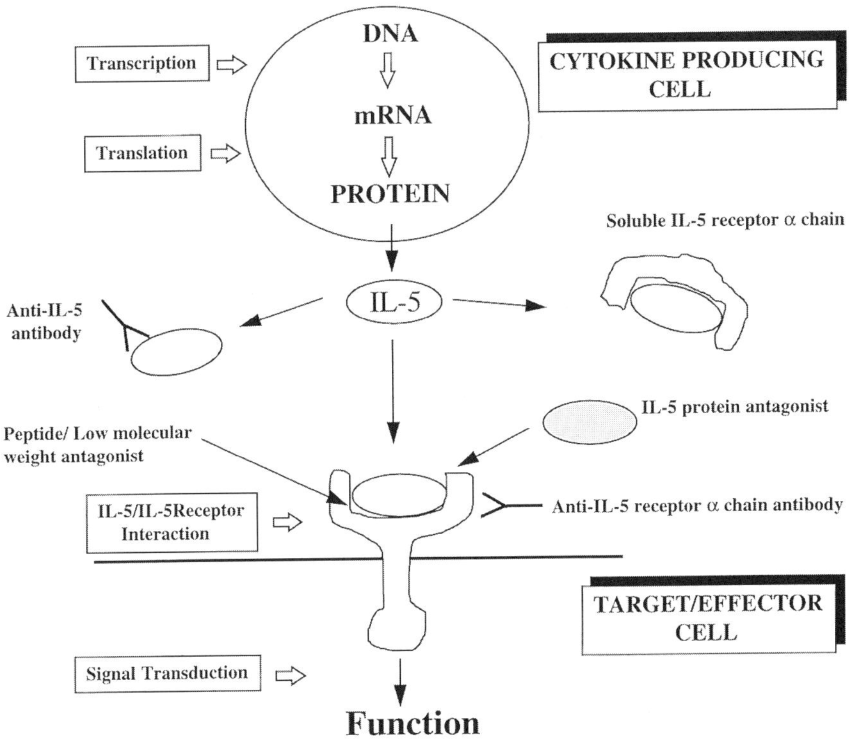


**Figure 1** Potential cellular and molecular levels for inhibition of cytokine action, highlighting the variety of strategies that can be adopted for the inhibition of IL-5 binding to its receptor. (Figure adapted from Ref. 40.)

lular and molecular levels (Fig. 1). In IL-5-producing cells such as T cells, mast cells, or eosinophils, cytokine production can potentially be inhibited at the transcriptional or at the translational level. Following its cellular release, IL-5 action can be blocked by inhibiting the interaction with its specific cell surface receptor expressed on the target cell, in this case cells of the eosinophil lineage. Strategies for the identification of inhibitors of IL-5 action essentially fall into two general categories, those aimed at identifying low molecular weight antagonists and peptide/protein antagonists. Here we will describe both strategies, with particular emphasis on the assay systems and technologies which have been employed for the identification of specific IL-5 receptor antagonists. We will discuss the relative merits of these approaches, highlighting the successes and failures of each.

The IL-5 receptor is a heterodimeric complex composed of a 60 kDa α chain which binds IL-5 specifically, and a 150 kDa β chain which confers high-affinity ligand binding and is essential for signal transduction (27). This β chain is shared with the related cytokines IL-3 and GM-CSF. Consequently, antagonizing the actions of IL-5 selectively can be achieved through preventing IL-5 binding to its receptor α chain. The ideal cytokine antagonist is a small synthetic molecule that is orally bioavailable, thus presenting fewer problems in drug production, administration, and stability than do peptide or protein therapeutics. However, given the clinical and financial success of protein therapeutics such as erythropoietin, one cannot rule out the possibility of peptide/protein antagonists as anticytokine therapies should an appropriate route of administration be identified.

## III. High Throughput Random Screening for Low Molecular Weight Antagonists

Current drug discovery programs in pharmaceutical companies rely predominantly on high throughput random screening (HTS) for the identification of potential drug candidates. By establishing the appropriate assay system, high throughput screening has the ability to discover compounds that could inhibit the actions of IL-5 at any one of the multiple cellular or molecular levels as depicted in Figure 1. As a source of potential inhibitors these screening programs have traditionally focused on natural products, such as microbial fermentation, marine organisms, and plant extracts. In addition, proprietary compound collections and more recently combinatorial chemical libraries have greatly added to the diversity of compounds which can be included in a screening program. It is possible to configure the screening assay to search for inhibitors of one specific process, such as receptor-ligand binding. Alternatively one can search for inhibitors of a whole pathway by looking for inhibitors of an IL-5-dependent functional response in a cell-based assay.

For a successful high throughput screening program, rapid and reliable assays are an essential prerequisite. Speed is a significant advantage; an advanced high throughput screen should be capable of carrying out 10,000 assays in 24 hr in a cost-effective manner. To achieve these throughputs the assay should be in a format that has the capacity to handle many hundreds of thousands of samples and consequently should be suitable for assay automation. These types of screens include a range of whole cellular and biochemical assays employing membrane preparations, cell/tissue extracts, or recombinant proteins. Clearly the simpler the assay and the readout the more amenable it is to automation.

### A. Cell-Based Assays

Cellular assays have been used to find inhibitors of whole pathways and this is a particularly attractive approach when many of the components of the pathway are uncharacterized, the so-called black-box screen. For such a screen one could measure an IL-5-induced biological response such as proliferation in an IL-5-dependent cell line, for example, TF-1 cells. We have recently described a rapid and sensitive in vitro assay to quantify the effect of IL-5-induced eosinophil adhesion to ICAM- or VCAM-coated plastic wells (28). Such functional assays are attractive because they use a physiologically relevant readout, however, they usually suffer from a low rate of sample throughput. Alternatively, for greater ease and throughput, engineered cell lines can be prepared containing a reporter gene, usually an enzyme, whose expression is driven from a cytokine responsive promoter. Although such whole cell screens are simple to set up and generate many inhibitors, these types of screening assays can represent a challenge in the dissection of the mechanism of action of the inhibitor compound. The advantage of such a screen is that many potential targets along the pathway of interest are screened simultaneously. As this technology evolves these engineered reporter gene assays offer the hope of pharmacological resolution of the complex mechanisms which underpin cytokine signaling by generating specific inhibitors of each step in the pathway.

### B. Receptor Binding Assays

In contrast to cell-based high throughput screens, biochemical screens aim to target individual events such as the receptor-ligand interaction. These simple binding assays make ideal high throughput screens. The extracellular domains of many cytokine receptors exist as soluble forms which bind ligand with high affinity, and recombinant extracellular domains can be prepared in large quantities. In general these soluble extracellular domains of receptors are prepared as a fusion protein that not only facilitates receptor purification, but allows the receptor to be anchored to a support for use in solid-phase binding assays. Using a fusion protein between the extracellular domain of the IL-5 receptor $\alpha$ chain and human IgG C $\gamma3$, Devos et al. screened 67,500 compounds in a solid-phase binding assay and identified a small molecule inhibitor, isothiazolone A (29). This method required a washing step in the procedure to separate bound from free ligand, a process that is not easily automated. Ideally, to automate this type of assay a homogeneous format should be used. Scintillation proximity assays allow homogeneous measurement of receptor-bound ligand without the need to separate free from bound ligand (see Fig. 2). We have designed a fully automated assay using scintillation proximity technology for measuring the interaction of IL-5 with the IL-5 receptor $\alpha$ chain (30). In this assay we used a recombinant soluble human IL-5 receptor $\alpha$ chain fused to the IgG binding domain of protein A (IL-5R-zz). Briefly antirabbit IgG is covalently attached to a plastic bead containing a fluor. This bead is then incubated with rabbit IgG and IL-5R-zz, thus coupling the receptor to the bead; this receptor bead complex is

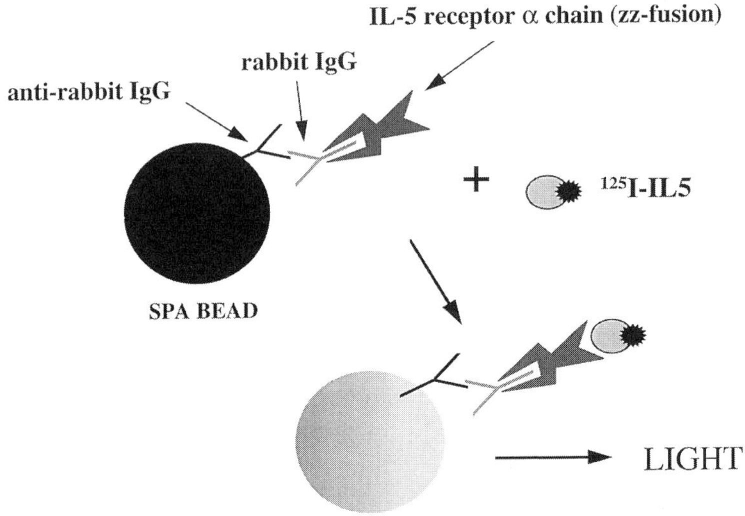


**Figure 2** Principle of the IL-5 receptor α-chain SPA assay. The basic principle of the assay depends on the two Auger electrons released when $^{125}$I decays. Free ligand in solution is too distant from the plastic bead to excite the enclosed fluor and therefore no light is emitted. However, receptor-bound ligand being in close proximity to the bead will excite the fluor; the emitted light being proportional to the amount of bound ligand.

stable at 4°C for 24 hr. The stability of reagents is an important consideration when automated screening on a continuous production scale is used. In this assay, compounds and natural product extracts were preprepared in microtiter plates together with controls to monitor the nonspecific binding and the maximum bound signals.

*Typical Robotic HTS for IL-5*

Typically, high throughput robotic screens of 100,000 to 200,000 compounds are run over a two week period. The robotic system used to run the IL-5 high throughput screen was the Robolab 9600 (Robocon Gesmb H, Austria) (see Fig. 3). The hardware consisted of a CRS A255 articulated robotic arm mounted on a 6 m track. The various instruments were arranged around this track with the A255 arm moving plates between the modules. The predispensed compounds were manually loaded into a static random access hotel. The [$^{125}$I]-IL-5 was dispensed from a bank of eight Cavro syringes, driven by a single stepper motor, into the assay plate and, like the receptor bead complex, maintained at 4°C in a large reservoir. The receptor bead complex was continuously circulated to a small reservoir on the deck of a Multiprobe 104 (Canberra Packard, USA) and then dispensed from this small reservoir into the assay plate. After incubation at room temperature the plates were transferred to a TopCount scintillation counter (Canberra Packard, USA).

During a typical screening campaign of 104,000 samples quality control microtiter plates were included in the run at approximately every 15,000 samples to monitor the progress of the screen. Such quality control (QC) analysis indicated that the screen was highly robust and reproducible; the typical variation in the screen is shown in Figure 4. The "hit" rate from the initial screen was very low from all the different samples that were tested (see Table 1). Some extracts gave false positive results because they were highly colored or contained nonspecific inhibitors. Highly colored extracts quench the light from the scintillation proximity bead, and even after quench correction can indicate a false positive result. Tannins and other polyphenolic natural product compounds were also found to be nonselective inhibitors.

While the identification of IL-5 receptor antagonists by high throughput random screening is dependent on serendipity, the chances of success can be increased significantly through the design of reliable and robust assays, allied with the ability to screen large numbers of diverse molecular entities in an automated fashion. Our screening technology systems meet these requirements and it is hoped that this approach will identify novel compounds which antagonize the IL-5/IL-5 receptor interaction.

## IV. Low Molecular Weight Antagonists

This section will concentrate on published compounds known to act as IL-5 inhibitors/receptor antagonists and strategies for the discovery of novel receptor antagonists. Small molecule inhibitors of cytokine activity which interfere at stages other than the ligand-receptor interaction have previously been reviewed (31).

### A. Protein-Protein Interactions

Inhibition of protein-protein interactions, such as the binding of IL-5 to its receptor, present a challenging opportunity for those interested in novel opportunities for drug discovery. The majority of traditional drug-macromolecule interactions are based on the drug mimicking a natural ligand which is similar in size to the eventual drug molecule. Protein-protein interactions present a difficult challenge when designing molecules to interfere with the interaction, since there is usually a large surface area of contact involved. Typically the surface area involved is in excess of 1250 $Å^2$ (32) (the area involved in the interaction of IL-5 is approximately 700 $Å^2$), whereas a small drug-like molecule would have in the region of only 300 $Å^2$ available if the whole surface was used. The

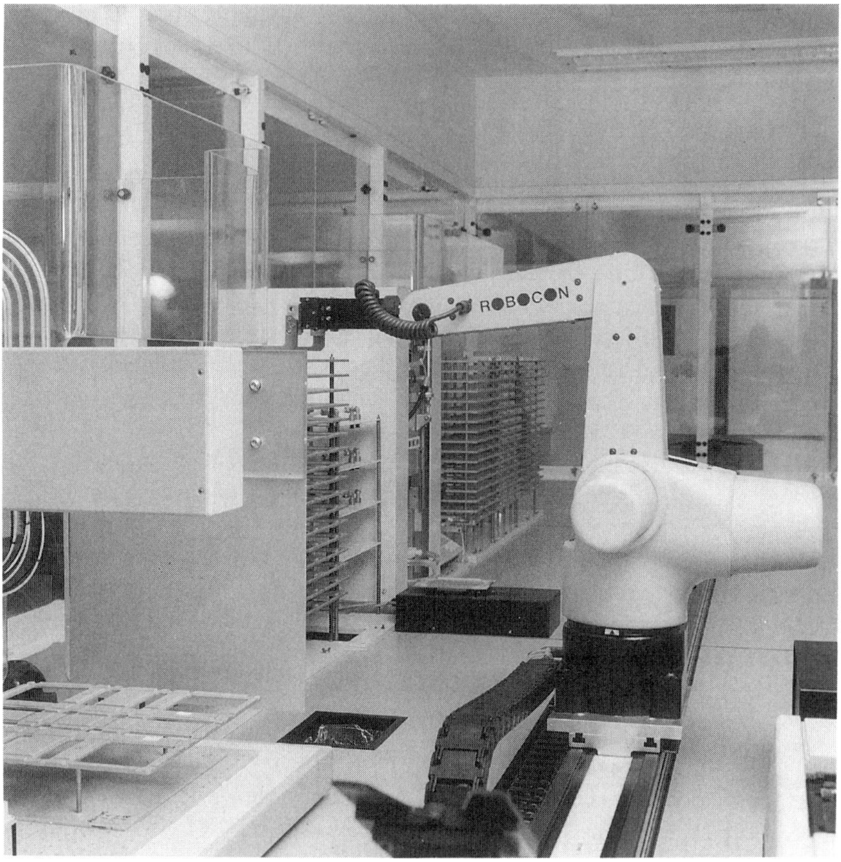


(a)

**Figure 3** (a) Robolab 9600 in action and (b) schematic layout of hardware modules.

shape of a small molecule also means that it cannot use its available surface area when competing with an extended (i.e., "flat") surface. This may explain why screening of collections of drug-like molecules have not been particularly successful at identifying leads for inhibiting protein-protein interactions.

The notable exceptions to the above generalizations are (1) where the protein-protein interaction is more localized (as in integrin interactions such as fibrinogen, VCAM, and ICAM, for which there are several examples of nonpeptide inhibitors) and (2) where X-ray analysis shows a large contact area (structural epitope), but site-directed mutagenesis reveals that the major part of the binding affinity (functional epitope) is localized to a few residues such as prolactin (33) and growth hormone (34,35) binding to the growth hormone receptor. In the latter case no small molecule agonists/antagonists have been de-

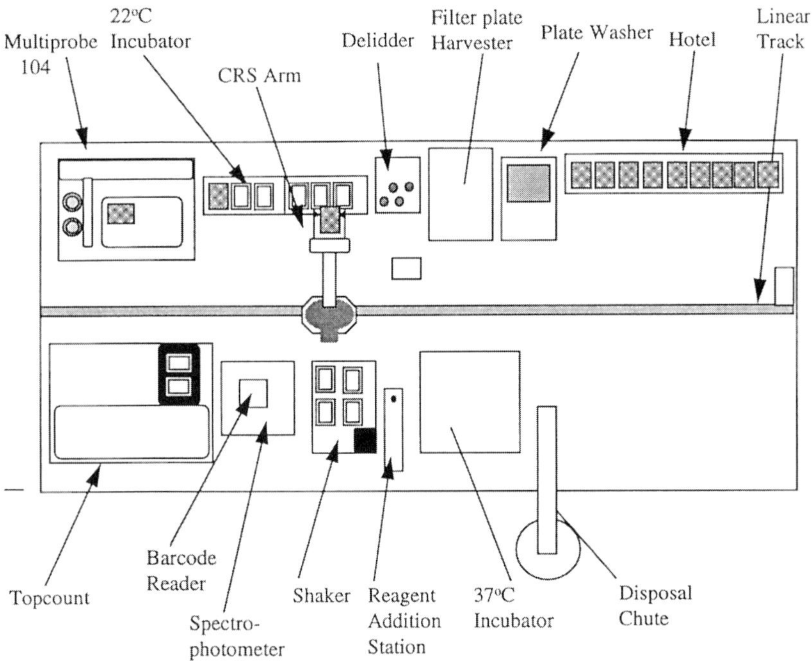


(b)

**Figure 3** Continued.

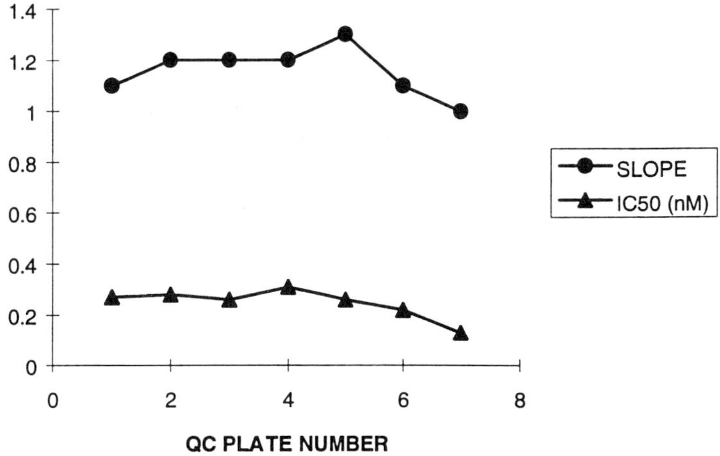


**Figure 4** Quality control (QC) data for typical IL-5 receptor α-chain high throughput screen showing the variation in the $IC_{50}$ and slope of the seven IL-5 standard curves included in a complete robot run.

**Table 1** Results of Typical IL-5 Receptor α Chain High Throughput Screen Showing the Percentage of Inhibitory Compounds Detected when Screening Natural Products and Compounds

| Sample type | Number tested | % Positive rate |
|---|---|---|
| Fungal extracts | 36,320 | 0.008 |
| Bacterial extracts | 33,360 | 0 |
| Plant extracts | 23,680 | 0.39 |
| Marine organism extracts | 1920 | 0 |
| Compounds | 5920 | 0.17 |

scribed but the prospects look promising, since the key residues are located in a compact region, provided the correct molecular entities are constructed. This may be of particular relevance to the structurally related interaction of IL-5 with its receptor. Indeed the X-ray crystal structure of human growth hormone has been utilized for the generation of models of the receptor interactions of IL-3 and GM-CSF (36).

### B. Known IL-5 Inhibitors

The first reported IL-5 antagonists were a class of isothiazolones discovered by Devos and coworkers at Roche (29) using a fusion protein of the human IL-5-receptor α chain (hIL-5Rα) and the human IgG Cγ3 chain, in a solid-phase assay for high throughput screening of compound collections. They reported the identification of isothiazolone derivatives (Fig. 5) as inhibitors of binding of IL-5 to the hIL-5Rα. The binding of human IL-4 and hGM-CSF to their respective receptors was not inhibited by the isothiazolones in similar assay systems. Scatchard analysis revealed that these compounds caused a decrease in affinity of the IL-5Rα for IL-5. The inhibition of IL-5 binding to its receptor by the isothiazolone derivatives was, however, shown to involve reaction with the sulfhydryl group of free cysteine residues in the hIL-5Rα. Mutation of Cys66 in hIL-5Rα led to a receptor which still bound IL-5, but which was insensitive to the inhibition by the isothiazolones. The use of radiolabeled isothiazolone confirmed that Cys66, present in the first domain of the receptor, was covalently

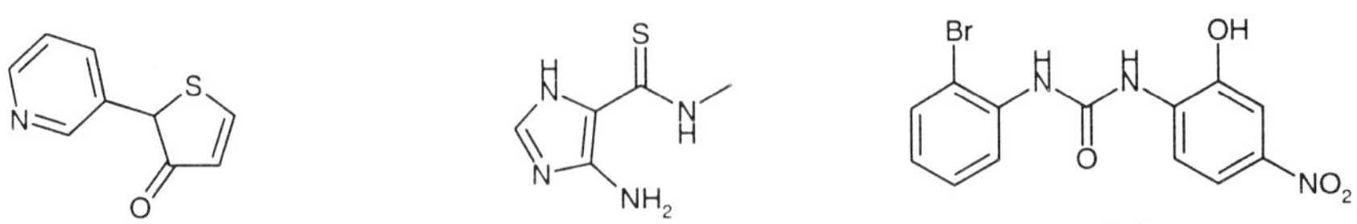


(1) (2) (3)

**Figure 5** Examples of small molecule inhibitors of cytokine and chemokine action.

modified by the isothiazolones, leading to a decrease in affinity. These compounds were therefore not progressed further.

A series of novel antiasthmatic agents based on 3-substituted 5-amino-1-[(methylamino)(thiocarbonyl)]-1H-1,2,4-triazole derivatives have been developed by the Green Cross Corporation (37). These compounds were evaluated in an eosinophilia model induced through IV injection of sephadex particles. After screening of several hundred compounds, a potent inhibitor of eosinophilia was identified, 5-amino-3-(4-chlorophenyl)-1-[(methylamino)(thiocarbonyl)]-1H-triazole (Fig. 5), which had $ID_{50}$ values of 0.3 and 0.07 mg/kg when administered orally and IP, respectively. This compound completely inhibited the airway hypersensitivity induced by ascaris inhalation at an IP dose of 1 mg/kg and exhibited low toxicity, with an $LD_{50}$ value of greater than 2.0 mg/kg in mice. This compound was shown to inhibit eosinophil survival induced by IL-5, but it had little or no effect on leukotriene D4 (LTD4) or platelet-activating factor (PAF)-induced responses. However, no evidence has been reported to confirm the site of action of this class of compounds. Further studies are reported to be under way.

Small molecule inhibitors of chemokines such as the Smith Kline Beecham IL-8 antagonist (Fig. 5) have been reported (38). However, the interaction of chemokines with their seven transmembrane-based receptors is of rather a different nature to that of cytokines with their receptors. Chemokine interactions may be more amenable to inhibition by small molecules due to more localized binding epitopes.

### C. Protein and Peptide Antagonists

The role of the WSXWS consensus motif in IL-5, IL-3, and GM-CSF receptor function has been studied using synthesized peptides encompassed within the WSXWS region (39). In a basophil mediator release assay, three peptides inhibited the priming effect of IL-3, IL-5, and GM-CSF on synthesis of leukotriene C4 induced by chemotactic peptides. The study suggests that, analogous to the integrin binding motif in extracellular matrix proteins (RGD), the WSXWS motif serves as a recognition site for functional protein-protein interaction of cytokine receptors. However, unlike the RGD motif the WSXWS region is unlikely to provide a major emphasis for drug discovery.

Other peptide and protein antagonists of IL-5, such as the point mutant E12K, have been developed and their use as antiasthma agents are discussed in section 5.

### D. Generation of IL-5 Selective Antagonists

There are three main methods available for the generation of small-molecule IL-5 selective antagonist, namely,

Lead discovery by random screening (see Section 3).
Lead discovery by random screening, followed by lead optimization via structure-based combinatorial library design.
Lead generation directly via structure-based combinatorial libraries and compound set generation.

General approaches for inhibition of cytokine action, strategies for the discovery of cytokine receptor antagonists, random screening, and rational design have previously been reviewed (40).

### Random Screening

As with any target, random screening of company databases and commercially available samples is of course possible (see section 3). The availability of high throughput SPA-based binding assays for IL-5 provide an excellent platform for such exercises. However, random screening is not generally an efficient process for protein-protein targets and the highly polar nature of the interaction of IL-5 with its receptor α chain, coupled with the large surface area of this interaction, suggests that most company proprietary compound collections may not contain many compounds that are potential noncovalent IL-5 antagonists. Targeted selection and synthesis of both compounds and combinatorial chemistry libraries may therefore be the most effective way forward.

### Targeted Sets and Compound Libraries

As an alternative to random screening of compounds, and usually allied to some knowledge of the interaction of a ligand with its receptor, is the use of targeted sets and compound libraries. These are typically either ligand-based or receptor-based sets.

#### Ligand-Based Design

The structures of many protein-protein interactions show them to have large generally flat interfaces, making the rational design of small molecule inhibitors a challenging area. However, if as with growth hormone (34,35), smaller functional epitopes can be identified, then the task of developing small molecule inhibitors could be greatly simplified.

IL-5 is an antiparallel homodimer constructed from two end-to-end four helical bundles (41,42). The two individual domains of the dimer are each related to the monomeric cytokines, GM-CSF, and IL-3, but are constructed from three helices from one dimer and a fourth from the second dimer (Fig. 6). The A and D′ helices constitute the major portion of the outer surface as presented to the receptor.

Site-directed mutagenesis studies and epitope mapping of neutralizing monoclonal antibodies have identified the charged residues of human IL-5 that

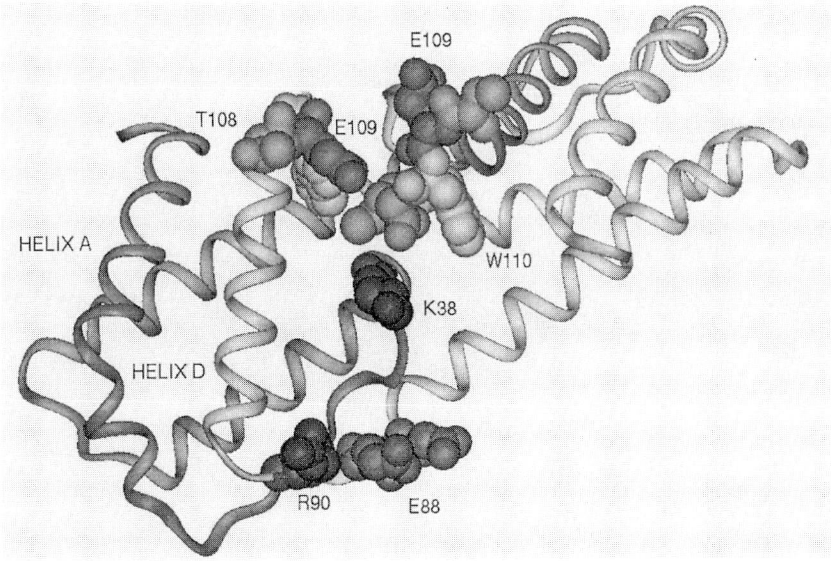


**Figure 6** Structure of IL-5 highlighting the key residues required for interaction with the receptor α chain.

are important in binding to its receptor α chain, and the subsequent cellular activation mediated via the receptor β chain (43–45). The key charged residue involved in binding to the β chain of the receptor is Glu-12. This residue is in an identical position to those previously identified in IL-3 and granulocyte-macrophage colony-stimulating factor (GM-CSF) and does not illustrate an area for the development of IL-5-specific small-molecule antagonists.

The α-chain binding site is composed of a region located close to the central symmetry axis of the dimer and principally involves the residues Arg-90 and Glu-109, located in the second beta sheet and after the end of the fourth helix, respectively. This site is unique to IL-5 and does not occur in IL-3 or GM-CSF and would therefore be a good target for the generation of IL-5-specific antagonists.

The key aspect for the rational design of IL-5 antagonists are that the major residues defined by site-directed mutagenesis, such as Arg-90 and Glu-109, are approximately 28 Å apart. This distance is rather long for typical "small molecule drugs," and therefore for combinatorial library design work and compound selections, the IL-5/IL-5 receptor α-chain contact area is more conveniently broken into two areas, based around Arg-90 and Glu-109, respectively. The profile of the surface to be scanned (Fig. 7) supports the division of the potential contact area into these two subgroups, with a plateau for the Arg-90-based

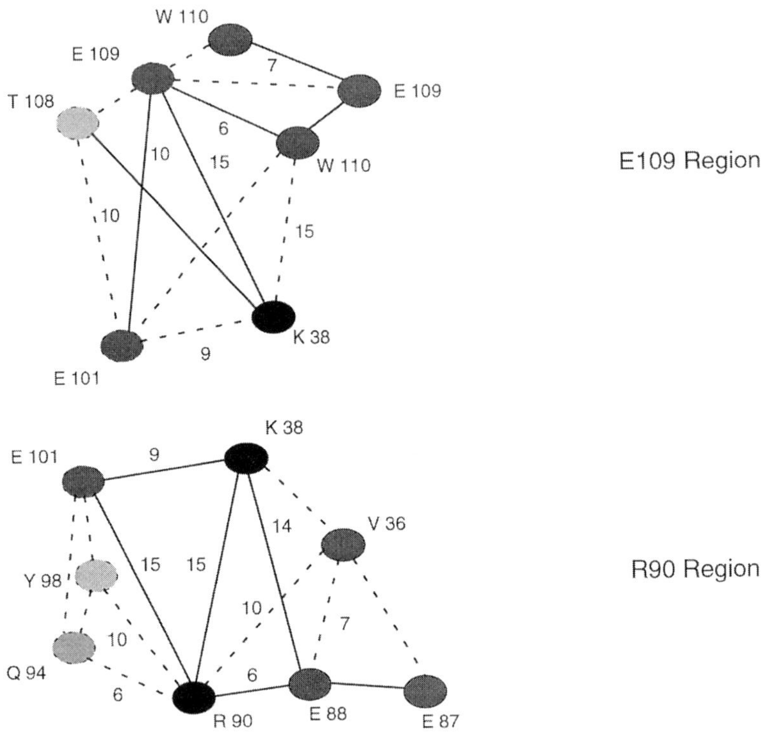


**Figure 7** Arg90 and E109 areas of IL-5.

search area and a substantial cavity for the Glu-109 area. Utilization of the detailed knowledge of the structure and likely contact residues of IL-5, derived from structural and site-directed mutagenesis experiments for the design of small molecule antagonists, depends critically on the development of ways to understand the importance of such data and how to interpret it. It is also likely that successful design of small-molecule inhibitors requires methods for the determination of the key areas of lipophilic interactions in the contact region between IL-5 and the receptor α chain, since these interactions are likely to be involved in the binding of high-affinity low molecular weight antagonist.

### Receptor-Based Design

A detailed knowledge at the molecular level of the IL-5/IL-5 receptor interaction is currently limited to identification of some of the key charged residues of IL-5 involved in the interaction with both the receptor α and β chains, and further information awaits the determination of the ligand/receptor cocrystal structure. Alternatively the interaction of human growth hormone is known (34,35) and models of the interaction of GM-CSF and IL-3 with their receptors have been made based on this structure (36). These models have provided insights into the binding of GM-CSF and IL-3 to their receptors, and this could also be a possible interim option for IL-5.

Species specificity for IL-5 is largely determined by the N-terminal module of the hIL-5R$\alpha$ chain. Based on homology and mutagenesis studies, a stretch of four amino acid residues (D55, D56, Y57, and E58) in the loop region that connects the C and D $\beta$ strands on the proposed tertiary structure of the N-terminal module, together with residue R188, have been identified as contributing to the ligand interaction (46). The ability to use this information requires a knowledge of the relative spatial distribution of these regions and their role in IL-5 binding.

While a range of peptide and protein IL-5 antagonists have been reported, no information on the identification of reversible small-molecule IL-5 antagonists has been published, and perhaps awaits the ligand-receptor cocrystal structure to provide a better understanding of the structural determinants required for the interaction of IL-5 with its receptor.

## V. Protein Antagonists

Protein-based antagonists of the IL-5/IL-5 receptor interaction fall into five distinct categories of molecular species, as depicted in Figure 1. These protein antagonists can be further divided into those that target the ligand, neutralizing IL-5 antibody or soluble IL-5 receptor, or those that target the IL-5 receptor directly, peptide antagonists, IL-5 mutant proteins, or neutralizing anti-IL-5 receptor $\alpha$-chain antibodies.

### A. Antibodies

Neutralizing monoclonal antibodies directed against human or mouse IL-5 have been identified (47,48). These antibodies have been characterized in a variety of cell-based in vitro assays and have been shown to specifically inhibit IL-5-dependent biological responses. The rat monoclonal antibody to mouse IL-5 (TRFK-5) has proved to be an extremely useful tool for probing the function of IL-5 in vivo since this antibody cross reacts with IL-5 from different species including mice, guinea pig, and human. As previously discussed, TRFK-5 has been shown to be very effective at blocking both systemic and lung eosinophilia and bronchial hyperreactivity in experimental models of allergic inflammation (21–25). Preliminary studies in a monkey model of allergic asthma suggest that these effects are long lasting, 3 to 6 months, even after a single dose of antibody (25). Significantly TRFK-5, either administered prophylactically or during an established eosinophilia, has been shown to be effective in blocking allergen-induced eosinophilic inflammation in the airways of sensitized mice (21). This result may have important clinical implications for the treatment of asthma since it suggests that inhibitors or antagonists of IL-5 action may be therapeutically effective when administered during an established eosinophil-driven lung inflammation.

Although neutralizing anti-IL-5 receptor α-chain antibodies have not been reported, theoretically this is an alternative means of specifically blocking IL-5 interacting with its receptor.

### B. Soluble Receptor

The extracellular domains of many membrane-bound cytokine receptors are produced as a soluble form either through differential splicing or through limited proteolysis (49). In human eosinophils and other IL-5 receptor expressing cells the most abundant IL-5 receptor α-chain transcript is the soluble variant (50). This soluble receptor is achieved through translation of alternatively spliced mRNAs, however, soluble receptor protein has not been detected physiologically. The extracellular domain of the IL-5 receptor α chain has been produced in a variety of expression systems (30,51) and this soluble protein binds IL-5 with similar affinity to the IL-5 receptor complex on cells. In contrast to the soluble human IL-6 receptor, which when bound to IL-6 leads to cell activation through association with gp130 (52), the soluble IL-5 receptor α chain does not associate with membrane-bound β chain. Consequently the soluble IL-5 receptor α chain competes with its membrane-bound counterpart for IL-5 and thus acts as a selective IL-5 antagonist, at least in in vitro bioassays (27,30). It has been postulated that the physiological role of soluble receptors released from cells is to act as local antagonists to limit the effect of cytokine action.

One of the potential problems of utilizing soluble receptors and antibodies therapeutically is that they may actually prolong cytokine activity by reducing clearance rates (53).

### C. Peptide Antagonists

As an intermediate between small molecule antagonists and large protein antagonists, such as antibodies or soluble receptors, emerging technologies such as phage display have facilitated the identification of small peptide agonists and antagonists of cytokine receptors. By extending the original work described by Smith (54) on the phage display, large libraries of peptides can be expressed on the surface of filamentous phage through fusion of oligonucleotides, encoding random peptides to the phage coat proteins gene III or gene VIII. This library of peptide-bearing phage is allowed to bind the extracellular domains of cytokine receptors and peptides are selected by affinity purification. This binding and selection procedure is employed in an iterative fashion to enrich for peptides of higher affinity. The identification of functional agonists or antagonists requires that these peptides are then screened in cell-based functional assays. Although this phage display technology has been employed successfully in the identification of peptide agonists of the erythropoietin (EPO) receptor (55) and peptide antagonists of the IL-1 receptor (56), such a process has not been described for the IL-5 receptor.

### D. IL-5 Mutant Protein

By a process of systematic replacement of charged residues with alanine, a process termed scanning alanine mutagenesis, a single-point mutant of IL-5 was identified, E12A, which was able to bind the IL-5 receptor with almost wild-type affinity but was a partial agonist in a TF-1 cell proliferation assay (43,44). Mutation of this acidic residue to the polar Gln (43) or the basic Lys (57) resulted in a mutant protein that was devoid of agonist activity and was a potent and specific IL-5 antagonist in a TF-1 cell proliferation assay. Although this mutant protein binds the receptor α chain, it appears to be capable of contacting but not activating the β chain, thereby preventing a proliferative signal in this erythroleukemia cell line.

Glutamic acid-12 resides on the amino terminal helix of IL-5 at an analogous position to E21 in GM-CSF and E22 in IL-3. Charge reversal mutations at these positions in IL-3 and GM-CSF similarly resulted in proteins which were unaltered in binding their respective α chains, but demonstrated an impaired ability to activate the common β chain. While IL-3 (E21R) retains agonist activity for TF-1 proliferation at 20,000-fold reduced potency relative to wild-type IL-3 (58), GM-CSF (E22R) lacks agonist activity and is a specific GM-CSF antagonist (59).

The antagonistic properties of IL-5 (E12K) are not restricted to inhibition of IL-5-induced cell proliferation. In human eosinophils IL-5 (E12K) was a selective antagonist of IL-5-induced eosinophil activation, as assessed by adhesion to immobilized IgG, exhibiting no effect on eosinophil activation induced by the related cytokines IL-3 and GM-CSF or the unrelated cytokine TNF-α. Somewhat surprisingly however, IL-5 (E12K) was a full agonist, albeit at reduced potency relative to wild-type IL-5, in an eosinophil survival assay (57). This apparent functional dichotomy in the actions of E12K in the eosinophil suggest that there may be distinct mechanisms of IL-5 receptor activation leading to different functional responses in the eosinophil. The dual agonist/antagonist properties of IL-5 (E12K) may preclude its use as a therapeutic.

## VI. Summary

In recent years it has become clear that cytokine networks regulate many of the body's host defense mechanisms and that inappropriate expression or overexpression of cytokines contributes to a number of pathological conditions. This realization led to great optimism that cytokines offered new opportunities to treat diseases, particularly chronic inflammatory diseases such as asthma and rheumatoid arthritis where there is still a great unmet medical need. Progress to this aim has been relatively slow, although cytokines such as erythropoietin and granulocyte colony-stimulating factor are successful therapeutics and are now making a significant impact on clinical practice. At present the scope of cytokine therapeutics is still limited to their administration as protein agonists, but the greatest clinical potential may be in the use of selective cytokine antagonists. In this respect there are encouraging results from a range of clinical trials with anticytokine antibodies, soluble receptors, or protein antagonists. However, there are major difficulties associated with the long-term administration of protein therapeutics for chronic disease. Clearly this is not impossible and diabetics administer daily injections of insulin to control their condition. The development of novel drug delivery systems may overcome the problems associated with the administration of proteins, thus making protein therapeutics more attractive. However, our goal is to develop low molecular weight cytokine antagonists which would offer a number of advantages over protein-based therpaeutics. These include their route of administration, their stability, and their cost. In addition there is still an unresolved question regarding the antigenicity of protein-based therapeutics during prolonged therapy.

We have outlined in this review the strategies we have adopted to find low molecular weight antagonists of IL-5 binding to the IL-5 receptor α chain. We believe that this represents an attractive target for diseases associated with mucosal inflammation resulting from the infiltration and activation of eosinophils, such as asthma. These strategies combine random high throughput screening and elements of "rational" design based on a functional understanding of the IL-5 structure. However, despite these significant efforts by us and many others, there are still very few examples of low molecular weight inhibitors of protein-protein interactions. Clearly there is still some way to go before we can deliver cheap, orally active cytokine antagonists to the clinic.

## References

1. Butterworth AE, Sturrock RF, Houba V, Mahmoud AAF, Sher A, Rees PK. Eosinophils as mediators of antibody-dependent damage to schistosomula. Nature 1975;256:727–729.
2. Butterworth AE, Wasson DL, Gleich GJ, Loegering DA, David JR. Damage to

schistosomula of *Schistosoma mansoni* induced by eosinophil major basic protein. J Immunol 1979;122:221–229.

3. Yazdanbakhsh M, Tai PC, Spry CJF, Gleich GJ, Roos D. Synergism between eosinophil cationic protein and oxygen metabolites in killing schistosomula of *Schistosoma mansoni*. J Immunol 1987;138:3443–3447.
4. Sanderson CJ. Interleukin-5, eosinophils, and disease. Blood 1992;79:3101–3109.
5. Kroegel C, Virchow JC Jr, Luttmann W, Walker C, Warner JA. Pulmonary immune cells in health and disease: the eosinophil leucocyte (part I). Eur Respir J 1994;7:519–543.
6. Kroegel C, Warner JA, Virchow JC Jr, Matthys H. Pulmonary immune cells in health and disease: the eosinophil leucocyte (part II). Eur Respir J 1994;7:743–760.
7. Bousquet JB, Chanez P, Lacoste JY, Barneon G, Ghavanian N, Enander I, Venge P, Ahlstedt S, Simony-Lafontaine J, Godard P, Michel FB. Eosinophilic inflammation in asthma. N Engl J Med 1990;323:1033–1039.
8. Laitinen L, Laitinen A, Neino M, Haahtela T. Eosinophilic airway inflammation during exacerbation of asthma and its treatment with inhaled corticosteroids. Am Rev Respir Dis 1991;143:423–427.
9. Gleich GJ. The role of the eosinophil leukocyte in bronchial asthma. Bull Eur Physiopathol Respir 1986;22:62–69.
10. Frigas E, Loegering DA, Solley GO, Farrow GM, Gleich GJ. Elevated levels of the eosinophil granular major basic protein in the sputum of patients with bronchial asthma. Mayo Clin Proc 1981;56:345–353.
11. Flavahan NA, Slifman NR, Gleich GJ, Vanhoutte PM. Human eosinophil derived major basic proteins cause hyperreactivity of respiratory smooth muscle. Am Rev Respir Dis 1988;138:685–688.
12. Coyle AJ, Ackerman SJ, Irvin CG. Cationic proteins induce airway hyperresponsiveness dependent on charge interactions. Am Rev Respir Dis 1993;147:896–900.
13. Clutterbuck EJ, Hirst EMA, Sanderson CJ. Human interleukin-5 (IL-5) regulates the production of eosinophils in human bone marrow cultures: comparison and interaction with IL-1, IL-3, IL-6 and GM-CSF. Blood 1989;73:1504–1512.
14. Denburg JA, Silver JE, Abrams JS. Interleukin-5 is a human basophilopoietin: induction of histamine content and basophilic differentiation of HL60 cells and of peripheral blood basophils. Blood 1991;77:1462–1468.
15. Plaut M, Pierce JH, Watson CJ, Hanley-Hyde J, Nordan RP, Paul WE. Mast cell lines produce lymphokines in response to cross-linkage of FcεRI or to calcium ionophores. Nature 1989;339:64–67.
16. Dubucquoi S, Desreumaux P, Janin A, Klein O, Goldman M, Tavernier J, Capron A, Capron M. Interleukin 5 synthesis by eosinophils: association with granules and immunoglobulin-dependent secretion. J Exp Med 1994;179:703–708.
17. Walsh GM, Hartnell A, Wardlaw AJ, Kurihara K, Sanderson CJ, Kay AB. IL-5 enhances the in vitro adhesion of human eosinophils, but not neutrophils, in a leucocyte integrin (CD11/18)-dependent manner. Immunology 1990;71:258–265.
18. Fujisawa T, Abu-Ghazaleh R, Kita H, Sanderson CJ, Gleich GJ. Regulatory effect of cytokines on eosinophil degranulation. J Immunol 1990;144:642–646.

19. Wang JM, Rambaldi A, Biondi A, Chen ZG, Sanderson CJ, Mantovani A. Recombinant human interleukin 5 is a selective eosinophil chemoattractant. Eur J Immunol 1989;19:701–705.
20. Yamaguchi Y, Hayashi Y, Sugama Y, Miura Y, Kasahara T, Kitamura S, Torisu M, Mita S, Tominaga A, Takatsu K, Suda T. Highly purified murine interleukin 5 (IL-5) stimulates eosinophil function and prolongs in vitro survival. IL-5 as an eosinophil chemotactic factor. J Exp Med 1988;167:1737–1742.
21. Kung TT, Stelts DM, Zurcher JA, Adams GK III, Egan RW, Kreutner W, Watnick AS, Jones H, Chapman RW. Involvement of IL-5 in a murine model of allergic pulmonary inflammation: prophylactic and therapeutic effect of an anti-IL-5 antibody. Am J Respir Cell Mol Biol 1995;13:360–365.
22. Blyth DI, Pedrick MS, Savage TJ, Hessel EM, Fattah D. Lung inflammation and epithelial changes in a murine model of atopic asthma. Am J Respir Cell Mol Biol 1996;14:425–438.
23. Van Oosterhout AJ, Landenius AR, Savelkoul HF, Van Ark I, Delsman KC, Nijkamp FP. Effect of an anti-IL-5 and IL-5 on airway hyperreactivity and eosinophils in guinea pigs. Am Rev Respir Dis 1993;147:548–552.
24. Akutsu I, Kojima T, Kariyone A, Fukuda T, Makino S, Takatsu K. Antibody against interleukin-5 prevents antigen-induced eosinophil infiltration and bronchial hyperreactivity in the guinea pig airways. Immunol Lett 1995;45:109–116.
25. Mauser PJ, Pitman AM, Fernandez X, Foran SK, Adams GK III, Kreutner W, Egan RW, Chapman TW. Effects of an antibody to interleukin-5 in a monkey model of asthma. Am J Respir Crit Care Med 1995;152:467–472.
26. Foster PS, Hogan SP, Ramsay AJ, Matthaei KI, Young IG. Interleukin 5 deficiency abolishes eosinophilia, airway hyperreactivity, and lung damage in a mouse asthma model. J Exp Med 1996;183:195–201.
27. Tavernier J, Devos R, Cornelis S, Tuypens T, Van der Heyden J, Fiers W, Plaetinck G. A human high affinity interleukin-5 receptor (IL5R) is composed of an IL5-specific $\alpha$ chain and a $\beta$ chain shared with the receptor for GM-CSF. Cell 1991;66:1175–1184.
28. Fattah D, Page KR, Bezbaruah S, Priest R, Horgan CM, Solari R. A rapid activation assay for human eosinophils based on adhesion to immobilised ICAM-1, VACM-1 and IgG. Cytokine 1996;8:248–259.
29. Devos R, Guisez Y, Plaetinck G, Cornelis S, Tavernier J, Van der Heyden J, Foley LH, Scheffler JE. Covalent modification of the interleukin-5 receptor by isothiazolones leads to inhibition of the binding of interleukin-5. Eur J Biochem 1994;225:635–640.
30. Banks M, Graber P, Proudfoot AEI, Arod CY, Allet B, Bernard AR, Sebille E, McKinnon M, Wells TNC, Solari R. Soluble interleukin-5 receptor $\alpha$-chain binding assays: use for screening and analysis of interleukin-5 mutants. Anal Biochem 1995;230:321–328.
31. Cooper K, Masamune H. Cytokine modulation as a medicinal chemistry target. Annu Rep Med Chem 1992;27:209–218.
32. Janin J, Chothia C. The structure of protein-protein recognition sites. J Biol Chem 1990;265:16027–16030.

33. Somers W, Ultsch M, De Vos AM, Kossiakoff AA. The x-ray structure of a growth hormone-prolactin receptor complex. Nature 1994;372:478–481.
34. Ultsch MH, Somers W, Kossiakoff AA, de Vos AM. The crystal structure of affinity-matured human growth hormone at 2 Å resolution. J Mol Biol 1994;236:286–299.
35. Clackson T, Wells JA. A hot spot of binding energy in a hormone-receptor interface. Science 1995;267:383–386.
36. Lyne PD, Bamborough P, Duncan D, Richard WG. Molecular modeling of the GM-CSF and IL-3 receptor complexes. Protein Sci 1995;4:2223–2233.
37. Naito Y, Akahoshi F, Takeda S, Okada T, Kajii M, Nishimura H, Sugiura M, Fukaya C, Kagitani Y. Synthesis and pharmacological activity of triazole derivatives inhibiting eosinophilia. J Med Chem 1996;39:3019–3029.
38. Widdowson KL, Veber DF, Jurewicz AJ, Rutledge MC Jr, Hertzberg RP. Preparation of N,N′-diphenylurea derivatives as interleukin-8 receptor antagonists. PCT Int. Appl., WO 9625157 A1 960822, Smithkline Beecham Corporation.
39. Bischoff SC, De Weck AL, Dahinden CA. Peptide analogs of consensus receptor sequence inhibit the action of cytokines on human basophils. Lymphokine Cytokine Res 1992;11:33–37.
40. McKinnon M, Proudfoot AEI, Wells TNC, Solari R. Strategies for the discovery of cytokine receptor antagonists. Drug News Perspect 1996;9:389–398.
41. Milburn MV, Hassell AM, Lambert MH, Jordan SR, Proudfoot AEI, Graber P, Wells TNC. A novel dimer configuration revealed by the crystal structure at 2.4 Å resolution of human interleukin-5. Nature 1993;363:172–176.
42. Wells TNC, Graber P, Proudfoot AEI, Arod CY, Jordan SR, Lambert MH, Hassel AM, Milburn MV. The three-dimensional structure of human interleukin-5 at 2.4 Å resolution: Implication for the structures of other cytokines. Ann NY Acad Sci 1994;725:118–127.
43. Tavernier J, Tuypens T, Verhee A, Plaetinck G, Devos R, Van der Heyden J, Guisez Y, Oefner C. Identification of receptor-binding domains on human interleukin 5 and design of an interleukin 5-derived receptor antagonist. Proc Natl Acad Sci USA 1995;92:5194–5198.
44. Graber P, Proudfoot AE, Talabot F, Bernard A, McKinnon M, Banks M, Fattah D, Solari R, Peitsch MC, Wells TN. Identification of key charged residues of human interleukin-5 in receptor binding and cellular activation. J Biol Chem 1995;270:15762–15769.
45. Dickason RR, Huston MM, Huston DP. Delineation of the IL-5 domains predicted to engage the IL-5 receptor complex. J Immunol 1996;156:1030–1037.
46. Cornelis S, Plaetinck G, Devos R, Van der Heyden J, Tavernier J, Sanderson CJ, Guisez Y, Fiers W. Detailed analysis of the IL-5/IL-5Rα interaction: characterization of crucial residues on the ligand and the receptor. EMBO J 1995;14:3395–3402.
47. McNamee LA, Fattah DF, Baker TJ, Bains SK, Hissey PH. Production, characterisation and use of monoclonal antibodies to human interleukin-5 in an enzyme-linked immunosorbent assay. J Immunol Meth 1991;141:81–88.
48. Schumacher JH, O'Garra A, Shrader B, van Kimmenade A, Bond MW, Mosman

TR, Coffman RL. The characterisation of four monoclonal antibodies specific for mouse interleukin (IL-)-5 and development of mouse and human enzyme-linked immunosorbent. J Immunol 1988;141:1576–1581.
49. Rose-John S, Heinrich PC. Soluble receptors for cytokines and growth factors: generation and biological function. Biochem J 1994;300:281–290.
50. Tavernier J, Tuypens T, Plaetinck G, Verhee A, Fiers W, Devos R. Molecular basis of the membrane-anchored and two soluble isoforms of the human interleukin 5 receptor α subunit. Proc Natl Acad Sci USA 1992;89:7041–7045.
51. Devos R, Guisez Y, Cornelis S, Verhee A, Van der Heyden J, Manneberg M, Lahm HW, Fiers W, Tavernier J, Plaetinck G. Recombinant soluble interleukin-5 (hIL-5) receptor molecules. J Biol Chem 1993;268:6581–6587.
52. Yawata H, Yasukawa K, Natsuka S, Murakami M, Yamasaki K, Hibi M, Taga T, Kishimoto T. Structure-function analysis of human IL-6 receptor: dissociation of amino acid residues required for IL-6 binding and IL-6 signal transduction through gp130. EMBO J 1993;12:1705–1712.
53. Sato TA, Widmer MB, Finkelman FD, Madani H, Jacobs CA, Grabstein KH, Malizewski CR. Recombinant soluble murine IL-4 receptor can inhibit or enhance IgE responses in vitro. J Immunol 1993;150:2717–2723.
54. Smith GP. Filamentous fusion phage: novel expression vectors that display cloned antigens on the virion surface. Science 1985;228:1315–1317.
55. Wrighton NC, Farrell FX, Chang R, Kashyap AK, Barbone FP, Mulcahy LS, Johnson DL, Barrett RW, Joliffe LK, Dower WJ. Small peptides as potent mimetics of the protein hormone erythropoietin. Science 1996;273:458–463.
56. Yanofsky SD, Baldwin DN, Butler JH, Holden FR, Jacobs JW, Balasubramanian P, Chinn JP, Cwirla SE, Peters-Bhatt E, Whitehorn EA, Tate EH, Akeson A, Bowlin TL, Dower WJ. High affinity type I interleukin 1 receptor antagonists discovered by screening recombinant peptide libraries. Proc Natl Acad Sci 1996;93:7381–7386.
57. McKinnon M, Page K, Uings IJ, Banks M, Fattah, D, Proudfoot AEI, Graber P, Arod C, Fish R, Wells TNC, Solari R. An interleukin-5 mutant distinguishes between two functional responses in human eosinophils. J Exp Med 1997; 186:121–129.
58. Barry SC, Bagley CJ, Phillips J, Dottore M, Cambareri B, Moretti P, D'Andrea R, Goodall GJ, Shannon MF, Vadas MA, Lopez AF. Two contiguous residues in human interleukin-3, Asp21 and Glu22, selectively interact with the α- and β-chains of its receptors and participate in function. J Biol Chem 1994;269:8488–8492.
59. Hercus TR, Bagley CJ, Cambareri B, Dottore M, Woodcock JM, Vadas MA, Shannon MF, Lopez AF. Specific human granulocyte-macrophage colony-stimulating factor antagonists. Proc Natl Acad Sci USA 1994;91:5838–5842.

# 18

# Pulmonary Biology of Anti-Interleukin-5 Antibodies

**ROBERT W. EGAN, CHUAN-CHU CHOU, RICHARD W. CHAPMAN, CHUNG-HER JENH, TED T. KUNG, and PETER J. MAUSER**

Schering-Plough Research Institute
Kenilworth, New Jersey

**DILJEET ATHWAL, J. SPENCER EMTAGE, and MARK W. BODMER**

CellTech Therapeutics
Slough, Berkshire, United Kingdom

There is strong but circumstantial evidence for a role of IL-5 in asthma, because IL-5 is an essential cytokine for the maturation of eosinophil precursors to eosinophils and it is those eosinophils that accumulate in the lungs during pulmonary inflammation (1). Inhibiting the actions of IL-5 should, therefore, block the maturation of eosinophil precursors to eosinophils and remove at least one of the major causes of asthma. We have investigated the effects of anti-IL-5 antibodies on allergic responses in mice, in guinea pigs, and in monkeys and will be extending this experimental paradigm into man using a humanized antibody against IL-5. Using that antibody, we will acquire a good deal of concrete information regarding the role of IL-5 in asthma.

The concept behind using an antibody to inhibit the action of a cytokine is that it binds the ligand, making it inaccessible to its receptor. It should, therefore, bind cytokine with a higher affinity than the receptor itself and, in the case of the antibodies described herein, such is the case. TRFK-5 antibody was raised against purified murine IL-5 (2) and has an $IgG_1$ isotype. We have also prepared a CDR grafted humanized antibody against IL-5 named Sch 55700. Both of them have $K_d$ values of about $10^{-10}$ M and both of them neutralize IL-5 from a variety of species.

In our monkey model of asthma, adult cynomolgus monkeys were tranquilized with ketamine, injected intravenously with the antibody of choice, anesthetized, and intubated with an endotracheal tube through which we inserted a pediatric bronchoscope in order to conduct broncheoaveolar lavage with two 10 ml saline washes (3). At the same time, we evaluated the responsiveness of the lungs to a dose response of aerosol histamine. These monkeys were naturally sensitive to aerosol ascaris antigen, which was used as the allergic stimulus. After 24 hr, bronchoalveolar lavage and airway hyperreactivity were evaluated such that each monkey served as its own control. In a set of six monkeys, airway hyperreactivity and bronchoalveolar lavage eosinophils were measured in the absence of the antibody. Two weeks later, when the pulmonary parameters in this set of monkeys had returned to baseline, the experiment was repeated in the presence of the antibody, such that this set of monkeys was internally controlled.

To quantitate airway hyperreactivity, we measured the histamine concentration required to cause a 40% decrease in dynamic compliance, the $C_{Dyn40}$, and defined a shift ratio, as the $C_{Dyn40}$ before divided by the $C_{Dyn40}$ after ascaris challenge. A shift greater than one indicates hyperreactivity, while a shift of one indicates that the status of the lungs is the same before and after the allergic challenge.

Using this experimental protocol, we examined the effects of 0.3 mg/kg of the TRFK-5 antibody on ascaris-induced pulmonary eosinophilia and airway hyperreactivity in monkeys (Table 1) (Figure 1) (3). In the control experiment, we treated the six animals with histamine to establish the pre-ascaris $C_{Dyn40}$, which turned out to be 0.04% histamine. Subsequent to the allergic challenge, we measured the response to histamine again and established a shift ratio of 7.6-fold. In these monkeys, lavage eosinophil levels were $14 \times 10^3$/ml before the allergic challenge and four- to five-fold higher after the ascaris challenge. Two weeks later when these animals had largely returned to normal, the same experiment was performed in the presence of 0.3 mg/kg TRFK-5 antibody. The pre-ascaris $C_{Dyn40}$ was 0.03%, virtually the same as before. However, instead of the shift of seven- to eight-fold, the shift ratio was 0.74, indicating that the

**Table 1** Effect of 0.3 mg/kg of TRFK-5 on Antigen-Induced Eosinophilia and Reactivity in Monkeys

| | $C_{Dyn40}$ (% histamine) | | EOS ($10^3$/cells/ml) | |
|---|---|---|---|---|
| Treatment | Pre-ascaris | Shift | Pre-ascaris | Increase (%) |
| Control | 0.039 ± 0.009 | 7.63 ± 3.72 | 13.8 ± 9.6 | 460 ± 145 |
| TRFK-5 | 0.032 ± 0.016 | 0.74 ± 0.41 | 52.6 ± 36.6 | 96 ± 39 |

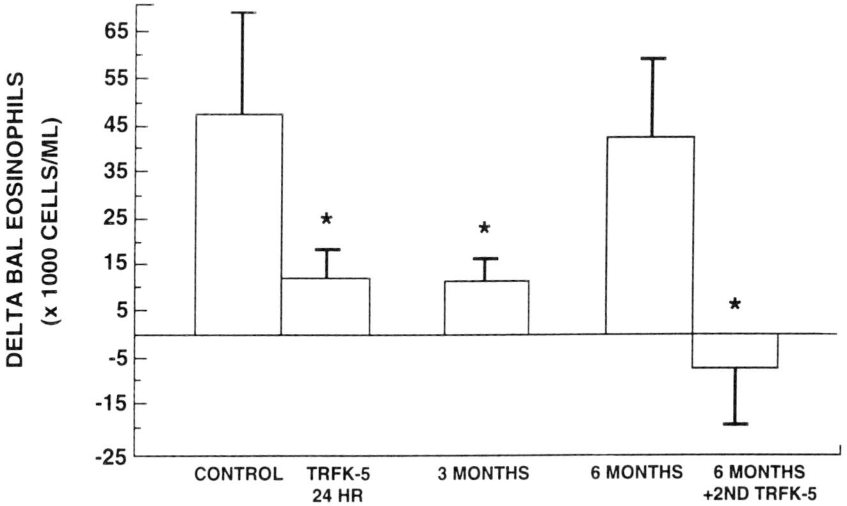


**Figure 1** The effect over six months of a single dose of 0.3 mg/kg of TRFK-5 on monkey eosinophilia. *Statistically significant from control monkeys.

monkey's lungs were not hyperreactive. Baseline eosinophils were about 52,000/ml, but there was only about a two-fold increase. Irrespective of whether the decrease in lung eosinophilia caused the reduced hyperreactivity, anti-IL-5 treatment inhibited airway hyperreactivity and this physiology should translate into meaningful results in human asthma.

In Figure 2 these data are shown in bar graph format instead of tabular form, where the difference in the eosinophils is the number of bronchoalveolar lavage eosinophils after the allergic challenge minus the number before. The bar on the left represents the untreated animals, where there was a difference of 45,000 eosinophils/ml. As in Table 1, when these animals were treated acutely with the TRFK-5 antibody there was about 75% inhibition of the eosinophil infiltration. Despite treating these monkeys with TRFK-5 antibody only once, eosinophilia in these animals was still suppressed as extensively 3 months later as for the acute treatment. After 6 months the eosinophil response largely recovered to normal and the eosinophilia was blocked by a second treatment with the TRFK-5 antibody. This phenomenon was not unique to the eosinophilia, because after 3 and 6 months the animals had not reestablished their hyperreactivity response to the control level of airway hyperreactivity. However, at 6 months they did respond to a second treatment with the TRFK-5 antibody.

In order to determine whether this phenomenon was peculiar to the monkey and to extend the experimental paradigm into a species that is more experi-

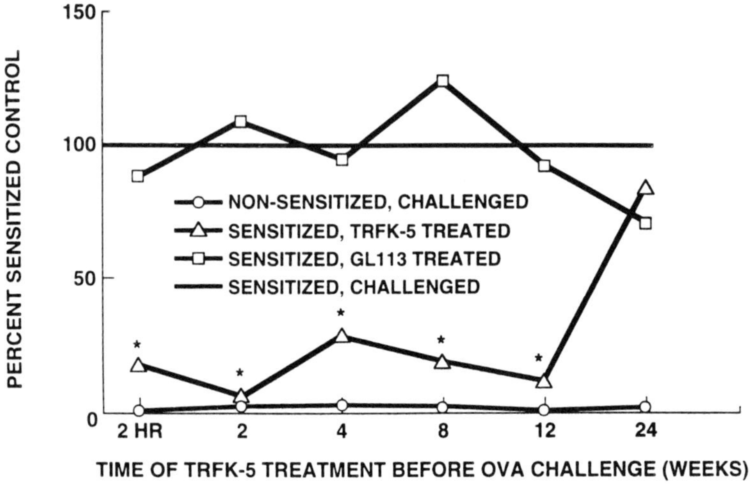


**Figure 2** The effect over six months of a single dose of 1 mg/kg of TRFK-5 on BAL eosinophilia in allergic mice.

mentally tractable, we have studied the extended duration of action of the TRFK-5 antibody in the B6D mouse. Mice were sensitized to alum-precipitated ovalbumin by a single 8 μg intraperitoneal injection. Five days later they were boosted with the same dose to enhance the responsiveness. After 12 days, when IgE levels had increased about seven-fold, they were challenged with aerosol ovalbumin, causing an allergic response. Twenty-four hours after the challenge, the mice were sacrificed and specimens of lavage fluid, lung tissue, blood, and bone marrow were analyzed for total cells and eosinophils. Antibody was administered 2 hr prior to the ovalbumin challenge.

Using this model we examined the effect of a single intraperitoneal dose of 1 mg/kg of the TRFK-5 antibody on bronchoalveolar lavage eosinophilia over an extended period of time (Fig. 2) (4). Each time point was normalized to the sensitized challenged animals (100%) to avoid age-related changes in the response. Throughout the study the nonsensitized mice had virtually no lavage eosinophils. At the 2 hr time point, the sensitized challenged mice treated with TRFK-5 antibody had their eosinophil response attenuated about 80%, while the mice treated with the isotype-matched control antibody, GL113, continued to show an eosinophil infiltrate. The same pattern was observed at 2 weeks, 4 weeks, 8 weeks, and 12 weeks, but at 24 weeks the mice largely returned to normal with TRFK-5 no longer inhibiting the eosinophil infiltrate. Therefore, as with the monkey, it took several months for the effect of a single dose of the TRFK-5 antibody to dissipate in the mouse.

During this interval we also examined bone marrow eosinophils in the femur, because the TRFK-5 antibody is known to inhibit release of mature eosinophils into the circulation, which is why they never appeared in the bronchoalveolar lavage fluid (Fig. 3) (5). Normalized to the sensitized challenged animals, the bone marrow eosinophils in the nonsensitized mice were significantly higher, because the sensitized challenged mice released eosinophils from their bone marrow more rapidly than it could replace them. Starting from a baseline of about 200,000 eosinophils per femur, the sensitized challenged animals dropped to about half that value. The TRFK-5 antibody blocked the change, while the GL-113 antibody had no impact. This effect continued for 2, 4, 8, and possibly 12 weeks, but the mice returned to normal by 24 weeks. Although we have not yet resolved the mechanism for this observation, it certainly will have an impact on the design of clinical trials with the humanized antibody.

To conduct similar studies in the human we would need a humanized antibody against IL-5 to facilitate multiple dosing and to reduce immunogenicity. We, therefore, performed CDR grafting based on the 39D10 antibody. The CDRs from 39D10 were grafted onto an otherwise human framework with an $IgG_4$ isotype and a few framework residues in the region of the CDRs in order to achieve maximum binding affinity. This antibody, named Sch 55700, was first tested for its innate activity to bind human IL-5 compared to 39D10 (6). Using a BIAcore binding assay, the on rates for both 39D10 and Sch 55700

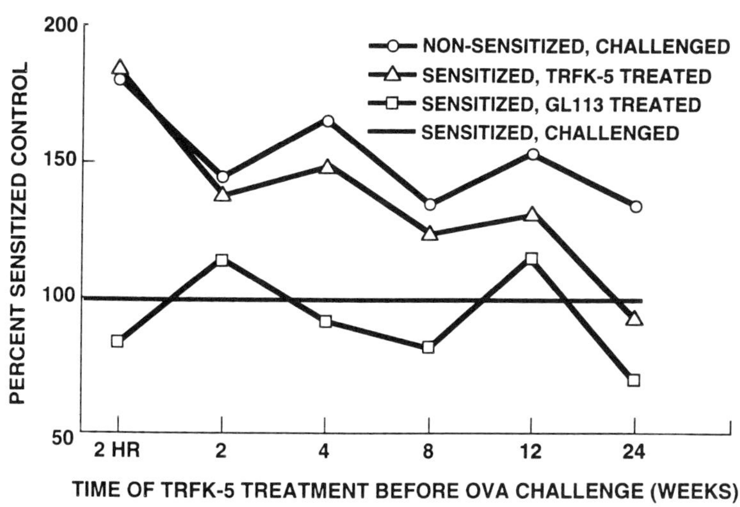


**Figure 3** The effect over six months of a single dose of 1 mg/kg of TRFK-5 on bone marrow eosinophilia in allergic mice.

were virtually identical at $5 \times 10^5$/M/sec. The off rates were between 3 and 4 $\times 10^5$/sec and gave $K_d$ values of 5 and $8 \times 10^{-11}$ M, respectively. To evaluate the neutralizing capacity, we tested antibody-based inhibition of IL-5-induced proliferation of the TF-1 human erythroleukemic cell line. Again, both antibodies were active in the range of $4 \times 10^{-11}$ M. Hence SCH 55700 is as potent as 39D10, and this binding affinity is stronger than the association between IL-5 and its high-affinity receptor, which has a $K_d$ of about $25 \times 10^{-11}$ M.

As with TRFK-5, intravenous Sch 55700 was examined in the monkey model of eosinophilia described previously (Fig. 4). In the control period, these monkeys had a pulmonary eosinophilic response of about 225,000 eosinophils/ml in the lavage. Following treatment with 0.3 mg/kg Sch 55700, the acute response was reduced to 40,000 eosinophils/ml, about 80% inhibition of the eosinophil infiltrate. This reduced response continued for six months following a single treatment of Sch 55700, as it did with TRFK-5.

Sch 55700 was also active against lung eosinophlia in allergic mice using the experimental protocol described previously (Fig. 5). When challenged, mice that were not previously sensitized did not mount an eosinophilic response, while those that were both sensitized and challenged gave a massive eosinophil infiltrate that was blocked by 1 mg/kg IP Sch 55700 or 1 mg/kg IP 39D10, but not by lower doses of either antibody.

Sch 55700 was also examined in guinea pigs, because it was possible to study both pulmonary eosinophilia and airway hyperreactivity in that species. The experimental paradigm was very similar to the mouse. The guinea pigs were sensitized to intraperitoneal ovalbumin then challenged with aerosol ovalbumin following treatment with the antibody or with a sham injection. We then examined lung tissue eosinophilia, lavage eosinophilia, and reactivity of the guinea

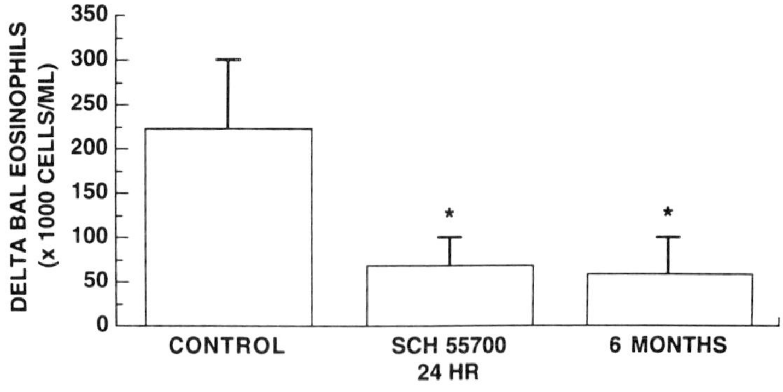


**Figure 4** The effect over six months of a single dose of 0.3 mg/kg of Sch 55700 on monkey eosinophilia. *Statistically significant from control monkeys.

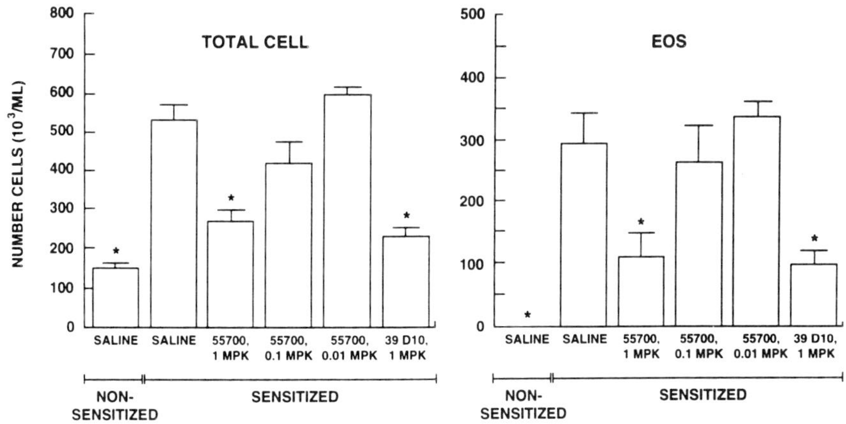


**Figure 5** Inhibition by Sch 55700 of the total cells and eosinophils from the BAL of allergic mice. *Statistically significant from nonsensitized, saline-pretreated mice.

pigs airways to substance P. Figure 6 shows the effects of intraperitoneal Sch 55700 on both eosinophil infiltration and airway hyperreactivity as indicated by either $C_{Dyn40}$ or specific lung resistance ($R_{L100}$). The eosinophil infiltrate was inhibited by 0.03 mg/kg, while it took 1 mg/kg before the physiology was altered. Both the eosinophil infiltration and the airway hyperreactivity were blocked completely at high doses of Sch 55700.

Selective inhibition of IL-5 by an antibody should be less immunosuppressive than steroid treatment and that can be measured by comparing the impact of Sch 55700 compared to steroids on circulating lymphocyte and granulocyte

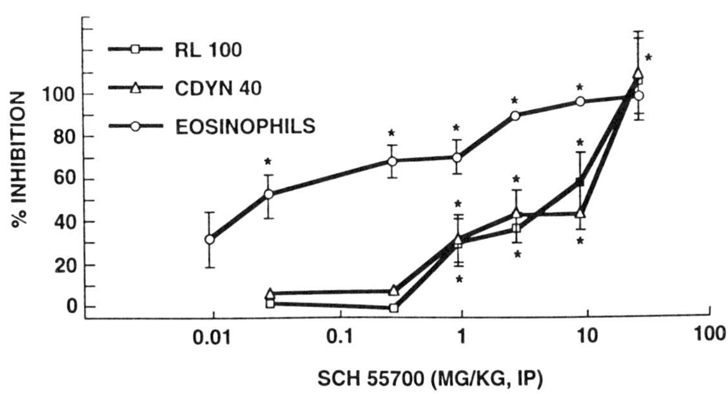


**Figure 6** Inhibition by Sch 55700 of the bronchial hyperresponsiveness and the pulmonary eosinophilia in allergic guinea pigs. *Statistically significant from ovalbumin sensitized challenged guinea pigs.

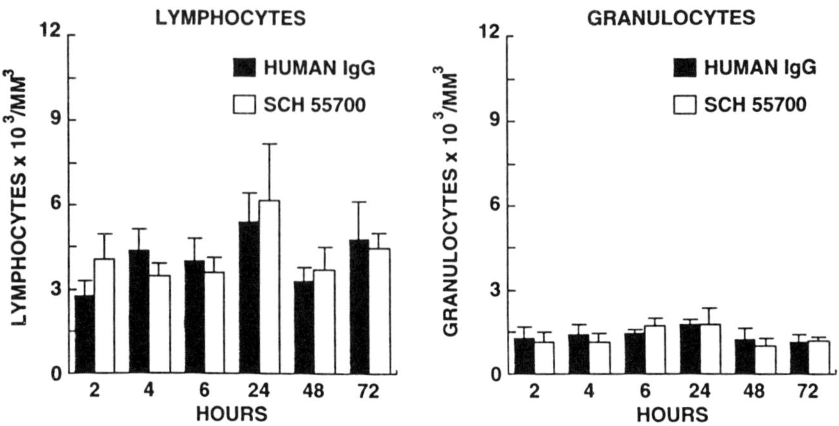


**Figure 7** The effect of Sch 55700 on circulating lymphocytes and granulocytes.

counts in guinea pigs. In guinea pigs, intraperitoneal betamethasone doubled the granulocyte counts and halved the lymphocyte counts over a period of 4 hr following treatment. Betamethasone is a systemically active steroid and such immunosuppression probably does not apply to topical steroids, but it indicates that steroids in general have the potential to cause immunosuppression. On the other hand, Sch 55700 did not alter either granulocyte or lymphocyte numbers for at least 3 days after intraperitoneal administration at the very high dose of 30 mg/kg (Fig. 7). Therefore, as opposed to steroids, Sch 55700 does not even have the potential to cause the immunosuppression seen with steroids in the guinea pig.

In summary, we have measured eosinophilia and airway hyperreactivity in monkeys, mice, and guinea pigs in response to an allergic challenge. Antibodies to IL-5 can completely inhibit the eosinophilia and the airway hyperreactivity. When we started these studies it was thought that GM-CSF or IL-3 could substitute in eosinophilopoiesis if IL-5 was inhibited, but certainly that is not the case. The duration of action of the antibodies is between 3 and 6 months, and we are working on the mechanism of extended duration. Nevertheless, this simple empirical observation will certainly help dictate our clinical protocol. Anti-IL-5 antibodies inhibit release of eosinophils from the bone marrow and that mechanism holds for the 3 to 6 months of biological activity. Lastly, Sch 55700 is a CDR-grafted humanized antibody against IL-5 that will proceed for testing against clinical asthma.

## References

1. Gleich GJ, Kita H, Adolphson CR. Eosinophils. In: MN Frank, Austen KF, Cloman HN, Unanue ER, eds. Santers Immunologic Diseases. Boston: Little Brown, 1995:205–245.
2. Schumacher JH, O'Garra A, Shrader B, van Kimmenade A, Bond MW, Mosmann TR, Coffman RL. The characterization of four monoclonal antibodies specific for mouse IL-5 and development of mouse and human IL-5 enzyme-linked immunosorbent. J Immunol 1988;141:1576–1581.
3. Mauser PJ, Pitman AM, Fernandez X, Foran SK, Adams GK III, Kreutner W, Egan RW, Chapman RW. Effect of an antibody to interleukin 5 in a monkey model of asthma. Am J Respir Crit Care Med 1995;152:467–472.
4. Egan RW, Wang P, Garlisi C, Mauser P, Chapman RW, Kreutner W, Umland SP, Kung TT. Mechanism of extended duration of anti-IL-5 antibodies against pulmonary eosinophilia. J Allergy Clin Immunol 1997;99:S122.
5. Kung TT, Stelts D, Zurcher JA, Adams GK III, Egan RW, Kreutner W, Watnick AS, Jones H, Chapman RW. Involvement of IL-5 in a murine model of allergic pulmonary inflammation: prophylactic and therapeutic effect of an anti-IL-5 antibody. Am J Respir Cell Mol Biol 1995;13:360–365.
6. Egan RW, Athwahl D, Chou C-C, Emtage S, Jen C-H, Kung TT, Mauser PJ, Murgolo NJ, Bodmer MW. Inhibition of pulmonary eosinophilia and hyperreactivity by antibodies to interleukin-5. Int Arch Allergy Immunol 1995;107:321–322.

# AUTHOR INDEX

## A


Aarden, LA, 144, 145, 149
Abaitua, I, 97, 114
Abbas, AK, 145, 151
Abdel Meguid, SS, 168, 170, 171, 173, 174, 183, 185, 246, 247, 260
Abraham, GN, 128, 133
Abraham, S, 248, 262
Abrahams, C, 14, 33
Abrams, J, 97, 112
Abrams, JS, 56, 57, 65, 66, 83, 92, 97, 102, 113, 117, 138, 146, 300, 317
Abu-Ghazaleh, R, 52, 63, 300, 317
Abu-Ghazeleh, RI, 20, 35
Acharakis, B, 254, 265
Ackerman, SJ, 2, 3, 13, 17, 18, 23, 24, 29, 30, 33, 34, 36, 75, 84, 85, 90, 97, 99, 100, 101, 113, 127, 131, 245, 259, 300, 317
Ackerman, ST, 98, 110, 114
Adachi, H, 193, 201
Adachi, M, 9, 32
Adams, GK, 27, 36, 37, 70, 82, 87, 154, 158, 162, 163, 244, 259, 300, 313, 314, 318, 322, 325, 329
Adcock, IM, 59, 67, 156, 158, 164
Adelroth, E, 58, 67
Adkinson, NF, 40, 48
Adolphson, CR, 2, 3, 4, 73, 29, 96, 98, 114, 127, 131, 321, 329
Adt, M, 18, 35
Agaki, K, 245, 250, 259, 264
Agosti, JM, 8, 32
Aguirre, V, 158, 165
Ahlstedt, S, 51, 62, 127, 131, 242, 257, 299, 317
Ahmed, T, 17, 34
Ahuja, SS, 294, 297
Aiuti, F, 102, 116
Akagi, M, 171, 187, 247, 260
Akahoshi, F, 309, 318
Akeson, A, 206, 220, 315, 320
Akira, S, 145, 151, 249, 251, 262
Akutsu, I, 127, 132, 244, 259, 300, 313, 318
Alam, R, 102, 117, 249, 263

Alberola-Ila, J, 277, 284
Alcami, A, 217, 222
Aldrich, TB, 207, 220
Aldrich, TH, 196, 203
Alevizopoulos, A, 294, 297
Alexander, AB, 54, 59, 60, 64, 67
Alexander, AG, 281, 287
Alexander, J, 144, 149
Alexander, WS, 144, 150
Allen, RC, 250, 263
Allet, B, 303, 314, 318
Alonso-Vega, C, 277, 284
Alouani, S, 144, 145, 150
Alpert, A, 208, 221
Altin, JG, 290, 291, 296
Altman, LC, 8, 32
Alum, R, 43, 49
Alumets, J, 4, 31
Aman, MJ, 144, 150
American Thoracic Society, 51, 61
Anan, S, 103, 117
Anderson, D, 208, 221
Anderson, GP, 21, 35
Anderson, M, 80, 85, 91
Anderson, SJ, 277, 284
Andersson, E, 80, 91
Andersson, J, 277, 280, 284
Andersson, M, 80, 91
Andersson, U, 277, 284
Andrade, S, 143, 149
Andrews, RK, 191, 196, 197, 201
Angel, P, 279, 285
Angelichio, M, 168, 170, 171, 173, 174, 183, 185, 246, 247, 260
Anguita, J, 140, 147
Aoki, I, 2, 29
Appella, E, 170, 186
Applebaum, E, 168, 170, 171, 173, 174, 183, 185, 246, 247, 260
Applebaum, ER, 246, 260
Appleby, MW, 251, 264, 277, 284
Arai, K, 60, 68, 90, 144, 150, 189, 191, 196, 200, 203, 206, 219, 225, 226, 227, 228, 229, 230, 231, 232, 234, 235, 236, 237, 238, 242, 251, 252, 257, 264, 271, 272, 274, 283, 293, 296
Arai, KI, 247, 249, 261, 268, 278, 282
Arai, N, 142, 148, 225, 227, 229, 236, 268, 271, 272, 274, 278, 282, 283, 293, 296
Arai, T, 75, 90
Arakawa, KC, 2, 29
Aritomi, M, 218, 223
Arm, JP, 130, 135
Armour, CL, 280, 287
Arod, C, 197, 198, 203, 315, 320
Arod, CY, 175, 177, 178, 180, 181, 182, 187, 195, 202, 303, 310, 314, 318, 319
Asakura, Y, 269, 280, 281, 283
Assal Melianai, A, 121, 125
Assenmacher, M, 140, 147
Assoufi, B, 51, 53, 54, 55, 56, 57, 58, 61, 62, 63, 64, 65, 67, 127, 128, 132, 280, 286
Athwahl, D, 70, 87, 325, 329
Atkins, PC, 102, 116
Attisano, L, 217, 222
Aubry, JP, 143, 149
Aud, D, 228, 237
Auphan, N, 294, 297
Austen, KF, 39, 48, 52, 62, 76, 90, 98, 99, 110, 115, 130, 135
Auwerx, J, 278, 285
Aversa, G, 142, 148
Ayala, LE, 17, 34
Ayars, GH, 32
Azuma, C, 52, 62, 154, 161, 168, 185, 241, 256
Azuma, S, 228, 237

Azzawi, M, 51, 53, 54, 63, 64, 69, 83, 85, 127, 128, 132, 154, 162, 244, 259

## B

Baba, M, 156, 164
Bachmann, M, 128, 129, 133, 139, 144, 146
Bachurski, CJ, 228, 237
Bacon, KB, 155, 163
Badalian, TM, 281, 287
Baggiolini, M, 155, 163
Bagley, CJ, 175, 187, 190, 191, 196, 197, 200, 201, 206, 219, 254, 265, 315, 320
Bains, SK, 313, 319
Bajaj, SP, 2, 29
Baker, C, 5, 32
Baker, CB, 8, 32
Baker, E, 70, 86, 207, 208, 221
Baker, TJ, 313, 319
Balasubramanian, C, 206, 220
Balasubramanian, P, 199, 203, 315, 320
Baldwin, AS, 294, 297
Baldwin, DN, 206, 220, 315, 320
Baltimore, D, 251, 264
Bamborough, P, 308, 313, 318
Ban, G, 217, 223
Banchereau, J, 52, 63, 119, 124, 142, 144, 148, 150, 227, 236
Banks, C, 175, 187
Banks, M, 171, 172, 174, 175, 176, 186, 187, 194, 197, 198, 202, 203, 303, 311, 314, 315, 318, 319, 320
Bao, S, 129, 134
Barandun, J, 104, 117
Baraniuk, J, 20, 35
Barberis Maino, L, 141, 147
Barbone, FP, 199, 203, 206, 220, 315, 320
Bardin, PG, 98, 114
Barkans, J, 41, 45, 48, 49, 53, 55, 56, 57, 59, 63, 64, 65, 83, 92, 119, 125
Barker, PA, 207, 220
Barker, RL, 2, 3, 16, 29, 30, 31, 34
Barneon, G, 51, 61, 69, 85, 127, 131, 242, 257, 299, 317
Barnes, NC, 54, 59, 64, 67, 281, 287
Barnes, PJ, 15, 17, 33, 34, 59, 67, 127, 130, 132, 279, 286
Baron-Hay, MJ, 124, 126
Barrett, R, 250, 264
Barrett, RW, 199, 203, 206, 220, 315, 320
Barry, SC, 169, 175, 186, 187, 191, 194, 201, 202, 206, 219, 315, 320
Barsoumian, EL, 278, 285
Bascom, R, 40, 48, 102, 117
Bashian, G, 280, 286
Basten, A, 52, 62
Bates, ME, 249, 263
Bauchamp, M, 81, 91
Bauden, R, 168, 185
Baum, CM, 73, 89
Baumann, MA, 245, 259
Baumbach, WR, 208, 221
Baumhueter, S, 73, 89
Bazan, JF, 155, 163, 190, 200, 241, 246, 250, 256, 259, 263
Beach, D, 235, 239
Beagley, KW, 129, 134
Beasley, R, 21, 22, 24, 36, 51, 62, 69, 85, 127, 131
Beaudry, P, 218, 223
Beck, LA, 279, 286
Beckmann, MP, 208, 221
Bedalac, A, 140, 147
Beeson, PB, 52, 62
Befus, AD, 76, 78, 80, 90

Begley, CG, 168, 185, 208, 221
Behm, CA, 128, 134, 245, 259, 289, 295
Behrmann, I, 206, 219
Beintema, JJ, 3, 30
Belda, A, 70, 76, 78, 83, 86, 90
Bell, MP, 2, 3, 4, 29, 30, 31
Belmont, JW, 250, 263
Belosevic, M, 120, 121, 125, 126
Bennett, B, 143, 149
Bennett, D, 168, 170, 171, 173, 174, 183, 185, 246, 247, 260
Bennett, DB, 246, 260
Bennett, L, 217, 223
Bennett, MJ, 178, 180, 188
Ben-Sasson, SZ, 139, 144, 146
Bentley, A, 128, 132, 280, 286
Bentley, AM, 45, 49, 53, 55, 56, 57, 58, 64, 66, 67, 83, 92, 119, 125, 127, 128, 132, 133
Ben-Yaakov, M, 57, 66, 102, 117
Bergstedt-Lindqvist, S, 52, 62, 128, 133, 168, 185, 241, 256
Berhee, A, 207, 208, 214, 221
Berkman, N, 156, 158, 164
Bernard, A, 168, 171, 172, 174, 175, 176, 185, 186, 194, 202, 311, 315, 319
Bernard, AR, 303, 314, 318
Bernasconi, S, 143, 149
Berndt, MC, 191, 196, 197, 201
Berns, A, 233, 238
Bernstein, I, 73, 89
Bertcs, PJ, 249, 263
Bertho, JM, 73, 90
Bertrand, C, 21, 35, 56, 65
Bettleheim, P, 76, 90
Betz, S, 103, 117
Beutner, U, 290, 291, 296
Bezbaruah, S, 303, 318
Bhattacharrya, S, 120, 125
Bhogal, B, 97, 112
Biagiotti, R, 52, 63
Bickel, C, 154, 162
Bickel, CA, 43, 49, 128, 134, 279, 286
Bidaud, C, 144, 150
Bienenstock, J, 76, 78, 80, 83, 90, 92, 103, 117
Bierer, BE, 281, 287
Biffi, M, 141, 147
Bilimoria, Y, 19, 35
Billah, MM, 271, 272, 274, 281, 283
Billian, G, 142, 148
Biondi, A, 155, 163, 300, 318
Bird, TA, 291, 296
Birkland, TP, 99, 115
Biron, CA, 139, 146
Bischoff, SC, 52, 63, 309, 318
Biswas, P, 52, 63, 138, 146
Bjorksten, B, 119, 120, 124, 125
Blake, JS, 14, 33
Blaser, K, 53, 55, 57, 58, 64, 65, 66, 104, 117, 127, 128, 130, 132, 134, 291, 296
Blasey, H, 143, 149
Bleuthmann, H, 128, 129, 133, 139, 144, 146
Bloom, BR, 56, 65, 138, 146
Bloom, ET, 144, 145, 150
Bluethjmann, H, 144, 149
Blume, R, 278, 284
Blyth, DI, 300, 313, 318
Bobrow, M, 250, 263
Bochner, BS, 17, 34, 98, 114, 127, 128, 130, 131, 134, 154, 155, 161, 279, 286
Bode, E, 57, 65, 130, 134, 291, 296
Bodmer, MW, 325, 329
Boer, C, 99, 115
Boer, L, 57, 65, 99, 115, 130, 134, 291, 296
Boguneiwicz, M, 104, 118
Bohjanen, PJ, 278, 285

Bohm, A, 241, 256
Boieje, LC, 144, 145, 149
Bollag, G, 230, 234, 235, 237
Bolles, L, 81, 91
Bond, MW, 52, 63, 138, 146, 243, 258, 313, 319, 321, 329
Bondadaa, S, 251, 264
Bonnefoy, JY, 143, 144, 145, 149, 150
Bonner, TI, 156, 164
Bonnin, O, 144, 150
Boone, T, 217, 223
Borego, L, 97, 105, 107, 113
Borlat, F, 177, 178, 180, 181, 182, 187, 195, 202
Borriello, F, 141, 147
Bos, JD, 277, 284
Boswell, HS, 278, 285
Bottomly, K, 139, 144, 146, 274, 283
Boumpas, DT, 294, 297
Bourke, PF, 271, 272, 274, 283, 291, 292, 293, 296
Bousquet, J, 51, 61, 69, 85, 127, 131, 242, 257
Bousquet, JB, 299, 317
Bouwmeester, T, 217, 222
Bower, J, 97, 112
Bowles, CA, 97, 113
Bowlin, TL, 206, 220, 315, 320
Boyce, JA, 76, 90
Boyd, A, 167, 184, 243, 244, 258
Boyd, G, 57, 66
Boyd, SD, 141, 147
Boyle, WJ, 217, 223
Bradding, P, 47, 50, 56, 65, 98, 114, 154, 162
Bradley, B, 53, 54, 63, 64, 69, 85, 127, 132, 154, 162, 244, 259
Bradley, BL, 51, 53, 57, 62, 66, 128, 132
Bradley, NJ, 73, 89
Bradley, TR, 72, 89
Brailly, H, 207, 221
Brannan, CI, 235, 239
Braun, C, 280, 286
Braun, P, 53, 64, 127, 128, 132
Braun, RK, 99, 115
Brenneise, IE, 154, 163
Bretscher, BA, 139, 146
Brewer, JM, 144, 149
Breyer, S, 97, 112
Briere, F, 142, 148
Britten, KM, 56, 58, 65, 66, 127, 131, 154, 162
Brofman, JD, 14, 33
Broide, DH, 57, 66, 83, 92, 127, 131, 154, 162
Brombacher, F, 128, 134, 245, 259, 289, 295
Bronson, RT, 228, 237
Brooks, I, 168, 170, 171, 173, 174, 183, 185, 246, 247, 260
Brooks, K, 70, 86
Brooks, MW, 248, 261
Brouwer, M, 277, 279, 284
Brovall, C, 72, 89
Brown, C, 218, 223
Brown, CR, 58, 59, 67
Brown, DR, 140, 147
Brown, J, 73, 89
Brown, JA, 141, 147
Brown, KD, 138, 142, 146, 147
Brown, MA, 124, 126
Brown, PH, 281, 287
Brown, SC, 175, 187
Bruijnzeel, PL, 103, 117
Bruijnzeel, PLB, 52, 53, 62, 64, 154, 161
Bruijnzeel-Koomen, CA, 103, 117
Bruijnzeel-Koomen, CAFM, 52, 63
Bruner, T, 143, 149
Bruno, E, 73, 89
Brusselle, G, 207, 208, 221
Bucay, N, 217, 223

Buckle, AM, 73, 89
Buckley, TL, 168, 185
Buday, L, 248, 261
Buhring, H, 73, 89
Buller, RM, 217, 222
Buller, RML, 217, 222
Bungre, J, 60, 68
Burakoff, SJ, 281, 287
Burch, R, 13, 33
Burd, PR, 140, 143, 147
Burgeon, E, 281, 287
Burgess, AW, 168, 185
Burgess, C, 21, 22, 24, 36, 252
Burgess, GS, 278, 285
Burton, LE, 170, 186
Buse, G, 207, 220
Bush, A, 53, 64
Businco, L, 102, 116
Busse, WW, 57, 66, 102, 117, 127, 131, 249, 263
Butler, JH, 315, 320
Butterfield, J, 143, 149
Butterfield, JH, 2, 29, 97, 112, 113
Butterworth, AE, 299, 316

C

Caldenhover, E, 249, 262
Calderon, MA, 58, 67
Calhoun, WJ, 57, 66, 102, 117
Callard, RE, 167, 184, 243, 244, 258
Callen, DF, 70, 86
Cambareri, B, 175, 187, 315, 320
Cameron, R, 84, 92
Campanelli, D, 2, 29
Campbell, HD, 52, 62, 63, 70, 86, 87, 128, 133, 142, 148, 154, 161, 167, 184, 242, 257, 271, 272, 274, 279, 283, 286, 289, 291, 295, 296
Campbell, P, 217, 223
Campos, L, 73, 89
Campos, MG, 17, 34
Capron, A, 56, 65, 84, 92, 128, 133, 300, 317
Capron, M, 56, 65, 128, 133, 300, 317
Caput, D, 142, 143, 144, 148, 149, 150
Carabelli, AA, 21, 36
Carayon, P, 142, 148
Cardell, BS, 21, 35
Carew, JA, 281, 287
Caristo, V, 129, 134
Carlson, MGCh, 4, 31
Carmichael, J, 58, 67
Carmini, D, 102, 116
Carr, S, 168, 170, 171, 173, 174, 183, 185, 246, 247, 260
Carrigan, PE, 154, 163
Carroll, M, 228, 237
Carson, RT, 145, 151
Cartier, A, 57, 66
Casellas, P, 142, 148
Castle, BE, 250, 264
Cato, AC, 294, 297
Caux, C, 73, 89, 227, 236
Cavallo, F, 248, 261
Celestin, J, 156, 164
Chaiken, I, 168, 170, 171, 172, 173, 174, 176, 177, 178, 179, 180, 181, 182, 183, 185, 186, 187, 188, 194, 195, 202, 246, 247, 260
Chaiken, IM, 176, 187, 246, 260
Chalmers, R, 103, 117
Chalon, P, 142, 148
Chan, CH, 119, 125
Chand, N, 61, 68, 127, 130, 132, 154, 162
Chand, RL, 70, 87
Chandrasekharappa, SC, 70, 86, 142, 148
Chanez, P, 51, 61, 69, 85, 127, 131, 242, 257, 299, 317
Chang, MS, 217, 223

Chang, R, 199, 203, 206, 220, 315, 320
Chaouat, G, 121, 125
Chapman, RW, 27, 37, 154, 158, 163, 244, 259, 300, 313, 314, 318, 322, 324, 325, 329
Chapman, V, 250, 263
Charlesworth, EN, 102, 103, 117
Charlesworth, MG, 102, 117
Chavanian, N, 69, 85
Cheavens,MD, 99, 115
Checkel, JL, 3, 16, 30, 34
Cheever, AW, 140, 147
Chelea,CJ, 45, 49
Chen, D, 278, 285
Chen, JX, 196, 203
Chen, KR, 97, 107, 108, 110, 113
Chen, X, 127, 130, 132
Chen, Y, 156, 164
Chen, YW, 70, 86
Chen, ZG, 155, 163, 300, 318
Cheng, G, 251, 264
Cherwinski, H, 52, 63, 138, 146
Cherwinski, HM, 138, 146
Chester, HM, 70, 86
Chevalier, S, 207, 220
Chi, EY, 19, 20, 35
Chiba, T, 228, 237
Chida, D, 228, 237
Chien, S, 251, 264
Chihara, J, 84, 92
Chinn, JP, 206, 220, 315, 320
Chiu, R, 279, 285
Choe, H, 156, 164
Chomarat, P, 144, 150
Chomienne, C, 84, 92
Chothia, C, 305, 318
Chou, C, 70, 87
Chou, CC, 199, 203, 325, 329
Chretien, I, 52, 63, 119, 124
Chu, C, 145, 151
Chu, CC, 243, 258
Chu, HM, 279, 285
Chung, CW, 170, 186
Chung, KF, 127, 130, 132
Church, MK, 17, 18, 34, 35, 107, 118
Civin, C, 72, 73, 76, 89, 90
Clackson, T, 306, 310, 318
Clark, RA, 98, 115
Clarke, AR, 233, 238
Clark Lewis, I, 156, 164
Clayberger, C, 56, 65, 138, 146
Clore, GM, 170, 186, 241, 256
Clutterbuck, E, 243, 244, 258
Clutterbuck, EJ, 39, 48, 52, 62, 70, 87, 119, 125, 128, 133, 154, 161, 167, 184, 289, 295, 300, 317
Coburn, DA, 83, 92, 127, 131
Cocks, BG, 142, 148
Coeffier, E, 154, 161
Coffer, P, 249, 262
Coffman, RL, 52, 63, 98, 114, 128, 133, 138, 141, 143, 145, 146, 147, 149, 154, 162, 242, 243, 247, 257, 258, 290, 296, 313, 319, 321, 329
Cogswell, PC, 294, 297
Cohen, H, 73, 90
Cohen, HM, 128, 133
Cohen, L, 250, 263
Cohn, AZ, 3, 30
Cohn, L, 274, 283
Colamonici, OR, 217, 222
Colby, TV, 61, 68, 97, 114
Coles, LS, 275, 284
Collin, M, 143, 149
Collins, JV, 9, 17, 32, 51, 52, 53, 54, 61, 62, 63, 64, 127, 128, 131, 132, 154, 162, 244, 259
Collins, PD, 54, 64, 70, 84, 88, 155, 156, 157, 158, 163
Colombel, JF, 56, 65
Colombero, A, 217, 223
Colotta, F, 143, 149
Comb, MJ, 279, 285

Combadiere, C, 156, 164
Conacher, M, 144, 149
Conley, ME, 250, 263
Conn, DL, 97, 113
Conni, M, 143, 149
Conroy, DM, 156, 164
Conscience, JF, 248, 249, 261
Consler, T, 177, 178, 180, 181, 182, 187, 195, 202
Constant, S, 139, 144, 146
Conteras, R, 168, 185, 279, 286
Convit, J, 56, 65, 138, 146
Cook, R, 168, 170, 171, 172, 173, 174, 176, 177, 178, 179, 180, 181, 182, 183, 185, 186, 187, 188, 194, 202, 246, 247, 260
Cooke, RM, 170, 186
Cookson, WO, 120, 125
Cooper, K, 305, 318
Cooper, MD, 250, 263
Copeland, N, 158, 165
Copeland, NA, 155, 163
Copeland, NG, 142, 148, 232, 235, 238, 239, 247, 248, 250, 260, 263
Corey, EJ, 98, 110, 115
Cornelis, S, 60, 67, 71, 85, 88, 93, 167, 171, 174, 185, 186, 187, 189, 190, 191, 192, 200, 201, 206, 207, 209, 218, 219, 220, 220, 221, 242, 246, 247, 248, 249, 252, 254, 257, 260, 262, 302, 303, 308, 313, 314, 318, 319, 320
Corrigan, C, 119, 125
Corrigan, CJ, 52, 53, 54, 55, 56, 57, 59, 63, 64, 65, 69, 83, 85, 154, 162, 162, 244, 259, 278, 280, 281, 285, 286, 287
Cory, DB, 130, 134, 140, 147
Cosman, D, 208, 221
Costello, RW, 17, 34
Cotnet, J, 279, 286
Coulam, CB, 2, 29
Cox, G, 83, 91
Coyle, AJ, 13, 21, 33, 35, 56, 65, 158, 165, 300, 317
Crabtree, G, 59, 67, 281, 287
Crane, J, 21, 22, 24, 36, 252
Cressman, DE, 278, 285
Crispe, IN, 207, 220
Crompton, GK, 58, 67
Cromwell, O, 52, 62, 70, 87, 98, 110, 115, 154, 155, 161
Crooks, GM, 73, 89
Cross, BA, 218, 223
Crotty, TB, 61, 68
Crowley, WF, 217, 222
Culpepper, J, 143, 149
Culpepper, JA, 142, 148
Cumberworth, V, 45, 49
Cunningham, BC, 171, 187
Cuomo, AJ, 83, 92, 127, 131
Curan, T, 294, 297
Curtis, R, 207, 220
Cusimano, D, 168, 170, 171, 173, 174, 183, 185, 246, 247, 260
Cusimano, DM, 246, 260
Cutler, RL, 70, 86
Cwirla, SE, 199, 203, 206, 220, 315, 320
Czech, W, 98, 102, 107, 114, 116, 118

## D

Dahinden, C, 45, 49, 143, 149
Dahinden, CA, 52, 63, 155, 163, 309, 318
Dahl, R, 3, 30
Dahlback, M, 81, 83, 91
Dahreine, TS, 278, 285
Dai, WJ, 128, 134, 245, 259, 289, 295
Dalloul, AH, 73, 90
Damen, JE, 228, 237

D'Andrea, A, 206, 219
D'Andrea, AD, 218, 223, 228, 237
D'Andrea, R, 175, 187, 315, 320
D'Andrea, RJ, 191, 201
Dang, W, 142, 143, 148, 149, 250, 264
Daniels, SE, 120, 125
Daoud, MS, 97, 113
Darnell, JE, 249, 262
Daugherty, BL, 156, 164
Davey, RT, 20, 35
David, JR, 299, 316
David, M, 249, 262
Davies, A, 250, 263
Davies, JG, 169, 186
Davis, MDP, 97, 113
Davis, S, 196, 203, 207, 220
Davy, E, 217, 223
De Boer, M, 277, 284
de Bos, J, 52, 63
Debre, P, 73, 90
De Bries, JE, 142, 148
De Carli, M, 52, 63, 138, 146
DeCastro, F, 97, 113
De Crescenzo, G, 18, 35
Dede, K, 177, 178, 187, 195, 202
Defrance, T, 142, 148
deGroot, C, 52, 63
De Groot, RP, 278, 285
DeGudicubus, SJ, 248, 261
De Jong, R, 277, 279, 284
De Jseu-Escobar, JM, 217, 222
Dekker, CA, 3, 30
DeLamarter, JF, 168, 185
Delaporte, E, 128, 133
Deleuran, B, 145, 150
Deleuran, M, 145, 150
Delia, D, 73, 89
Del Prete, G, 52, 58, 119, 124, 138, 146
Del Prete, GF, 52, 63
Delsman, KC, 27, 36, 154, 162, 300, 313, 318
Delvaux, A, 277, 284
DeMartino, J, 156, 164
De Monchy, JG, 127, 130, 131
Denburg, J, 47, 50
Denburg, JA, 70, 76, 78, 80, 81, 82, 83, 84, 86, 90, 91, 92, 300, 317
De Nevasquez, S, 21, 36
Dennin, R, 97, 113
Dent, L, 272, 283
Dent, LA, 52, 62, 70, 84, 87, 92, 154, 155, 163, 271, 283
Denzler, KL, 154, 163
Derby, P, 217, 223
D'Ercole, M, 272, 273, 278, 279, 283, 293, 297
Derig, HG, 278, 285
De Robertis, EM, 217, 222
Derocq, JM, 142, 148
DeRose, M, 217, 223
Desreumaux, P, 56, 65, 128, 133, 300, 317
DesRoches, L, 145, 151
De Vos, AM, 171, 187, 306, 310, 318
Devos, AM, 190, 192, 200
Devos, G, 311, 315, 319
Devos, R, 60, 67, 68, 71, 85, 88, 93, 167, 168, 169, 170, 171, 174, 175, 185, 186, 187, 189, 190, 191, 194, 197, 200, 201, 202, 205, 206, 207, 208, 209, 214, 219, 220, 221, 242, 246, 247, 248, 249, 252, 254, 257, 259, 260, 262, 277, 284, 302, 303, 308, 313, 314, 318, 319, 320
DeVries, IJ, 99, 115
de Vries, J, 52, 63, 119, 124
De Vries, JE, 142, 148
De Vries, K, 127, 130, 131
De Vriew, JE, 143, 149
De Waal Malefyt, R, 142, 143, 148, 149
Dewald, B, 155, 163

De Weck, AL, 52, 63, 309, 318
Dhand, R, 230, 234, 237
Diamantis, W, 61, 68, 127, 130, 132, 154, 162
Diaz, P, 58, 67
Dickason, R, 56, 65
Dickason, RA, 244, 258
Dickason, RR, 180, 181, 188, 195, 202, 311, 319
Dickersin, GR, 228, 237
DiDonato, JA, 294, 297
Diepgen, T, 102, 116
Dighe, AS, 141, 147
Dimantis, W, 57, 62
DiPersio, JF, 191, 196, 201
Direstein, GS, 57, 66
DiStefano, PS, 207, 220
Dixon, CM, 17, 34
Djousso, O, 144, 150
Djukanovic, R, 53, 56, 58, 59, 60, 64, 65, 67, 127, 131, 154, 162
Doherty, PC, 145, 151
Doherty, TM, 143, 149
Doi, S, 154, 162, 280, 286
Dolganov, GM, 142, 148
Dolovich, J, 23, 26, 27, 36, 78, 80, 83, 84, 85, 90, 91, 92, 103, 117
Domanski, P, 217, 222
Domen, J, 233, 238
Dor, PJ, 23, 24, 36
Doshi, P, 191, 196, 201
Dottore, M, 175, 187, 227, 236, 315, 320
Douglas, JG, 58, 67
Dover, JS, 97, 112
Dower, WJ, 190, 199, 200, 203, 206, 220, 315, 320
Downing, JR, 207, 220
Downward, J, 230, 234, 237
Doyle, AG, 143, 149
Doyle, EL, 142, 148
Doyle, M, 168, 170, 171, 173, 174, 180, 181, 183, 185, 188, 246, 247, 260
Doyle, ML, 195, 202
Drage, LA, 97, 113
Dranoff, G, 229, 237
Drazen, JM, 130, 135, 158, 165
Dresch, C, 84, 92
Druker, B, 249, 262
Dryden, P, 248, 262
Dubart, A, 228, 237
Dubucquoi, S, 128, 133, 300, 317
Duddle, JM, 58, 67
Duff, DW, 207, 220
Duffin, DJ, 199, 203
Duffy, J, 97, 113
Dul, E, 168, 170, 171, 173, 174, 183, 185, 246, 247, 260
Dumenil, D, 228, 237
Dumont, FJ, 281, 287
Dumont, X, 142, 148
Duncan, D, 308, 313, 318
Dunnette, S, 9, 17, 32, 51, 61, 62, 102, 117
Dunnette, SL, 97, 114, 127, 131
Dunnill, MS, 21, 36
Dunstan, CRJ, 217, 223
Durack, DT, 3, 30, 31
Duran, WN, 8, 32, 98, 110, 115
Durham, S, 53, 64, 102, 104, 116, 119, 125, 127, 128, 132, 280, 286
Durham, SR, 9, 32, 40, 41, 43, 44, 45, 48, 49, 50, 51, 53, 54, 55, 56, 57, 58, 59, 60, 61, 62, 63, 64, 65, 66, 67, 68, 71, 83, 88, 92, 119, 125, 128, 132, 133, 154, 162, 218, 223, 244, 259, 280, 286
Duronio, V, 248, 262
Duschl, AL, 144, 150
Dusserre, Y, 294, 297
Dutton, RW, 70, 86, 168, 185

Duvert, V, 73, 89
Dvorak, AM, 107, 118
Dvorak, HF, 99, 115
Dybdal, N, 73, 89

## E

Ebisawa, M, 154, 155, 161, 162
Eckmann, CM, 4, 31
Eder, M, 196, 202, 227, 230, 236, 238, 251, 252, 264
Edgerton, MD, 177, 178, 180, 181, 182, 187, 195, 202
Edmonson, JH, 97, 112
Edwards, BF, 170, 186
Efthimiadis, A, 23, 26, 27, 36
Egan, RW, 8, 27, 32, 36, 37, 70, 82, 84, 87, 92, 98, 110, 115, 154, 158, 162, 163, 244, 259, 271, 272, 274, 281, 283, 300, 313, 314, 318, 322, 324, 325, 329
Egan, SE, 248, 261
Egesten, A, 4, 31
Eguchi, M, 70, 87, 154, 161
Eidelman, DH, 84, 92
Eisenberg, D, 178, 180, 188
Elbert, BL, 75, 84, 85, 90
Elbon, CL, 16, 17, 34
El-Fakahany, EE, 16, 34
Elias, JA, 279, 285
El-Lati, SG, 18, 35, 107, 118
Elliot, J, 121, 125
Elliott, MJ, 60, 68, 71, 88, 191, 201
Elliott, R, 217, 223
Ellis, AG, 1, 21, 28
Ellis, N, 2, 29
Ellis, R, 81, 83, 91
Ellis, S, 206, 219
Elovic, A, 99, 115
Elsner, J, 98, 114
Elson, G, 144, 145, 150
Ely, B, 193, 201
Ema, H, 76, 90
Emerson, SG, 279, 285
Emilie, D, 56, 65
Emmi, L, 52, 63, 138, 146
Emtage, S, 70, 87, 325, 329
Enander, I, 51, 61, 69, 85, 127, 131, 242, 257, 299, 317
Endo, T, 168, 185, 232, 238
Engel, AG, 97, 113
Engel, JD, 228, 237
Engels, P, 242, 257, 273, 275, 283, 293, 297
English, JSC, 97, 112
English, M, 70, 86, 128, 133
Enver, T, 73, 89
Erard, F, 21, 35, 56, 65
Erdel, A, 243, 258
Erle, DJ, 130, 134
Ernst, TJ, 196, 202, 227, 236
Espinosa, R, 142, 148
Espiritu, BR, 18, 19, 35
Essayan, D, 280, 286
Etoh, T, 277, 280, 284
Eugster, HP, 144, 145, 150
Eum, SY, 127, 130, 132
Evan, CM, 17, 34
Evans, S, 23, 26, 27, 36

## F

Fabbri, LM, 57, 66
Faccioli, LH, 155, 163
Fache, I, 168, 185, 191, 201, 209, 221, 249, 252, 254, 262
Fackler, MJ, 72, 73, 89
Fame, TM, 15, 34
Fanales-Belasio, E, 102, 116
Farina, AR, 294, 297
Farmer, SC, 154, 163
Farrell, FX, 199, 203, 206, 220, 315, 320

Farrow, G, 51, 61
Farrow, GM, 5, 8, 17, 23, 24, 31, 299, 317
Farruggella, T, 207, 220
Farzan, M, 156, 164
Fattah, D, 168, 171, 172, 174, 175, 176, 185, 186, 187, 194, 197, 198, 202, 203, 300, 303, 311, 313, 315, 318, 319, 320
Fattah, DF, 313, 319
Fauci, AS, 99, 115
Faux, JA, 120, 125
Favre, C, 73, 89
Feather, IH, 98, 114
Federman, EC, 83, 92, 127, 131
Feger, F, 228, 237
Feldman, GM, 249, 262
Felli, MP, 294, 297
Feng, NP, 144, 145, 150
Ferguson, EL, 217, 222
Fernandez, X, 27, 36, 37, 61, 68, 70, 87, 154, 162, 300, 313, 314, 318, 322, 329
Ferrara, M, 102, 116
Ferrara, P, 142, 143, 144, 148, 149, 150
Fiers, W, 60, 67, 68, 71, 88, 167, 168, 171, 174, 185, 186, 187, 189, 190, 191, 194, 200, 201, 202, 206, 207, 208, 209, 214, 218, 219, 220, 221, 242, 246, 247, 248, 249, 252, 254, 257, 259, 260, 262, 279, 286, 302, 313, 314, 318, 319, 320
Figdor, C, 143, 149
Fikrig, E, 140, 147
Filley, WV, 24, 36
Filutowicz, HI, 168, 185
Fina, L, 73, 89
Finbloom, DS, 249, 262
Finidori, J, 209, 221
Finkelman, F, 127, 130, 132, 143, 149
Finkelman, FD, 128, 133, 139, 144, 146, 218, 223, 314, 320
Firak, TA, 70, 86, 142, 148
Firestein, GS, 154, 162
Fischkoff, S, 191, 201
Fish, R, 175, 177, 178, 180, 181, 182, 187, 195, 197, 198, 202, 203, 315, 320
Fisher, JA, 292, 296
Flavahan, NA, 14, 33, 127, 131, 300, 317
Flavell, RA, 140, 147, 242, 257, 277, 284
Fleischer, B, 52, 62
Fleischer, S, 52, 62
Fleissner, S, 278, 280, 285, 286
Fleit, HB, 128, 133
Flinter, F, 250, 263
Foley, LH, 191, 201, 220, 246, 260, 303, 308, 318
Foley, R, 76, 81, 82, 84, 90, 91
Folkerts, G, 27, 36, 70, 87
Folkesson, HG, 130, 134
Foran, SK, 27, 37, 70, 87, 300, 313, 314, 318, 322, 329
Ford, J, 268, 283
Fores-Romo, L, 143, 149
Forni, G, 248, 261
Forray, C, 16, 34
Foster, DW, 98, 110, 115
Foster, P, 280, 286
Foster, PS, 27, 37, 61, 68, 70, 84, 88, 128, 129, 130, 134, 135, 154, 158, 163, 165, 289, 295, 300, 318
Fowell, DJ, 140, 147
Francke, U, 142, 148
Fransway, AF, 97, 112
Frantz, C, 73, 90
Fraser, JD, 278, 285, 290, 296
Frati, L, 294, 297
Frazer, J, 52, 62
Freed, J, 13, 33

Freeman, GJ, 141, 147
Frew, AJ, 43, 49, 53, 63, 69, 85, 127, 132, 281, 287
Frick, WE, 127, 131
Frickhofen, N, 52, 62
Friedman, M, 144, 145, 150
Friedmann, FC, 144, 150
Frieling, J, 207, 221
Friend, D, 76, 90, 158, 165, 208, 221
Frigas, E, 5, 7, 8, 17, 21, 23, 24, 31, 32, 36, 51, 61, 127, 131, 299, 317
Frith, PA, 57, 66
Fruman, DA, 281, 287
Fryer, AD, 9, 15, 16, 17, 32, 33, 34
Fujisawa, T, 19, 35, 52, 63, 97, 100, 101, 102, 103, 112, 113, 127, 131, 300, 317
Fujita, T, 232, 238
Fukaya, C, 309, 318
Fukuda, T, 127, 130, 131, 132, 300, 313, 318
Fukuda, Y, 102, 117
Fukul, H, 207, 218, 221

## G

Gabay, J, 2, 29
Gabriele, L, 143, 149
Gaga, M, 43, 49, 102, 104, 116
Galdwin, ET, 170, 186
Gale, K, 73, 89
Galis, B, 208, 221
Galizzi, JP, 142, 148
Galli, SJ, 56, 65, 99, 115, 140, 147
Gamble, JR, 52, 63, 70, 87, 128, 133, 154, 161, 167, 184, 227, 236, 289, 295
Ganser, A, 196, 202
Ganser, J, 227, 236
Gao, J, 156, 164
Garcia Zepeda, EA, 156, 164
Garfein, E, 141, 145, 147
Garlisi, C, 324, 329
Garrett, DS, 170, 186
Gartner, S, 156, 164
Gascan, H, 207, 220
Gasson, J, 279, 286
Gatanaga, M, 207, 220
Gatanaga, T, 207, 220
Gates, CM, 199, 203
Gauchat, JF, 143, 144, 145, 149, 150
Gauldie, J, 83, 91, 103, 117
Gavett, SH, 127, 130, 132
Gazzinelli, RT, 139, 146
Gearing, DP, 227, 236
Geha, RS, 142, 148
Geich, GJ, 3, 19, 30
Gelfand, EW, 15, 27, 34, 37, 154, 163
Gemou Engesaeth, V, 53, 64, 154, 162, 280, 286
Genovese, A, 18, 35
George, T, 97, 102, 105, 107, 113, 117
George, TJ, 107, 118
Gerard, C, 156, 164, 277, 284
Gerard, NP, 156, 164
Gerhartz, C, 206, 219
Gerritsen, ME, 10, 17, 32, 33, 103, 117
Gesser, B, 145, 150
Ghavanian, N, 51, 61, 127, 131, 242, 257, 299, 317
Gibson, PG, 80, 84, 85, 91
Giddings, BW, 248, 261
Gieldin, MA, 52, 63, 58, 138, 146
Gilbert, DJ, 232, 238, 247, 248, 260
Gillis, D, 191, 201
Gimbrone, MA, 128, 134
Gimpel, SD, 208, 221
Girgis-Gabardo, A, 80, 85, 91
Giudice, GJ, 107, 118
Gleich, G, 27, 37

Gleich, GJ, 1, 2, 3, 4, 5, 6, 7, 8, 9, 10, 11, 12, 14, 15, 16, 17, 18, 19, 20, 21, 23, 24, 26, 27, 28, 29, 29, 31, 32, 33, 34, 34, 35, 35, 36, 51, 57, 58, 61, 62, 63, 66, 68, 95, 96, 97, 98, 99, 100, 101, 102, 103, 105, 107, 108, 110, 112, 113, 114, 115, 117, 127, 128, 131, 133, 299, 300, 316, 317, 321, 329
Glimcher, LH, 141, 147
Glitz, DG, 3, 30, 31
Glynn, AA, 21, 36
Go, NF, 250, 264
Godard, P, 51, 62, 127, 131, 242, 257, 299, 317
Goldberg, NC, 97, 113
Goldman, M, 128, 133, 277, 284, 300, 317
Goldstein, H, 56, 65, 138, 146
Gollob, KJ, 141, 145, 147
Gome, Z, 45, 49
Goncalves, F, 228, 237
Gonchoroff, N, 97, 112
Gonda, T, 206, 219
Gonzalo, J, 156, 158, 164, 165
Goodall, GJ, 175, 187, 190, 191, 196, 197, 200, 201, 206, 219, 227, 236, 315, 320
Goodwin, RG, 217, 222
Gordon, ACH, 58, 67
Gordon, J, 167, 184, 243, 244, 258
Gordon, JR, 56, 65, 140, 147
Gordon, MH, 3, 30
Gordon, S, 143, 149
Gorman, CM, 189, 191, 200
Gorman, DM, 227, 236, 242, 247, 248, 257, 260
Goube de Laforest, P, 73, 90
Gough, J, 21, 36
Gough, NM, 227, 236
Goujon, L, 209, 221
Gounni, AS, 128, 133
Gout, I, 230, 234, 237
Graber, P, 70, 86, 169, 171, 172, 174, 175, 176, 177, 178, 180, 181, 182, 186, 187, 193, 194, 195, 197, 198, 202, 203, 241, 256, 303, 310, 311, 314, 315, 318, 319, 320
Grabstein, KH, 218, 223, 314, 320
Graeve, L, 206, 207, 219, 220
Granger, G, 207, 220
Grant, IWB, 58, 67
Grant, JA, 102, 117
Grant, TA, 43, 49
Gratas, C, 84, 92
Graves, J, 15, 34
Gray, BH, 19, 35, 97, 102, 103, 112
Greaves, DR, 155, 163
Greaves, MD, 72, 89
Greaves, MF, 73, 89
Greaves, MW, 97, 112
Greiff, L, 80, 91
Griffin, JD, 196, 202, 227, 230, 236, 238, 251, 252, 264
Griffith, J, 2, 29
Griffiths-Johnson, DA, 54, 64, 70, 84, 88, 155, 156, 157, 158, 163, 164
Grigis-Gabardo, A, 80, 84, 91
Grignani, F, 248, 261
Grimaldi, JC, 250, 263
Gronenborn, AM, 170, 186, 241, 256
Gronhoj Larsen, C, 145, 150
Grosveld, F, 73, 89
Grosveld, P, 145, 151
Groth, CJ, 277, 284
Groth, DW, 97, 113
Grotzer, M, 58, 66
Gruart, V, 84, 92
Gruart-Gouilleux, V, 242, 257, 273, 275, 283, 293, 297
Grusby, MJ, 145, 151
Grutter, MG, 170, 186
Guba, SC, 279, 285
Gubler, U, 141, 147

Guilbert, L, 120, 125
Guilbert, LJ, 120, 121, 125, 126
Guillemot, JC, 142, 148
Guisez, Y, 71, 85, 88, 93, 169, 170, 171, 174, 175, 176, 186, 187, 191, 201, 205, 206, 209, 219, 220, 221, 246, 247, 248, 249, 252, 254, 260, 262, 311, 313, 314, 315, 319, 320
Gulbenkian, AR, 70, 87, 154, 162
Gulino, A, 294, 297
Gundel, RH, 10, 11, 12, 16, 17, 32, 33, 34, 51, 61, 103, 117
Gupta, S, 141, 145, 147
Gutierrez Ramos, J, 156, 158, 164, 165

## H

Haahtela, T, 299, 317
Habre, W, 120, 121, 122, 123, 125, 126
Hackett, RH, 249, 262
Haczku, A, 127, 130, 132, 154, 162, 163, 280, 286
Hafner, D, 57, 66
Haile, S, 127, 130, 132
Hallgren, R, 3, 30
Halonen, MJ, 124, 126
Hamann, KJ, 3, 16, 30, 31, 34
Hamelmann, E, 27, 37
Hamid, Q, 53, 54, 55, 56, 57, 58, 59, 60, 63, 64, 65, 66, 67, 68, 69, 82, 83, 85, 91, 92, 102, 104, 116, 118, 119, 125, 128, 132, 133, 154, 162, 218, 223, 244, 259, 280, 286
Hamid, QA, 40, 41, 43, 48, 49, 50, 52, 59
Hamilton, SA, 58, 67
Hammarstrom, L, 154, 161, 168, 185, 250, 263
Hanai, M, 249, 252, 253, 263
Hanley-Hyde, J, 300, 317
Hannemann, J, 206, 219
Hansel, TT, 57, 65, 99, 115, 130, 134, 291, 296
Hao, QL, 73, 89
Hara, T, 205, 206, 219, 227, 232, 236, 238, 250, 263
Harada, H, 142, 148
Harada, K, 142, 148
Harada, N, 52, 62, 70, 86, 87, 144, 150, 154, 161, 168, 171, 185, 187, 193, 201, 226, 232, 236, 238, 241, 249, 254, 256, 262, 262
Harada, S, 156, 164
Hardiman, G, 155, 163
Hardy, RR, 243, 258
Hargreave, FE, 23, 26, 27, 36, 57, 66, 80, 85, 91, 103, 117
Harris, P, 3, 30
Harrison, JE, 61, 68, 127, 130, 132, 154, 162
Hart, CE, 207, 220
Hartland, RM, 217, 222
Hartnell, A, 39, 48, 52, 54, 63, 70, 87, 128, 134, 154, 161, 300, 317
Hartnell, AH, 53, 64
Hasbold, J, 250, 264
Hashimoto, K, 235, 238
Haskell, MD, 19, 35
Haslett, C, 52, 62
Hassell, AM, 70, 86, 169, 186, 193, 202, 241, 256, 310, 319
Hastie, AT, 8, 32
Hatada, M, 241, 256
Hattevig, G, 119, 124, 125
Haugen, HS, 97, 99, 100, 101, 113
Hauquier, G, 168, 185
Havlik, MH, 230, 237, 251, 264
Hawk, JLM, 97, 112
Hayakawa, K, 243, 258
Hayashi, N, 228, 237
Hayashi, Y, 128, 133, 154, 161, 244, 258, 289, 295, 300, 318

Hayashida, K, 189, 191, 196, 200, 203, 242, 247, 257, 260
He, J, 156, 164
Healy, L, 73, 89
Heesel, B, 206, 219
Heimann-Weitschat, I, 278, 285
Heimpel, H, 52, 62
Heinrich, P, 206, 219
Heinrich, PC, 207, 220, 314, 320
Heise, MT, 3, 31
Helander, SD, 97, 114
Heldin, CH, 196, 202
Helmberg, A, 294, 297
Hemmerich, S, 73, 89
Henchoz, S, 143, 149
Henderson, WR, 4, 19, 20, 31, 35
Hendriks, T, 207, 221
Hennessy, L, 73, 90
Hensley, P, 168, 170, 171, 173, 174, 180, 181, 183, 185, 188, 195, 202, 246, 247, 260
Henzel, W, 73, 89
Her, E, 52, 62
Herbein, G, 143, 149
Hercus, TR, 175, 187, 254, 265, 315, 320
Herdman, MJ, 58, 67
Hermann, K, 102, 116
Hermanns, H, 206, 219
Herman-Weitschat, I, 280, 286
Herrmann, JM, 206, 219
Herron, LR, 243, 258
Herst, EMA, 70, 87
Hertzberg, RP, 309, 318
Herzenberg, LA, 243, 258, 281, 287
Hessel, EM, 300, 313, 318
Heusser, C, 128, 133
Heusser, CH, 56, 65, 98, 114, 154, 162
Hey, YW, 144, 150
Hibi, M, 196, 203, 248, 251, 261, 264, 314, 320
Hieshima, K, 156, 164
Higuchi, S, 167, 171, 185
Hill, D, 217, 223
Hill, M, 15, 34
Hill, MR, 120, 125
Hilsmeier, KA, 102, 117
Hilton, DJ, 144, 150
Hinton, LM, 142, 148
Hirabayashi, Y, 228, 237
Hirai, H, 242, 258, 273, 274, 283, 293, 296
Hirai, K, 99, 115
Hirano, N, 242, 258, 273, 274, 283, 293, 296
Hirano, T, 248, 261
Hirata, Y, 248, 261
Hirokawa, K, 249, 254, 262
Hirose, S, 243, 258
Hirst, EM, 52, 62, 119, 125
Hirst, EMA, 39, 48, 300, 317
Hissey, PH, 313, 319
Hitoshi, Y, 70, 87, 154, 162, 167, 171, 185, 187, 208, 221, 227, 228, 236, 241, 242, 243, 244, 246, 247, 248, 250, 251, 256, 258, 260, 261, 264
Ho, AM, 281, 287
Ho, AS, 119, 125
Hochstetter, R, 98, 114
Hocker, P, 73, 89
Hodes, RJ, 278, 285
Hodgkin, PD, 128, 134, 245, 259, 289, 295
Hoelzer, D, 196, 202, 227, 236
Hoffman, R, 73, 89
Hofman, G, 168, 185
Hofsteenge, J, 3, 30
Hogan, PG, 281, 287
Hogan, S, 280, 286
Hogan, SP, 27, 37, 61, 68, 70, 88, 128, 129, 130, 134, 135, 154, 158, 163, 289, 295, 300, 318

Holden, FR, 206, 220, 315, 320
Holgate, ST, 51, 53, 56, 58, 62, 64, 65, 66, 69, 85, 98, 114, 127, 131, 154, 162
Holland, J, 250, 263
Holley, KE, 24, 36
Holley, SA, 217, 222
Holt, BJ, 120, 121, 122, 123, 124, 125, 126
Holt, PG, 119, 120, 121, 122, 123, 124, 125, 126
Honda, H, 242, 258, 273, 274, 283, 293, 296
Hong, YM, 2, 29
Honjo, T, 52, 62, 154, 161, 241, 247, 256, 260
Honma, M, 154, 162
Hood, AF, 103, 117
Hoogland, H, 98, 115
Hooper, ML, 233, 238
Hordinsky, MD, 97, 113
Horgan, CM, 303, 318
Horie, S, 98, 114
Horn, BR, 51, 61
Horn, F, 206, 219
Horner, DL, 208, 221
Hort, Y, 52, 62, 128, 133, 154, 161, 167, 184, 279, 286, 289, 295
Horton, MA, 2, 29, 154, 163
Hoshi, H, 154, 162
Hoshino, A, 269, 280, 281, 282, 283, 287
Hosoya, Y, 243, 244, 258
Houba, V, 299, 316
Houston, JC, 21, 36
Howard, M, 250, 263, 264
Howarth, PH, 53, 56, 58, 59, 60, 64, 65, 66, 98, 114, 127, 131, 154, 162
Howie, K, 76, 78, 81, 82, 83, 90, 92
Hozumi, M, 208, 221
Hruby, DE, 217, 222
Hsieh, CS, 139, 146, 242, 257
Hsu, JC, 278, 285
Hsuan, JJ, 155, 156, 158, 163
Hu, FQ, 217, 222
Hu, J, 16, 34
Huang, S, 154, 162, 280, 286
Huber, BT, 290, 291, 296
Huber, HL, 1, 21, 28
Hudak, S, 70, 87, 154, 162
Huerre, M, 127, 130, 132
Huez, G, 279, 286
Hughes, DPM, 207, 220
Hughes, JM, 280, 287
Hughes, TM, 217, 223
Huijbens, R, 143, 149
Hu Li, J, 140, 147
Humbert, M, 55, 56, 57, 60, 64, 65, 68, 71, 88, 218, 223
Humbles, AA, 156, 164
Hunninghake, GW, 19, 35
Hunt, LW, 61, 68
Hurata, H, 75, 90
Husband, AJ, 129, 134
Huston, DP, 180, 181, 188, 195, 202, 243, 244, 258, 311, 319
Huston, MM, 243, 244, 258, 311, 319
Huston, D, 56, 65, 244, 258
Hutson, G, 128, 133
Huyghe, B, 144, 150
Hwang, C, 207, 220
Hyman, BA, 61, 68

## I

Ichihara, M, 71, 88, 228, 232, 236, 238, 250, 263
Idzerda, RL, 208, 221
Igarashi, H, 249, 262
Iglesias, L, 97, 105, 107, 113
Ihle, J, 251, 252, 264
Ihle, JN, 145, 151, 230, 231, 237, 238, 249, 262

Iijima, M, 9, 32
Ikuta, I, 244, 245, 259
Ikuta, K, 154, 158, 163
Illei, P, 143, 149
Imai, T, 156, 164
Inagaki, N, 70, 87, 154, 162
Ingley, E, 167, 185
Inhorn, R, 196, 202, 227, 236
Inhorn, RC, 230, 238, 251, 252, 264
Inman, MD, 81, 82, 83, 91
Inoue, M, 107, 118, 249, 262
Inoue, S, 269, 280, 281, 283
Inoue, T, 228, 237
Ip, NY, 196, 203, 207, 220
Irani, AM, 128, 132
Irani, AMA, 40, 41, 45, 48, 49, 51, 53, 62
Ireland, R, 191, 201
Irie, M, 3, 30
Irvin, CG, 13, 33, 300, 317
Iryo, K, 107, 118
Isakson, P, 70, 86
Ishii, A, K, 189, 200
Ishii, N, 144, 150
Ishikawa, Y, 294, 297
Isobe, M, 245, 259
Ito, K, 99, 115, 269, 277, 280, 281, 283, 284
Itoh, N, 189, 200, 227, 236, 247, 248, 260
Itoh, T, 227, 230, 231, 234, 236, 237, 238
Iwakura, Y, 228, 237
Iwama, M, 3, 30
Izukkura, R, 102, 116

## J

Jabara, HH, 142, 148
Jackson, J, 70, 87, 154, 162, 208, 221
Jacobs, CA, 218, 223, 314, 320
Jacobs, JW, 206, 220, 315, 320
Jacobsen, NG, 141, 147
Jacobsen, SEW, 143, 149
Jacobson, M, 41, 43, 49, 50, 51, 53, 62, 128, 132
Jacobson, MR, 40, 41, 43, 45, 48, 49, 50
Jacobson, SEW, 85, 92
Jacoby, D, 141, 147
Jacoby, DB, 8, 15, 16, 17, 32, 33, 34
Jacyk, WK, 97, 113
Jain, J, 281, 287, 294, 297
Jakob, T, 102, 116
Jakubicki, R, 127, 130, 132, 154, 162
Jamal, N, 70, 76, 86
James, A, 120, 125
James, W, 143, 149
Janeway, CA, 268, 282
Janin, A, 56, 65, 128, 133, 300, 317
Janin, J, 305, 318
Jansen, HM, 52, 63, 127, 130, 131, 277, 280, 284, 286
Janzen, C, 206, 219
Jeannin, P, 56, 65, 144, 145, 150
Jeffery, PK, 21, 36, 51, 52, 53, 54, 57, 62, 63, 64, 66, 69, 85, 127, 128, 132, 154, 162, 244, 259
Jen, CH, 325, 329
Jenh, C, 70, 87
Jenh, CH, 199, 203
Jenkins, BJ, 206, 219
Jenkins, MK, 277, 284
Jenkins, NA, 142, 148, 155, 158, 163, 165, 232, 235, 238, 239, 247, 248, 250, 260, 263
Jenkins, RB, 3, 31
Jhalli, N, 58, 67
Jia, G, 158, 165
Jinquan, T, 145, 150
Jkubicki, R, 61, 68
Johanson, K, 168, 170, 171, 173, 174, 183, 185, 246, 247, 260
Johanson, KO, 246, 260

Johansson, SA, 58, 67
John, S, 144, 145, 150
Johnson, DL, 190, 199, 200, 203, 206, 220, 315, 320
Johnson, GR, 168, 185
Johnson, JG, 277, 284
Johnson, PW, 53, 64
Joliffe, LK, 190, 199, 200, 203, 206, 220, 315, 320
Joller-Jemelka, H, 102, 116
Jones, B, 268, 282
Jones, H, 27, 36, 70, 87, 154, 158, 162, 163, 244, 259, 300, 313, 314, 318, 325, 329
Jones, K, 206, 219
Jones, KA, 294, 297
Jones, S, 70, 86
Jong, EC, 4, 19, 31, 35
Jongeneel, CV, 170, 186
Jordan, SE, 58, 67
Jordan, SR, 70, 86, 169, 186, 193, 202, 241, 256, 310, 319
Jordana, M, 83, 91
Jordon, RE, 103, 117
Jose, PJ, 54, 64, 70, 84, 88, 155, 156, 157, 158, 163, 164
Joseph, D, 16, 17, 34, 154, 161
Jubinsky, PT, 196, 202, 227, 236
Juhlin, L, 102, 116
Julisson, S, 45, 49, 50
Jurewicz, AJ, 309, 318
Justement, L, 249, 263
Jutel, M, 45, 49

## K

Kadonaga, JT, 294, 297
Kaegi, MK, 53, 59, 64, 127, 128, 132
Kagey-Sobotka, A, 103, 117, 280, 286
Kaghad, K, 142, 148
Kaghad, M, 144, 150
Kagi, MK, 102, 104, 116, 117
Kagitani, Y, 309, 318
Kagley-Sobotka, A, 40, 48
Kaiser, J, 43, 49, 128, 134
Kajii, M, 309, 318
Kakizaki, MM, 156, 164
Kaliner, MA, 20, 35
Kalthoff, FS, 52, 63
Kam, JC, 58, 59, 67
Kamada, AK, 58, 67
Kamen, R, 279, 286
Kamimura, K, 102, 116
Kaminuma, O, 269, 277, 280, 281, 282, 283, 284, 287
Kamiya, A, 235, 238
Kamiya, T, 246, 260
Kanai, Y, 243, 244, 258
Kanazawa, H, 71, 88, 154, 158, 163, 196, 203, 206, 219, 244, 245, 248, 249, 253, 254, 259, 262, 262
Kaneda, A, 142, 148
Kaneko, M, 128, 133, 154, 162
Kanekura, Y, 232, 238
Kanofsky, JR, 98, 115
Kanters, D, 249, 262
Kaplan, MH, 145, 151
Kapp, A, 98, 102, 103, 107, 114, 116, 117, 118
Kapsenberg, ML, 52, 63, 277, 284
Karin, M, 279, 285, 294, 297
Kariyone, A, 244, 259, 300, 313, 318
Karlen, S, 272, 273, 278, 279, 283, 293, 297
Karlsson, G, 45, 50
Karperien, M, 278, 285
Karplus, PA, 241, 256
Kasahara, T, 70, 87, 99, 115, 128, 133, 154, 161, 244, 258, 289, 294, 295, 297, 300, 318
Kashiwamura, S, 145, 151
Kashyap, AK, 199, 203, 206, 220, 315, 320

Kassman, N, 156, 164
Kastelein, R, 143, 149, 250, 264
Kastelein, RA, 206, 219
Katagiri, T, 248, 251, 261
Katayama, T, 193, 201
Kato, K, 102, 107, 116, 118
Kato, M, 154, 155, 161
Kato, T, 218, 223
Katoh, S, 243, 244, 258
Katona, IM, 128, 133
Katz, F, 72, 89
Katz, H, 158, 165
Katzen, DR, 97, 112
Kauffman, HF, 127, 130, 131
Kaushansky, K, 218, 223
Kawahara, A, 278, 285
Kawai, M, 206, 219
Kawashima, E, 168, 185
Kawashima, EH, 168, 185
Kay, AB, 9, 17, 21, 32, 36, 39, 40, 41, 43, 45, 48, 49, 50, 51, 52, 53, 54, 55, 56, 57, 58, 59, 60, 61, 62, 63, 64, 65, 66, 67, 68, 70, 83, 87, 92, 98, 99, 102, 104, 110, 114, 115, 116, 119, 125, 127, 128, 131, 132, 133, 134, 154, 155, 161, 162, 163, 218, 223, 278, 280, 281, 285, 286, 287, 300, 317
Kaye, J, 268, 282
Kaziro, Y, 248, 262
Keating, A, 72, 74, 89
Keegan, AD, 144, 150
Kees, UR, 268, 283
Keller, JR, 85, 92
Kelley, M, 217, 223
Kelly, PA, 209, 221
Kelly, TJ, 294, 297
Kelner, GS, 155, 163
Kennedy, J, 2, 29, 155, 163
Kephart, GM, 17, 24, 34, 36, 61, 68, 95, 97, 110, 112, 114
Kerner, JD, 251, 264
Kerppola, TK, 294, 297
Kerr, IM, 249, 262
Kiguchi, T, 232, 238
Kikuchi, Y, 71, 88, 154, 162, 167, 184, 189, 193, 200, 201, 207, 221, 243, 246, 247, 248, 249, 250, 251, 254, 258, 259, 260, 261, 262, 262, 264, 280, 286
Kikutani, H, 129, 134, 289, 295
Kilbourne, EM, 97, 114
Kim, SH, 217, 222
Kim, SM, 145, 151
Kim, YK, 83, 92
Kim J, 281, 287
Kimmig, D, 98, 114
Kimmitt, P, 57, 64
Kimoto, M, 250, 264
Kinashi, T, 52, 62, 154, 158, 161, 163, 168, 185, 241, 244, 245, 256, 259
Kincade, PW, 70, 86
King, JA, 227, 236
Kinjyo, I, 232, 238, 250, 263
Kinnon, C, 250, 263
Kinoshita, T, 231, 232, 233, 234, 235, 238, 250, 263
Kips, J, 205, 219
Kirayama, F, 218, 223
Kirkuchi, Y, 70, 86
Kishi, A, 228, 237
Kishi, K, 143, 149
Kishimoto, T, 145, 151, 196, 203, 207, 218, 221, 248, 249, 251, 261, 262, 264, 314, 320
Kita, H, 2, 3, 4, 73, 20, 27, 29, 35, 36, 52, 57, 63, 66, 96, 97, 98, 102, 107, 113, 114, 117, 118, 128, 133, 300, 317, 321, 329
Kitamura, D, 248, 251, 261
Kitamura, S, 128, 133, 154, 161, 244, 258, 289, 295, 300, 318

Kitamura, T, 60, 68, 71, 88, 172, 186, 189, 191, 200, 201, 209, 221, 226, 232, 233, 234, 236, 238, 242, 247, 250, 253, 257, 261, 263
Kitaura, M, 156, 164
Kitoshi, Y, 154, 162
Kjellman, B, 119, 124, 125
Klaus, GGB, 70, 86, 250, 264
Klebanoff, SJ, 3, 4, 19, 20, 31, 35
Klee, DB, 281, 287
Klein, O, 128, 133, 300, 317
Klen, B, 207, 221
Kleng, DA, 43, 49
Kleyensteruber, S, 155, 163
Klinberg, D, 278, 285
Klisak, I, 250, 263
Klunk, D, 154, 162
Klunk, DA, 128, 134
Knaff, W, 73, 89
Knapp, A, 102, 116
Knepel, W, 278, 284
Knowles, G, 69, 85, 127, 132
Knowles, GK, 53, 63
Knox, B, 124, 126
Kobata, A, 168, 185
Kobayashi, H, 9, 32
Kobierski, LA, 279, 285
Kobza-Black, A, 97, 112
Kodama, S, 168, 185, 193, 201
Koeffler, HP, 279, 286
Koenderman, L, 52, 62, 249, 262
Koessler, KK, 1, 21, 28
Koeter, GH, 127, 130, 131
Kofoed, MA, 154, 160
Kohler, G, 128, 129, 133, 134, 139, 142, 144, 146, 149, 245, 259, 289, 295
Kohler, PF, 9, 32, 97, 98, 110, 112
Koike, M, 71, 88, 249, 250, 252, 253, 263, 264
Koishihara, Y, 207, 218, 221
Kojima, K, 244, 259
Kojima, T, 300, 313, 318
Kok, PTM, 52, 62
Koker, PJ, 10, 32
Komiya, S, 232, 238
Kon, OM, 60, 67
Konderman, L, 154, 161
Kondo, M, 144, 150
Konishi, M, 52, 62, 154, 161, 168, 185, 241, 256
Kopf, M, 128, 129, 133, 134, 139, 142, 144, 146, 149, 158, 165, 245, 259, 289, 295
Kopf, MA, 140, 147
Koprak, SL, 281, 287
Korman, N, 104, 118
Korpelainen, E, 191, 201
Korpelainen, EI, 227, 236
Kortsik, C, 57, 66
Koshino, T, 99, 115
Koskinen, A, 129, 130, 134, 135, 280, 286, 289, 295
Kossiakoff, AA, 171, 187, 190, 192, 200, 306, 310, 318
Kossover, S, 73, 90
Kotanides, H, 145, 151
Kotsimbos, ATC, 60, 68
Kotsimbos, TC, 71, 88, 218, 223
Kotzin, BL, 243, 258
Kouro, T, 249, 252, 253, 254, 262, 262, 263
Kovach, JS, 97, 113
Koyama, N, 243, 244, 258
Koyanho-Nakagawa, N, 268, 278, 282
Kozak, CA, 70, 86, 142, 148
Krafft, H, 275, 284
Krajewski, AS, 58, 67
Krammer, PH, 275, 284
Kraulis, P, 192, 194, 203
Kreknief, J, 52, 62
Kreutner, W, 27, 36, 37, 70, 87, 154, 158, 162, 163, 244, 259, 300, 313, 314, 318, 322, 325, 329

Krinks, M, 217, 222
Krishnan, L, 120, 121, 125, 126
Krishnaswamy, G, 154, 162
Kristensen, T, 2, 29
Kroegel, C, 57, 66, 299, 317
Krouwels, GH, 280, 286
Kruger, M, 278, 284
Kruijer, W, 278, 285
Krutmann, J, 102, 116
Kruys, V, 279, 286
Krystal, G, 228, 231, 237, 238
Ku, H, 218, 223
Kubagawa, H, 250, 263
Kuchroo, VK, 141, 147
Kueppers, F, 2, 8, 29, 32
Kuhn, R, 140, 142, 143, 147, 149
Kuijper, PH, 103, 117
Kuijper, PHM, 154, 161
Kuiper, HM, 277, 279, 284
Kumai, M, 154, 162
Kumura, Y, 245, 259
Kung, J, 27, 36
Kung, S, 70, 82, 87
Kung, T, 70, 87, 154, 162
Kung, TT, 70, 87, 154, 158, 163, 244, 259, 300, 313, 314, 318, 324, 325, 329
Kuo, TT, 97, 114
Kupfer, A, 56, 65
Kupfer, H, 56, 65
Kurata, H, 228, 237
Kurihara, K, 39, 48, 52, 62, 63, 70, 87, 128, 134, 154, 155, 161, 300, 317
Kuszewski, J, 170, 186
Kyle, C, 73, 89

## L

Labit, C, 142, 148
Lacey, DL, 217, 223
Lacoste, JY, 51, 61, 62, 69, 85, 127, 131, 242, 257, 299, 317
Lacout, C, 228, 237
Ladenius, AR, 27, 36
Ladenius, RS, 154, 162
Lahm, HW, 171, 174, 186, 194, 202, 206, 219, 314, 320
Lahm, W, 247, 248, 260
Lai, CK, 119, 125
Lai, JH, 277, 284
Lai, KN, 119, 125
Laing, TD, 218, 223
Laird, PW, 233, 238
Laitinen, A, 21, 36, 299, 317
Laitinen, L, 299, 317
Laitinen, LA, 21, 36
Lambert, JN, 294, 297
Lambert, MH, 70, 86, 169, 186, 193, 202, 241, 256, 310, 319
Lamers, MC, 128, 129, 133, 139, 144, 146
Lamkhioued, B, 128, 133
Lammers, JJ, 154, 155, 161
Lammers, JW, 17, 34, 249, 262
Lammers, K, 277, 279, 284
Landenius, AR, 300, 313, 318
Lane, SJ, 59, 67
Lane, WS, 281, 287
Lanfrancone, L, 248, 261
Langhorne, J, 142, 149
Lappe e Silva, JR, 16, 17, 34
Larche, M, 56, 65
Largaespada, DA, 142, 148, 155, 163, 235, 239, 250, 263
Large, TH, 207, 220
Larner, AC, 249, 262
Larner, M, 217, 222
Larsen, GL, 13, 27, 33, 37
Larson, GL, 15, 34
Larson, KA, 2, 29, 154, 163
Larson, RA, 142, 148

Lasky, LA, 73, 89
Lathrop, GM, 120, 125
Laurent, P, 144, 150
Lautens, LL, 156, 164
Layton, J, 70, 86
Layton, MJ, 174, 187, 208, 221
Layton, ML, 218, 223
Leaves, NI, 120, 125
Le Beau, MM, 70, 86, 142, 148, 242, 257
Lecron, JC, 73, 90
Ledbetter, JA, 279, 285
Leder, P, 156, 158, 164, 165
Lederer, JA, 145, 151
Lee, BL, 142, 148
Lee, CW, 98, 110, 115
Lee, F, 225, 227, 229, 236
Lee, HJ, 268, 271, 272, 274, 278, 282, 283, 293, 296
Lee, J, 27, 37
Lee, JJ, 2, 29, 154, 163
Lee, JS, 70, 86, 142, 148
Lee, NA, 2, 29, 154, 163
Lee, R, 217, 223
Lee, TC, 98, 110, 115
Lee, TDG, 76, 90
Lee, TH, 59, 67
Leff, AR, 14, 15, 33
Lefort, J, 17, 34, 127, 130, 132
Lefort, S, 144, 150
Le Gros, G, 56, 65, 128, 129, 133, 139, 144, 146
Lei, JT, 97, 113
Leich, GJ, 5, 8, 17, 23, 24, 31
Leiferman, KM, 18, 19, 35, 95, 96, 97, 99, 100, 101, 102, 103, 105, 107, 108, 110, 112, 113, 115, 117, 118
Leikauf, GD, 154, 163
Leland, P, 144, 150
Lelias, JM, 144, 150
Lemons, RS, 142, 148, 242, 257
Lenihan, DJ, 98, 110, 115
Lens, L, 217, 222
Lentz, V, 279, 285
Leonard, WJ, 144, 145, 150, 170, 186
Leonor, N, 232, 238
Leplatois, P, 142, 148
Le Souef, PN, 120, 125
Letts, LG, 11, 12, 17, 33, 51, 61
Leung, DY, 58, 59, 67, 280, 286
Leung, DYM, 97, 104, 112, 118, 142, 148
Leung, JC, 119, 125
Levin, SD, 277, 284
Levinsky, R, 250, 263
Levi-Schaffer, F, 56, 65, 98, 99, 114
Lewis, A, 71, 88, 191, 201
Lewis, DB, 140, 147
Lewis, DM, 2, 4, 29, 31
Lewis, JC, 4, 31
Lewis, RA, 98, 110, 115
Leyden zu Konigsberg, E, 21, 36
Li, B, 56, 65
Li, J, 170, 172, 174, 176, 177, 178, 179, 180, 181, 182, 183, 186, 187, 188, 194, 195, 202
Li, T, 230, 237, 251, 264
Li, X, 142, 148
Liauzun, P, 142, 148
Libol, E, 228, 237
Lichtenstein, L, 280, 286
Lichtenstein, LM, 40, 48, 102, 103, 117, 127, 130, 131, 154, 155, 161
Lichtman, A, 158, 165
Lichtman, AH, 145, 151
Lida, M, 99, 115
Life, P, 143, 149
Lilly, CM, 158, 165
Lim, B, 70, 76, 86
Lin, AW, 235, 239

Lin, G, 158, 165
Lin, H, 120, 125
Lin, JX, 144, 145, 150
Lin, K, 217, 222
Linden, M, 58, 67, 80, 91
Lindstaedt, R, 278, 280, 285, 286
Lindsten, T, 279, 285
List, AF, 142, 148
Little, C, 4, 31
Liu, MC, 154, 155, 161
Liu, ZJ, 278, 285
Livnah, O, 190, 200
Li-Weber, M, 275, 284
Loader, J, 27, 37
Loader, JE, 15, 34
Lobb, RR, 16, 17, 34
Locati, M, 156, 164
Lock, P, 174, 187, 193, 201
Lock, SH, 60, 67
Locksley, RM, 130, 134, 140, 147
Lodi, PJ, 170, 186
Loegering, DA, 2, 3, 5, 8, 16, 17, 23, 24, 29, 30, 31, 32, 34, 51, 61, 99, 115, 127, 131, 299, 316, 317
Lofquist, AK, 294, 297
Logan, JS, 208, 221
Logun, C, 20, 35
Loh, R, 120, 121, 122, 125
Loison,G, 142, 148
Looney, RJ, 128, 133
Lopez, A, 60, 68
Lopez, AF, 52, 60, 63, 68, 70, 71, 87, 88, 128, 133, 154, 161, 167, 168, 175, 184, 185, 187, 190, 196, 200, 201, 206, 219, 227, 236, 254, 265, 289, 295, 315, 320
Lopez, IG, 39, 48
Lotz, M, 83, 92
Lovett, M, 142, 148
Lovino, S, 73, 89
Lowe, SW, 235, 239
Lowhagen, O, 41, 43, 49, 50
Lowhagen, R, 45, 49
Lu, B, 217, 222
Luchtel, DL, 5, 32
Luhowskyj, S, 191, 196, 201
Luksza, AR, 9, 32
Lund, V, 47, 50
Lundell, D, 199, 203
Lundgren, B, 20, 35
Lundgren, JD, 20, 35
Luo, C, 281, 287
Lupker, J, 142, 144, 148, 150
Luscinskas, FW, 128, 134
Luster, AD, 156, 158, 164, 165
Luthy, R, 217, 223
Lutter, R, 280, 286
Luttmann, W, 299, 317
Lux, G, 278, 284
Luyten, FP, 217, 222
Lyman, SD, 218, 223
Lyne, PD, 308, 313, 318


## M


Maare, H, 145, 150
Macatonia, SE, 139, 146, 242, 257
Macaubas, C, 120, 121, 122, 123, 125, 126
Macchia, D, 52, 63, 119, 124, 138, 146
Maclagan, J, 15, 33
MacIntyre, D, 57, 66
Mackay, CR, 156, 164
Mackay, IS, 40, 41, 43, 48
Mackiewicz, A, 207, 220
MacLean, JA, 158, 165
Madani, H, 218, 223, 314, 320
Madden, BJ, 2, 29
Maddow, DE, 2, 29
Maeda, K, 103, 117
Maestrelli, P, 57, 66
Maggi, E, 52, 63, 119, 124, 138, 146
Mahmoud, AAF, 299, 316

Mahoney, JR, 4, 31
Mahrer, S, 75, 84, 85, 90
Maikoe, T, 154, 155, 161
Majdic, O, 73, 89
Majumdar, S, 53, 64
Maki, K, 154, 158, 163, 244, 245, 259
Makino, S, 127, 130, 132, 244, 259, 300, 313, 318
Maldonado, JE, 2, 29
Malech, HL, 84, 92
Malek, TR, 144, 150
Maliszewski, CR, 217, 218, 222, 223, 251, 264, 314, 320
Malkowitz, L, 156, 164
Malone, B, 98, 110, 115
Mandler, R, 243, 258
Mangold, H, 215, 222
Manley, JL, 215, 222
Mann, KG, 2, 29
Manneberg, M, 71, 88, 194, 202, 206, 219, 247, 248, 260, 314, 320
Manneerg, M, 171, 174, 186
Manning, PJ, 80, 84, 91
Mano, H, 242, 258, 273, 274, 283, 293, 296
Manolitsas, ND, 58, 67
Mantovani, A, 143, 149, 155, 163, 300, 318
Manzini, S, 13, 33
March, CJ, 208, 221
Marcous, JP, 9, 32
Marcoux, JP, 97, 98, 110, 112
Marino, I, 18, 35
Mark, EL, 228, 237
Marleau, S, 54, 64, 70, 84, 88, 155, 156, 157, 158, 163, 164
Maroder, M, 294, 297
Marom, Z, 20, 35
Marone, G, 18, 35
Marsh, DG, 154, 162
Marshall, JD, 45, 49
Marshall, JS, 83, 92
Martal, J, 121, 125
Martin, G, 248, 249, 261
Martin, RJ, 58, 59, 67, 280, 286
Martin, RW, 97, 113
Martinez, FD, 124, 126
Martinotti, S, 294, 297
Martinson, ME, 52, 62, 70, 86, 128, 133, 154, 161, 167, 184, 279, 286, 289, 295
Masamune, H, 305, 318
Mastromauro, C, 52, 63
Masuda, ES, 271, 272, 274, 283, 293, 296
Masuhara, M, 232, 238, 250, 263
Masuyama, K, 41, 43, 49, 50
Mathaei, KI, 57, 62
Mathey-Prevot, B, 206, 219, 228, 237
Matico, R, 168, 170, 171, 173, 174, 183, 185, 246, 247, 260
Matico, RE, 246, 260
Matossian, K, 99, 115
Matsuda, F, 52, 62, 154, 161, 168, 185, 241, 256
Matsuda, I, 167, 171, 185
Matsuda, T, 248, 261
Matsumoto, A, 232, 238, 250, 263
Matsumoto, M, 70, 86, 145, 151, 193, 201
Matsumoto, R, 76, 90, 243, 244, 258
Matsumoto, S, 102, 116, 154, 162
Matsusaka, T, 249, 262
Matsushima, K, 170, 186, 294, 297
Matsuzaki, G, 277, 280, 284
Matteucci, C, 143, 149
Matthaei, KI, 27, 37, 61, 68, 70, 84, 88, 128, 129, 130, 134, 154, 158, 163, 165, 289, 292, 295, 296, 300, 318
Matthay, MA, 130, 134
Matthei, KI, 245, 259
Matthys, H, 57, 66, 299, 317
Mattila, PS, 281, 287

Mauser, P, 324, 329
Mauser, PJ, 27, 36, 37, 61, 68, 70, 87, 154, 162, 300, 313, 314, 318, 322, 325, 329
Max, EE, 140, 143, 147, 243, 258
May, G, 73, 89
Maynard, B, 97, 105, 107, 113
Mayo, G, 52, 62, 128, 133, 154, 161, 167, 184, 289, 295
Mazzei, G, 143, 149
McAulay, A, 58, 67
McCaffrey, PG, 281, 287, 294, 297
McCaig, DJ, 15, 33
McCormick, F, 230, 234, 235, 237
McCurrach, ME, 235, 239
McCusker, MT, 17, 34
McDonnell, P, 168, 170, 171, 173, 174, 183, 185, 246, 247, 260
McEvoy, MT, 97, 112
McFadden, G, 217, 222
McGarry, MP, 154, 163
McGlade, J, 248, 261
McGrogan, M, 2, 29
McIntyre, BW, 128, 134
McKean, DJ, 2, 3, 29, 30, 31
McKenzie, AN, 167, 169, 184, 186, 193, 194, 201, 202
McKenzie, ANJ, 142, 144, 148, 150
McKenzie, DT, 39, 48, 70, 86, 168, 185
McKinnon, M, 171, 172, 174, 175, 176, 177, 178, 180, 181, 182, 186, 187, 194, 195, 197, 198, 202, 203, 301, 303, 310, 314, 315, 318, 319, 320
McManus, MM, 8, 32
McMenamin, C, 120, 125
McNamee, LA, 313, 319
McNeil, T, 228, 237
McNulty, D, 168, 170, 171, 173, 174, 180, 181, 183, 185, 188, 246, 247, 260
McNulty, DE, 195, 202
McSweeney, PA, 81, 91
Meagher, L, 52, 62
Meco, D, 294, 297
Mee, PJ, 229, 237
Meeker, TC, 142, 148
Meglio, P, 102, 116
Mehregan, DR, 97, 112
Melino, MR, 281, 287
Mellor, AL, 52, 62, 70, 87, 154, 155, 163, 271, 283
Meng, Q, 43, 49, 55, 57, 58, 64, 66, 67, 128, 133
Mengelers, HJJ, 154, 161
Menichella, G, 73, 89
Menon, N, 139, 146
Menon, S, 142, 143, 148, 149
Menot, ML, 84, 92
Menz, G, 55, 56, 57, 60, 64, 65, 66, 68, 127, 132, 218, 223
Mermod, JJ, 168, 185
Mermod, N, 294, 297
Merritt, EA, 192, 194, 203
Messner, H, 70, 76, 86
Metcalf, D, 70, 72, 86, 89, 144, 150, 174, 187, 193, 201, 218, 223
Metters, H, 243, 244, 258
Metzger, WJ, 19, 35
Meuller, R, 154, 162
Meyers, DA, 40, 48
Mibourne, EA, 245, 259
Michaels, L, 21, 36
Michel, FB, 51, 62, 127, 131, 242, 257, 299, 317
Middleton, SA, 190, 200
Mietz, J, 144, 145, 150
Migita, M, 71, 88, 167, 171, 184, 185, 189, 200, 207, 221, 243, 244, 246, 258, 259, 260
Migone, TS, 144, 145, 150
Mihm, MC, 99, 107, 115, 118
Mikami, T, 281, 282, 287

Milatovich, A, 142, 148
Milbourne, EA, 128, 134, 289, 295
Milburn, MV, 70, 86, 169, 186, 193, 202, 241, 256, 310, 319
Miller, FD, 207, 220
Mills, FC, 140, 143, 147
Miloux, B, 142, 144, 148, 150
Milton, SE, 71, 88, 191, 201
Minami, M, 145, 151
Minami, Y, 278, 285
Minamitake, Y, 193, 201
Miner, Z, 294, 297
Minette, P, 15, 33
Minette, PA, 17, 34
Minicozzi, M, 84, 92, 98, 110, 115
Minnicozzi, M, 8, 32
Minowada, J, 246, 260
Minshall, E, 60, 68, 71, 84, 88, 92, 218, 223
Minty, A, 142, 143, 148, 149
Minty, C, 142, 148
Mio, M, 2, 29
Miossec, P, 144, 150
Misawa, H, 232, 238, 250, 263
Mita, S, 70, 86, 128, 133, 154, 161, 167, 171, 185, 187, 189, 193, 200, 201, 208, 221, 242, 243, 244, 246, 247, 253, 256, 258, 260, 261, 289, 295, 300, 318
Mitchell, S, 73, 90
Mitsui, K, 232, 238, 250, 263
Miura, Y, 70, 76, 87, 90, 128, 133, 154, 161, 289, 295, 300, 318
Miuri, Y, 244, 258
Miyajima, A, 60, 68, 71, 88, 144, 150, 172, 186, 189, 191, 196, 200, 201, 203, 206, 209, 219, 221, 225, 226, 227, 228, 229, 230, 231, 232, 234, 235, 236, 237, 238, 242, 247, 247, 248, 249, 250, 251, 252, 260, 261, 262, 263, 264
Miyake, K, 250, 264
Miyamasu, M, 99, 115
Miyamima, A, 205, 219
Miyasato, M, 102, 107, 116, 118
Miyatake, S, 225, 227, 229, 236
Miyazaki, H, 218, 223
Miyazaki, J, 154, 158, 163
Miyazaki, JI, 243, 244, 245, 250, 258, 259, 264
Miyazaki, T, 232, 238, 244, 245, 259, 278, 285
Miyazawa, K, 269, 280, 281, 283, 287
Mjuto, A, 251, 252, 264
Mochizuki, DY, 278, 285
Modi, W, 156, 164
Modi, WS, 144, 150
Modlin, RJ, 138, 146
Modlin, RL, 56, 65
Mohandas, T, 250, 263
Mohan-Peterson, S, 143, 149
Mohr, RN, 250, 263
Molgaard, HV, 73, 89
Moller, G, 128, 133
Monaghan, P, 73, 89
Monick, M, 19, 35
Montanier, LJ, 143, 149
Montefort, S, 56, 65, 154, 162
Moon, HB, 128, 133
Moore, JP, 243, 244, 258
Moore, KW, 155, 163, 250, 264
Moore, SB, 99, 115
Moos, M, 217, 222
Moqbel, R, 41, 45, 49, 53, 54, 56, 59, 60, 64, 65, 69, 83, 85, 98, 99, 102, 104, 110, 114, 115, 116, 119, 125, 127, 130, 132, 154, 155, 156, 158, 162, 163, 244, 259
Morawetz, RA, 143, 149
Moreau, JF, 206, 219
Moretti, P, 175, 187, 206, 219, 315, 320
Moretti, PA, 191, 201

Morgan, JC, 142, 148
Mori, A, 269, 277, 280, 281, 282, 283, 284, 287
Morikawa, Y, 227, 236
Morita, M, 294, 297
Morita, T, 3, 30
Morita, Y, 99, 115
Moriyama, M, 232, 238
Morla, AO, 248, 261
Morris, MM, 23, 26, 27, 36, 80, 85, 91
Morse, HC, 143, 149
Mortin, T, 170, 172, 174, 176, 186
Morton, T, 168, 170, 171, 173, 174, 183, 185, 194, 202, 246, 247, 260
Morton, TA, 246, 260
Moseley, P, 19, 35
Mosely, B, 208, 221
Moser, B, 155, 163
Moser, R, 144, 145, 150
Moskowitz, NH, 140, 147
Mosmann, T, 121, 125
Mosmann, TR, 52, 56, 60, 63, 65, 98, 114, 120, 121, 125, 126, 128, 133, 138, 142, 146, 147, 242, 247, 250, 257, 264, 290, 296, 313, 319, 321, 329
Mossalayi, MD, 73, 90
Mossman, K, 217, 222
Motojima, S, 5, 32, 127, 130, 131, 132
Mould, AM, 129, 134, 289, 295
Mould, AW, 70, 84, 88, 128, 134, 158, 165
Moy, JN, 3, 19, 21, 29, 98, 115
Moyer, TP, 97, 113
Moyiyama, M, 250, 263
Mudde, GC, 52, 63
Mueller, R, 56, 65
Mui, AL, 196, 203, 231, 238, 242, 247, 250, 257, 263
Mui, ALF, 225, 226, 228, 230, 232, 233, 234, 236, 238, 249, 262
Mukai, H, 102, 116
Mukaida, N, 294, 297
Mulcahy, LS, 190, 199, 200, 203, 206, 220, 315, 320
Mullberg, J, 207, 220
Muller, UR, 45, 49
Muller, W, 140, 142, 143, 147, 149
Mulligan, RC, 228, 237
Mullol, J, 20, 35
Munoz, E, 290, 291, 296
Munoz, NM, 14, 33
Murakami, M, 196, 203, 248, 251, 261, 264, 314, 320
Murata, K, 71, 88
Murata, Y, 167, 172, 184, 186, 189, 191, 200, 201, 207, 221, 245, 246, 248, 259, 260, 261
Murgolo, NJ, 325, 329
Murphy, GM, 97, 112
Murphy, KM, 139, 141, 146, 147, 242, 257
Murphy, MEP, 192, 194, 203
Murphy, PM, 156, 164
Murphy, RA, 207, 220
Murray, LJ, 73, 89
Murray, R, 228, 229, 237
Musk, AW, 120, 125
Muto, A, 196, 203, 206, 219, 227, 230, 231, 234, 236, 237
Muzio, M, 143, 149

## N

Nabavi, N, 141, 147
Naclerio, RM, 40, 48, 102, 117
Nadel, JA, 8, 32
Nagai, H, 70, 87, 154, 162
Nagareda, T, 102, 116
Nagata, S, 4, 31
Nagata, Y, 228, 237

Nagayoshi, K, 76, 90
Nagy, S, 277, 280, 284
Nahori, MA, 17, 34
Naito, Y, 268, 278, 282, 309, 318
Najjar, SM, 294, 297
Nakafuku, M, 248, 262
Nakagawa, H, 277, 280, 284
Nakagawa, N, 83, 92, 196, 203, 251, 264
Nakagawa, T, 251, 264
Nakahata, T, 228, 237
Nakai, S, 2, 29
Nakajima, T, 156, 164
Nakama, T, 107, 118
Nakamura, M, 144, 150
Nakamura, T, 140, 147
Nakamura, Y, 144, 150
Nakanishi, K, 145, 151
Nakauchi, H, 76, 90, 250, 264
Nakayama, N, 228, 237
Naomi, S, 171, 187
Naora, H, 271, 272, 283, 290, 291, 292, 293, 296
Narazaki, M, 207, 218, 221
Narula, S, 199, 203
Naruto, M, 249, 262
Nathan, C, 2, 29
Natsuka, S, 314, 320
Naugle, C, 249, 262
Nauseef, WM, 98, 115
Naylor, B, 21, 36
Neino, M, 299, 317
Nelson, D, 120, 125
Nelson, FC, 51, 52, 62
Neul, JL, 217, 222
Newman, W, 97, 105, 107, 108, 110, 113, 128, 134, 156, 164
Nguyen, HQ, 217, 223
Nicola, N, 208, 221
Nicola, NA, 70, 86, 144, 150, 174, 187, 193, 201, 218, 223, 227, 236
Nicoletti, I, 248, 261
Niedner, R, 102, 116
Nijkamp, FP, 27, 36, 154, 162, 168, 185, 300, 313, 318
Nikolaizik, WH, 58, 66
Nish, WA, 102, 117
Nishida, J, 242, 258, 268, 273, 274, 278, 282, 283, 293, 296
Nishida, T, 2, 29
Nishijima, I, 228, 237
Nishimura, H, 309, 318
Nishimura, M, 156, 164
Nishimura, N, 243, 258
Nishinakamura, R, 228, 229, 237
Nishio, Y, 249, 262
Nishioka, K, 102, 116
Nishiyama, S, 102, 116
Nishizaki, Y, 277, 280, 284
Nishizumi, M, 251, 264
Noben-Trauth, N, 143, 149
Noguchi, H, 97, 114
Noguchi, M, 144, 150
Noguchi, T, 102, 116
Nolan, K, 61, 68, 127, 130, 132, 154, 162
Noma, T, 154, 161, 168, 185
Nomiyama, H, 156, 164
Nordan, RP, 300, 317
Norman, PS, 103, 117
Norris, PG, 97, 112
North, J, 53, 55, 58, 64, 67, 119, 125, 128, 133
Nosaka, T, 145, 151
Notarangelo, LD, 144, 145, 150
Nourshargh, S, 155, 163
Novak, TJ, 278, 285
Numao, T, 127, 132

## O

Obiri, NI, 144, 150
O'Byrne, PM, 76, 78, 80, 81, 82, 83, 84, 90, 91

Occhiodoro, F, 275, 284
Ochiai, K, 128, 133
O'Connell, EJ, 9, 32, 97, 98, 110, 112
O'Connor, MB, 217, 222
O'Conor, R, 230, 237
O'Donnell, MC, 3, 17, 18, 29, 98, 110, 114
Oefner, C, 169, 170, 171, 174, 175, 176, 186, 206, 220, 311, 315, 319
Oetjen, E, 278, 284
O'Farrell, AM, 232, 238, 249, 262
O'Garra, A, 70, 86, 139, 146, 242, 257, 313, 319, 321, 329
Ogata, N, 249, 252, 253, 262, 263
Ogawa, M, 218, 223
Ogorochi, T, 225, 226, 228, 230, 236, 242, 247, 257
Ohagen, A, 156, 164
Ohashi, Y, 127, 130, 132
Ohgi, K, 3, 30
Ohkubo, T, 232, 238
Ohman, H, 139, 146
Ohmura, T, 269, 280, 281, 282, 283, 287
Ohnishi, M, 83, 92
Ohnishi, T, 102, 117
Ohno, I, 154, 162
Ohno, S, 14, 33
Ohsugi, Y, 207, 218, 221
Ohta, K, 99, 115
Ohta, S, 70, 87, 244, 258
Ohtoshi, T, 83, 91
Ohtsubo, M, 232, 238, 250, 263
Okada, S, 107, 118
Okada, T, 243, 258, 309, 318
Okajima, M, 278, 285
Okamoto, S, 294, 297
Okayama, Y, 18, 35, 107, 118
O'Keefe, P, 124, 126
Okkenhaug, C, 143, 149
Okudaira, H, 269, 277, 280, 281, 282, 283, 284, 287
Okumura, Y, 269, 280, 281, 283
Olsen, RL, 4, 31
Olsson, I, 3, 4, 30, 31
Olwell, E, 191, 201
O'Neal, KD, 254, 264
O'Neill, LA, 291, 296
Oohashi, M, 102, 116
Oshiba, A, 27, 37
Ostertag, W, 206, 219
Ota, Y, 218, 223
Otsuka, H, 78, 80, 90
Ott, NL, 97, 100, 101, 103, 113
Out, TA, 280, 286
Ovington, KS, 128, 134, 245, 259, 289, 295
Owczarek, CM, 208, 221
Owen, WF, 39, 48, 52, 62, 76, 90
Ownbey, RT, 156, 164
Oxvig, C, 2, 29

## P

Paganelli, R, 102, 116
Page, CP, 19, 35
Page, K, 175, 187, 197, 198, 203, 315, 320
Page, KR, 303, 318
Paine, MM, 154, 162
Paliogianni, F, 294, 297
Pallavicini, MG, 142, 148
Palmegren, M, 4, 31
Pan, L, 196, 203
Panayotatos, N, 207, 220
Pandrau, D, 73, 89
Paolini, A, 73, 89
Parish, CR, 137, 146
Park, H, 230, 237, 251, 264
Park, J, 281, 287
Park, LS, 191, 201, 208, 221
Parker, JW, 70, 86
Parks, WC, 107, 118
Parolini, O, 250, 263

Parronchi, P, 52, 63, 119, 124, 138, 146
Pasqualini, T, 139, 144, 146
Passini, N, 141, 147
Patel, N, 206, 219
Patella, V, 18, 35
Paterson, IC, 58, 67
Pattison, W, 217, 223
Paul, CC, 75, 84, 85, 90, 245, 259
Paul, WE, 128, 133, 139, 140, 144, 145, 146, 147, 150, 151, 243, 250, 258, 263, 300, 317
Pawson, T, 248, 261
Payvandi, F, 154, 162, 271, 273, 283
Pazdrak, K, 249, 263
Pearce, EJ, 140, 147
Pearce, N, 21, 22, 24, 36
Pearlman, E, 158, 165
Pearson, RSB, 21, 35
Pease, J, 156, 164
PEase, LR, 3, 30
Pease, LR, 2, 3, 16, 29, 30, 31, 34
Peault, B, 73, 89
Pedrick, MS, 300, 313, 318
Pehamberger, H, 97, 112
Peitsch, M, 177, 178, 180, 181, 182, 187
Peitsch, MC, 170, 171, 172, 174, 175, 176, 186, 187, 194, 195, 202, 311, 315, 319
Peleman, R, 205, 219
Pelicci, G, 248, 261
Pellicci, PG, 248, 261
Perez, GL, 97, 113
Perez, VL, 145, 151
Perlmutter, RM, 251, 264, 277, 278, 284, 285
Perniciaro, C, 97, 113
Pernis, A, 141, 145, 147
Peroni, SE, 268, 283
Perretti, F, 13, 33
Persson, AM, 3, 30
Persson, U, 128, 133
Peters, MS, 4, 31, 95, 97, 105, 107, 110, 112, 113, 114, 118, 127, 131
Peters-Bhatt, E, 206, 220, 315, 320
Petersen, J, 39, 48
Peterson, CG, 3, 30
Peterson, CGB, 3, 4, 31
Peterson, EA, 97, 100, 101, 103, 107, 112, 113
Petrangeli, E, 294, 297
Petreccia, DC, 98, 115
Petricoin, EF, 249, 262
Pfeiffer, C, 139, 144, 146
Pfister, R, 55, 56, 57, 60, 64, 65, 68, 218, 223
Phillips, J, 175, 187, 315, 320
Piccolo, S, 217, 222
Pichler, WJ, 45, 49
Pickup, DJ, 217, 222
Pieper, W, 154, 160
Pierce, JH, 300, 317
Pierelli, L, 73, 89
Pillar, J, 61, 68, 127, 130, 132, 154, 162
Pincus, SH, 99, 115
Pipkorn, U, 40, 45, 48, 49, 102, 117
Pircher, H, 56, 65
Pitman, A, 27, 36, 154, 162
Pitman, AM, 27, 37, 61, 68, 70, 87, 300, 313, 314, 318, 322, 329
Pittlekow, MR, 97, 107, 108, 110, 113
Pizzichini, E, 23, 26, 27, 36
Pizzichini, MMM, 23, 26, 27, 36
Plaetinck, G, 60, 67, 68, 71, 85, 88, 93, 167, 169, 170, 171, 174, 175, 185, 186, 187, 189, 190, 191, 194, 197, 200, 202, 205, 206, 207, 208, 209, 214, 218, 219, 220, 221, 242, 246, 247, 248, 249, 252, 254, 257, 259, 260, 262, 265, 302, 303, 308, 311, 313, 314, 315, 318, 319, 320

Plaut, M, 300, 317
Ploysongsang, Y, 60, 68, 71, 88, 218, 223
Plumas, J, 56, 65, 84, 92
Pluznik, DH, 71, 88
Polentarutti, N, 143, 149
Ponath, PD, 156, 164
Porcelli, S, 268, 282
Posada, M, 97, 114
Post, TW, 156, 164
Postel-Vinay, MC, 209, 221
Poupart, P, 279, 286
Poznansky, MC, 58, 67
Power, CA, 156, 158, 164
Prabhu Das, M, 141, 147
Prendergasst, FG, 2, 29
Prescott, SL, 120, 121, 122, 123, 125, 126
Presky, DH, 141, 147
Pretolani, M, 16, 17, 34
Priest, R, 303, 318
Prin, L, 56, 65, 84, 92
Prosser, D, 199, 203
Proud, D, 13, 33, 40, 48, 102, 117
Proudfoot, AE, 70, 86, 194, 197, 198, 202, 203, 241, 256
Proudfoot, AEI, 168, 169, 171, 172, 174, 175, 176, 177, 178, 180, 181, 182, 185, 186, 187, 193, 195, 202, 301, 303, 310, 314, 315, 318, 319, 320
Punonnen, J, 142, 148
Puri, RK, 144, 150

## Q

Qin, S, 156, 164
Qiuyu, S, 227, 236, 254, 265
Quan, S, 250, 263
Quelle, FW, 145, 151, 230, 238, 251, 252, 264
Quint, DJ, 54, 64, 154, 162

## R

Raaijimakers, JA, 249, 262
Raaijmakers, JAM, 154, 161
Radbruch, A, 140, 147
Raghavachar, A, 52, 62
Raghavan, A, 281, 287
Raghupathy, R, 121, 125
Rajarathnam, K, 217, 222
Rajewsky, K, 140, 142, 143, 147, 149
Rajka, G, 99, 115
Rak, S, 41, 43, 49
Rambaldi, A, 155, 163, 300, 318
Ramsay, AJ, 27, 37, 61, 68, 70, 88, 128, 129, 130, 134, 154, 158, 163, 289, 295, 300, 318
Ramsey, AJ, 245, 259
Ranford, PR, 268, 283
Ranger, AM, 141, 147
Rankin, JA, 3, 30
Rankin, SM, 156, 164
Rao, A, 281, 287, 294, 297
Rapoport, AP, 191, 196, 201
Raptis, A, 294, 297
Rashid, A, 228, 237
Raub, R, 278, 285
Rawlings, D, 250, 263
Rawlings, DJ, 250, 263
Ray, A, 271, 274, 283, 293, 296
Ray, P, 271, 274, 283, 293, 296
Re, F, 143, 149
Ream, B, 228, 237
Rebelsky, MS, 70, 86, 142, 148
Reda, AM, 97, 113
Reed, CE, 61, 68, 97, 112, 127, 131
Reed, JC, 230, 237
Rees, PK, 299, 316
Regiani, S, 4, 31
Reich, NC, 145, 151
Reiner, SL, 140, 147
Rennick, D, 70, 87, 154, 162
Renshaw-Gegg, L, 217, 223

Renz, H, 15, 34
Renz, M, 73, 89
Ricci, M, 52, 63, 119, 124, 138, 146
Rice, N, 294, 297
Richard, WG, 308, 313, 318
Richards, CL, 217, 222
Richardson, M, 76, 90
Richerson, HB, 19, 35
Rih, S, 99, 115
Rincon, M, 140, 147, 277, 284
Ring, J, 102, 116
Ringler, DJ, 156, 164
Rizzo, LV, 143, 149
Robb, LG, 208, 221
Robbins, SE, 142, 148
Roberts, AB, 85, 92
Roberts, JA, 51, 56, 62, 65, 69, 85, 127, 131, 154, 162
Roberts, R, 57, 66
Robertson, D, 73, 89
Robin, ED, 51, 61
Robinson, D, 128, 132, 280, 286
Robinson, DS, 40, 41, 48, 49, 51, 53, 54, 55, 56, 57, 58, 60, 61, 62, 63, 64, 65, 66, 67, 68, 83, 92, 119, 125, 127, 128, 132, 133
Roche, W, 21, 22, 24, 36
Roche, WR, 51, 58, 62, 66, 69, 85, 127, 131
Roddy, LL, 98, 110, 115
Rodriguez, M, 4, 31
Rodriguez-Viciana, P, 230, 234, 237
Rogers, KH, 140, 147
Rogge, L, 141, 147
Rohrbach, MS, 3, 19, 30, 98, 115
Rolfe, F, 281, 287
Rolfe, FG, 268, 280, 283, 287
Rolink, AG, 243, 258
Romagnani, S, 52, 63, 119, 124, 138, 146
Romioka, K, 128, 134
Rooney, S, 61, 68, 127, 130, 132, 154, 162
Roos, D, 4, 31, 299, 317
Rose-John, S, 207, 220, 314, 320
Rosen, SD, 73, 89
Rosenberg, HF, 3, 30
Rosenberg, M, 168, 170, 171, 173, 174, 183, 185, 246, 247, 260
Rosenfeld, PJ, 294, 297
Rosenhall, L, 58, 67
Rosette, C, 294, 297
Rossi, AG, 155, 163
Rothenberg, EV, 278, 285
Rothenberg, ME, 39, 48, 156, 158, 164, 165
Rothman, P, 141, 145, 147
Rouleau, KA, 81, 91
Roussel, MF, 207, 220
Rowley, JD, 142, 148
Roxwarski, DA, 241, 256
Rsukada, S, 250, 263
Rubin, JR, 170, 186
Ruffie, C, 16, 17, 34
Ruhno, J, 83, 92
Rumi, C, 73, 89
Rungger, D
Ruscetti, FW, 85, 92
Russell, AS, 120, 125
Russell, SM, 144, 150
Rutledge, MC, 309, 318
Rutschmann, SK, 144, 145, 149
Ryan, D, 73, 90
Ryan, DH, 128, 133
Ryan, GF, 120, 125
Ryan, GR, 275, 284
Rzucidlo, DA, 217, 222

## S

Sabin, EA, 140, 147
Sachs, MI, 9, 32, 97, 98, 110, 112
Sad, S, 56, 65, 138, 146

Sadelain, M, 228, 237
Saetta, M, 57, 66
Saffran, DC, 250, 263
Saito, T, 2, 29
Sakai, R, 242, 258, 273, 274, 283, 293, 296
Sakamaki, K, 4, 31, 225, 226, 227, 228, 230, 232, 234, 235, 236, 237, 242, 247, 257
Sakamaki, S, 247, 249, 261
Sakamoto, H, 232, 238
Sakamoto, K, 171, 187, 247, 260
Sakiyama, Y, 102, 116
Saklatvala, J, 291, 296
Saks, SL, 71, 88
Salgame, P, 56, 65, 138, 146
Salto, T, 207, 218, 221
Sampson, HA, 97, 99, 100, 101, 103, 113, 117
Samter, M, 154, 160
Sand, O, 2, 29
Sanda, T, 102, 116
Sander, S, 217, 223
Sanderson, CJ, 39, 48, 52, 55, 62, 63, 65, 70, 84, 86, 87, 92, 119, 125, 128, 133, 134, 142, 147, 154, 155, 160, 161, 163, 167, 169, 174, 184, 186, 187, 190, 191, 192, 193, 194, 200, 201, 202, 241, 242, 244, 246, 256, 260, 268, 271, 272, 273, 278, 279, 280, 282, 283, 286, 289, 293, 295, 297, 299, 300, 313, 317, 318, 319
Sangster, MY, 145, 151
Santoli, D, 230, 237
Sarawar, SR, 145, 151
Saris, CJ, 233, 238
Sarmiento, EU, 18, 19, 35
Sasai, Y, 102, 107, 116, 118, 217, 222
Sato, A, 142, 148
Sato, N, 60, 68, 189, 200, 227, 230, 231, 232, 234, 236, 238, 242, 247, 247, 249, 251, 252, 261, 264
Sato, S, 248, 251, 261
Sato, TA, 218, 223, 314, 320
Satoh, T, 248, 262
Satoskar, A, 144, 149
Satterthwaite, A, 230, 237, 251, 264
Sauerwein, R, 207, 221
Savage, TJ, 300, 313, 318
Savelkoul, HF, 27, 36, 300, 313, 318
Savelkoul, HFJ, 70, 87, 154, 162
Savill, J, 52, 62
Sawai, T, 102, 116
Scala, E, 102, 116
Schad, CR, 3, 31
Schall, TJ, 155, 163
Schaller, J, 107, 118
Schandene, L, 277, 284
Scheffler, JE, 191, 201, 246, 260, 303, 308, 318
Scheinman, RI, 294, 297
Scheman, AJ, 97, 113
Scherer, S, 207, 220
Schieven, GL, 3, 30
Schindler, C, 141, 145, 147
Schindler, U, 145, 151
Schlagenhauf, E, 144, 145, 150
Schlecht, H, 1, 28
Schleffer, JE, 206, 220
Schleimer, R, 84, 92
Schleimer, RP, 98, 114, 128, 134, 154, 155, 161, 162, 279, 286
Schlessinger, J, 248, 261
Schlunegger, MP, 170, 178, 180, 186, 188
Schmidt, J, 278, 280, 285, 286
Schmitz, A, 168, 185
Schmitz, J, 140, 147
Schmitz-Van der Leur, H, 206, 219
Schneyer, AL, 217, 222
Schofield, BH, 17, 34

Schoni, MH, 58, 66
Schooley, RJ, 99, 115
Schooltink, H, 207, 220
Schopf, E, 98, 102, 107, 114, 116, 118
Schrader, JW, 248, 262
Schragge, W, 76, 78, 81, 82, 90
Schreiber, M, 217, 222
Schreiber, SL, 59, 67, 281, 287
Schreurs, J, 189, 200, 227, 236, 248, 261
Schroeter, AL, 9, 32, 95, 97, 98, 103, 110, 112, 113, 117
Schumacher, JH, 138, 146, 313, 319, 321, 329
Schwaninger, M, 278, 284
Schwartz, JF, 72, 89
Schwartz, LB, 45, 49, 51, 53, 57, 62, 66, 102, 117, 127, 128, 131, 132
Schweibert, LM, 279, 286
Schweitzer, AN, 141, 147
Schweitzer, RC, 154, 155, 161
Schwenker, G, 1, 28
Schwiebert, LA, 279, 286
Sciacca, FL, 143, 149
Scott, R, 2, 29
Screpanti, L, 294, 297
Sealand, S, 73, 89
Sebille, E, 303, 314, 318
Secrist, H, 45, 49
Seder, R, 139, 144, 146
Sedgwick, JB, 57, 66, 102, 117, 127, 131
Sehmi, R, 51, 62, 70, 76, 78, 81, 82, 84, 87, 90, 91, 154, 155, 161, 163
Sekhsaria, S, 84, 92
Serrano, M, 235, 239
Sethna, MP, 141, 147
Sever, CE, 142, 148
Severinson, E, 52, 62, 128, 133, 154, 161, 168, 185, 241, 256
Sewell, W, 281, 287
Sewell, WA, 268, 280, 283, 287
Seymore, BWP, 154, 162
Seymour, BW, 70, 87
Shah, AJ, 73, 89
Shalit, M, 84, 92
Shannon, MF, 175, 187, 275, 284, 315, 320
Shaper, JH, 72, 89
Sharma, S, 281, 287
Sharpe, AH, 141, 147
Shaw, G, 279, 286
Shaw, KT, 281, 287
Shaw, RJ, 98, 110, 115
Shearer, WT, 254, 264
Shelhamer, JH, 20, 35
Sher, A, 299, 316
Sher, ER, 58, 59, 67, 280, 286
Sherr, CJ, 207, 220
Shi, W, 145, 151
Shi, X, 156, 164
Shields, JG, 167, 184, 243, 244, 258
Shier, KJ, 103, 117
Shiiba, M, 71, 88, 196, 203, 206, 219, 248, 249, 250, 253, 254, 262, 263
Shikama, Y, 249, 262
Shimamoto, G, 217, 223
Shimoda, K, 145, 151
Shindoh, Y, 2, 29
Shirai, T, 243, 258
Shirato, K, 154, 162
Shire, D, 142, 148
Shirouzu, M, 235, 238
Shleimer, RP, 43, 49
Shoemaker, S, 218, 223
Shoji, A, 102, 116
Shrader, B, 313, 319, 321, 329
Siciliano, SJ, 156, 164
Sideras, P, 52, 62, 168, 185, 241, 250, 256, 263
Sieff, CA, 249, 262
Siegel, MD, 174, 271, 283, 293, 296
Sifai, RD, 154, 162

Sigal, NH, 281, 287
Sigrist, KS, 14, 33
Sihra, BS, 60, 67
Siigaglia, S, 141, 147
Silberstein, DS, 39, 48
Silver, JE, 97, 112, 113, 300, 317
Sim, T, 43, 49
Sim, TC, 102, 117
Simon, HU, 58, 66
Simonelli, C, 52, 63, 138, 146
Simonet, WS, 217, 223
Simonin, G, 209, 221
Simonsen, C, 2, 29
Simony-Lafontaine, J, 51, 62, 127, 131, 242, 257, 299, 317
Simpson, EM, 141, 147
Simpson, RJ, 168, 185, 218, 223
Sims, JE, 208, 217, 221, 222
Simson, IW, 97, 113
Singer, MS, 73, 89
Singer, SC, 199, 203
Sironi, M, 143, 149
Sirontino, A, 156, 164
Sito, M, 248, 261
Sizeland, AM, 248, 261
Sjoerdsma, K, 19, 35
Skrbric, D, 45, 49
Slater, DN, 97, 113
Slifman, NR, 3, 14, 19, 30, 31, 33, 98, 115, 300, 317
Slovak, ML, 142, 148
Sluiter, JH, 127, 130, 131
Slungaard, A, 4, 31
Sluss, PM, 217, 222
Sly, PD, 120, 121, 122, 123, 124, 125, 126
Smallacombe, T, 120, 121, 122, 125
Smerz-Bertling, C, 144, 150
Smiley, ST, 145, 151
Smith, C, 208, 221
Smith, CA, 217, 222
Smith, CI, 168, 185
Smith, CIE, 154, 161, 250, 263
Smith, GL, 217, 222
Smith, GP, 314, 320
Smith, H, 156, 164
Smith, MR, 248, 261
Smith, RM, 129, 134
Smith, SH, 167, 184, 243, 244, 258
Smith, TD, 217, 222
Smith, WB, 227, 236
Smolak, P, 217, 222
Smorgorzewska, EM, 73, 89
Snapper, CM, 128, 133, 243, 258
Snoek, M, 52, 63, 277, 284
Snyder, MR, 3, 30
Sobel, RA, 141, 147
Sodhi, N, 97, 112
Sofia, D, 61, 68
Sofia, RD, 127, 130, 132
Sokoloski, T, 168, 170, 171, 173, 174, 183, 185, 246, 247, 260
Solari, R, 171, 172, 174, 175, 176, 186, 187, 194, 197, 198, 202, 203, 301, 303, 310, 311, 314, 315, 318, 319, 320
Soldevilla, L, 97, 114
Solley, G, 51, 61
Solley, GO, 5, 8, 17, 23, 24, 31, 99, 103, 115, 117, 299, 317
Solway, J, 14, 33
Somers, W, 190, 200, 306, 310, 318
Sonoda, E, 189, 200, 208, 221, 242, 243, 246, 250, 256, 258, 264
Sorrentino, S, 3, 31
Soter, NA, 99, 103, 115, 117
Sotiropoulos, A, 209, 221
Sottrup-Jensen, L, 2, 29
Spaethe, SM, 14, 33
Sparkes, RS, 250, 263
Spemann, H, 215, 222
Spriggs, MK, 217, 222
Springer, MS, 156, 164
Spry, CJF, 98, 110, 115, 154, 161, 299, 317

Spurr, NK, 73, 89
Squillace, D, 23, 26, 27, 36
St. Charles, R, 170, 186
Stacey, DW, 248, 261
Staels, B, 278, 285
Stafford, S, 249, 263
Stahl, N, 196, 203, 207, 220
Stahle-Backdahl, M, 107, 118
Standaert, RF, 281, 287
Stark, GR, 249, 262
Staruch, MJ, 281, 287
Steeber, DA, 17, 34
Steinmuller, D, 5, 8, 31
Stella, G, 279, 285
Stellato, C, 279, 286
Stellwagen, A, 279, 286
Stelts, D, 325, 329
Stelts, DM, 70, 82, 87, 154, 158, 163, 244, 259, 300, 313, 314, 318
Sterdinsky, SA, 43, 49
Stern, M, 52, 62
Stevens, RJ, 39, 48
Stewart, GA, 124, 126
Stobl, H, 73, 89
Stocking, C, 206, 219
Stomski, FC, 190, 191, 196, 197, 201, 219, 220200
Storz, C, 127, 132
Storz, CHR, 57, 66
Stoyan, T, 207, 220
Stranick, KS, 271, 272, 273, 274, 281, 283
Strath, M, 52, 62, 70, 84, 86, 87, 92, 154, 155, 160, 163, 167, 169, 184, 186, 194, 202, 271, 272, 279, 283, 286
Straus, D, 278, 285, 290, 296
Strauss, LC, 72, 89
Strebinsky, SA, 128, 134
Strek, ME, 14, 15, 33
Strob, R, 81, 91
Strom, TB, 141, 147
Stura, EA, 190, 200
Sturrock, RF, 299, 316
Su, S, 154, 162
Su, WPD, 97, 107, 108, 110, 113, 114
Suda, J, 154, 161
Suda, T, 70, 76, 87, 90, 244, 258, 300, 318
Sudderick, RM, 40, 41, 43, 48, 49
Sudo, T, 249, 262
Sugaamura, K, 144, 150
Sugai, T, 102, 116
Sugama, Y, 128, 133, 154, 161, 244, 258, 289, 295, 300, 318
Sugane, K, 128, 134, 289, 295
Sugaya, H, 154, 158, 163, 244, 245, 259
Sugiura, M, 309, 318
Sugiyama, RH, 3, 30
Sugo, T, 168, 185
Suko, M, 269, 277, 280, 281, 282, 283, 284, 287
Sulakvelidze, I, 83, 92
Sullivan, J, 217, 223
Sullivan, L, 154, 162
Sullivan, M, 242, 257, 273, 275, 283, 293, 297
Sumi, SM, 3, 31
Sun, J, 127, 130, 132
Sun, L, 154, 161
Sun, Q, 60, 68, 191, 196, 197, 201
Sun, XH, 232, 238
Sun, Z, 245, 259
Sunaga, S, 154, 158, 163, 244, 245, 259
Suphioglu, C, 124, 126
Sur, S, 20, 35, 61, 68, 97, 100, 101, 102, 103, 113, 117
Surs, W, 58, 59, 67
Sutherland, DR, 72, 73, 74, 76, 78, 81, 82, 89, 90
Sutherland, G, 207, 208, 221

Sutherland, GR, 70, 86
Suto, M, 277, 280, 281, 284, 287
Suzuki, R, 232, 238
Svensson, C, 80, 91
Swain, SL, 70, 86, 128, 133, 168, 185
Swanson, MC, 128, 133
Sweitzer, SM, 217, 222, 249, 262
Switzer, J, 76, 83, 90, 92
Symons, J, 217, 222
Symons, JA, 207, 220
Szabo, SJ, 141, 147
Szefler, SJ, 58, 59, 67, 280, 286
Szelenyi, I, 278, 280, 285, 286

## T

Taga, T, 196, 203, 207, 218, 221, 248, 249, 251, 261, 262, 264, 314, 320
Tahatsu, K, 244, 258
Tai, PC, 154, 161, 299, 317
Takafuji, S, 52, 63
Takagi, M, 154, 158, 163, 244, 245, 250, 259, 263
Takagi, S, 156, 164
Takahashi, K, 128, 133
Takahashi, M, 52, 62, 168, 185, 241, 256
Takahashi, T, 9, 32, 70, 86, 193, 201, 248, 261
Takahashi, Y, 99, 115
Takahiko, H, 71, 88
Takaishi, T, 99, 115
Takaki, S, 70, 71, 86, 88, 154, 158, 163, 167, 172, 184, 186, 189, 191, 196, 200, 201, 203, 206, 207, 208, 209, 219, 221, 227, 228, 236, 241, 242, 243, 244, 245, 246, 247, 248, 249, 251, 253, 254, 256, 258, 259, 260, 261, 262
Takamoto, M, 128, 134, 289, 295
Takatsu, K, 52, 62, 70, 71, 86, 87, 88, 128, 133, 154, 158, 161, 162, 163, 167, 168, 171, 172, 184, 185, 186, 187, 189, 191, 193, 196, 200, 201, 203, 206, 207, 208, 209, 219, 221, 227, 228, 230, 236, 237, 241, 242, 243, 244, 245, 246, 247, 248, 249, 250, 251, 253, 254, 256, 258, 259, 260, 261, 262, 262, 264, 280, 286, 289, 295, 300, 313, 318
Takatsu, L, 154, 161
Takeda, S, 309, 318
Takeda, T, 145, 151
Takeshita, T, 144, 150
Takimoto, M, 73, 89
Talabot, D, 143, 149
Talabot, F, 171, 172, 174, 175, 176, 186, 187, 194, 202, 311, 315, 319
Tamura, G, 154, 162
Tan, CL, 292, 293, 294, 296, 297
Tan, HL, 217, 223
Tan, TH, 277, 284
Tan, Y, 279, 285
Tanabe, T, 52, 62, 154, 161, 168, 185, 241, 256
Tanaka, N, 142, 148
Tanaka, S, 193, 201
Tanaka, T, 145, 151, 242, 258, 273, 274, 283, 293, 296
Tanaka, Y, 103, 117, 128, 133
Tang, J, 119, 125
Taniguchi, T, 142, 148, 232, 238, 278, 285
Tanimura, S, 232, 238
Tanno, Y, 76, 90, 154, 162
Taremi, S, 199, 203
Tarpley, J, 217, 223
Tasaka, K, 2, 29
Tate, EH, 206, 220, 315, 320

Tavana, G, 243, 244, 258
Tavernier, J, 60, 67, 68, 71, 84, 85, 88, 92, 93, 128, 133, 167, 168, 169, 170, 171, 174, 175, 185, 186, 187, 189, 190, 191, 194, 197, 200, 201, 202, 205, 206, 207, 208, 209, 214, 218, 219, 220, 221, 223, 242, 245, 246, 247, 248, 249, 252, 254, 257, 259, 260, 262, 265, 300, 302, 303, 308, 311, 313, 314, 315, 317, 318, 319, 320
Tayebi, N, 144, 150
Taylor, KJ, 9, 32
Tedder, TF, 17, 34
Telizyn, S, 70, 76, 78, 83, 86, 90
Ten, RM, 3, 30, 31, 97, 114
Tennen, DG, 245, 259
Teopili, L, 73, 89
Terada, N, 231, 232, 234, 238, 247, 249, 261
Test, ST, 4, 31
Teti, A, 98, 114
Thalmann, P, 243, 258
Theil, A, 140, 147
Theodore, J, 51, 61
Thestrup-Pedersen, K, 145, 150
Thiemann, FT, 73, 89
Thomas, GJ, 98, 110, 114
Thomas, JD, 250, 263
Thomas, LL, 3, 17, 18, 19, 21, 29, 34, 35, 98, 110, 114, 115
Thomas, WR, 124, 126
Thompson, CB, 279, 285
Thompson, J, 143, 149
Thompson, WC, 140, 143, 147
Thomson, NC, 57, 66
Thyresson, NH, 97, 113
Tiesman, J, 207, 220
Tiffany, HL, 156, 164
Tijan, R, 294, 297
Till, S, 56, 65
Timans, JC, 206, 219
Tindle, RW, 72, 89
Tiri, A, 52, 63, 119, 124, 138, 146
Tite, J, 268, 282
Tivol, EA, 141, 147
Tobler, A, 279, 286
Todokoro, K, 227, 228, 236, 237
Togias, AG, 40, 48
Tohya, K, 227, 236
Tokota, T, 268, 278, 282
Tolbert, M, 75, 84, 85, 90
Tomida, M, 208, 221
Tominaga, A, 52, 62, 70, 71, 86, 87, 88, 128, 133, 154, 161, 167, 168, 171, 172, 184, 185, 186, 187, 189, 191, 193, 200, 201, 207, 208, 209, 221, 241, 242, 243, 244, 246, 247, 250, 253, 256, 258, 259, 260, 261, 264, 289, 295, 300, 318
Tomioka, K, 43, 49
Tomonaga, M, 4, 31, 167, 171, 185
Tonkonogy, SL, 70, 86
Torigoe, T, 230, 237
Torisu, M, 128, 133, 154, 161, 244, 258, 289, 295, 300, 318
Torpier, G, 56, 65
Totty, NF, 155, 156, 158, 163
Toyoda, Y, 228, 237
Trail, G, 217, 223
Trifilieff, A, 21, 35
Trigg, CJ, 58, 67
Trinchieri, G, 242, 257
Tripp, CA, 139, 146
Tripp, CS, 242, 257
Tripp, RA, 145, 151
Trischman, T, 73, 89
Troon, JT, 144, 145, 149
Trounce, JR, 21, 36
Truong, O, 155, 156, 158, 163
Tsai, JJ, 281, 287

Tsai-Pflugfelder, M, 294, 297
Tsang, M, 144, 145, 150
Tsang, ML, 170, 186
Tsarbopoulos, A, 199, 203
Tsicopoulos, A, 55, 56, 64, 83, 92, 119, 125
Tsuda, S, 102, 107, 116, 118
Tsuda, T, 83, 92
Tsujimoto, M, 168, 185, 193, 201
Tsujimoto, Y, 278, 285
Tsukada, S, 230, 237, 248, 250, 251, 261, 263, 264
Tsukamoto, A, 73, 89
Tsukui, K, 4, 31
Tsuruoka, N, 70, 87, 154, 162, 168, 185, 246, 260, 277, 280, 284
Tsuyuki, J, 21, 35
Tsuyuki, S, 21 35
Tucker, GK, 3, 31
Tucker, WQ, 128, 133, 167, 184, 279, 286, 289, 295
Tucker, WQJ, 52, 62, 154, 161
Tunther, M, 207, 220
Tuntipopipat, S, 120, 125
Turcatti, G, 169, 186
Turka, LA, 279, 285
Tusujimoto, M, 246, 260
Tuypens, T, 60, 67, 68, 71, 88, 167, 169, 170, 171, 174, 175, 185, 186, 189, 190, 191, 194, 197, 200, 201, 202, 206, 206, 207, 208, 209, 214, 218, 220, 220, 221, 242, 245, 246, 257, 259, 302, 311, 314, 315, 318, 319, 320
Tybulewica, VLJ, 229, 237
Tye, MJ, 97, 113

**U**

Uchida, DA, 13, 33
Uehara, M, 102, 116
Ueki, IF, 8, 32
Uings, I, 177, 178, 180, 181, 182, 187, 195, 202
Uings, IJ, 175, 187, 197, 198, 203, 315, 320
Ullrich, A, 248, 261
Ultsch, M, 171, 187, 190, 192, 200, 306, 310, 318
Umetsu, DT, 45, 49
Umland, SP, 271, 272, 274, 281, 283, 324, 329
Undem, BJ, 127, 130, 131
Upham, JW, 124, 126
Upton, C, 217, 222
Urdal, D, 208, 221
Urwyler, A, 45, 49
Uss, AS, 271, 272, 274, 281, 283
Usuku, G, 243, 244, 258

**V**

Vacca, A, 294, 297
Vadas, M, 206, 219
Vadas, MA, 39, 48, 52, 60, 63, 68, 70, 71, 87, 88, 128, 133, 154, 161, 167, 175, 184, 187, 190, 191, 200, 201, 227, 236, 275, 284, 289, 295, 315, 320
Valent, P, 76, 90
Valentine, J, 281, 287
Valle, A, 73, 89
Valtier, S, 102, 117
Van Ark, I, 27, 36, 70, 87, 154, 162, 168, 185, 300, 313, 318
Vancheri, C, 83, 92
Van de Heyden, J, 206, 207, 209, 218, 220
Vandekerckhove, J, 168, 171, 185, 187
VandenBos, T, 208, 221
Van der Brugger, T, 249, 262

Van der Heijden, JF, 280, 286
van der Heyden, J, 60, 67, 71, 85, 88, 93, 167, 168, 169, 170, 171, 174, 175, 185, 186, 187, 189, 191, 194, 197, 200, 201, 202, 205, 206, 209, 219, 221, 242, 246, 247, 248, 249, 252, 254, 257, 260, 262, 302, 303, 308, 311, 313, 314, 315, 318, 319, 320
Van der Linde, HJ, 27, 36
Van der Linde, HL, 70, 87
van der Linden, C, 207, 221
Van Der Lugt, NM, 233, 238
Van der Pouw Kraan, TC, 144, 145, 149
Van der Weld, T, 142, 149
Van Deursen, J, 145, 151
Van Haelst-Pisani, C, 97, 113
Vanhaesebroeck, B, 230, 234, 237
Vanhoutte, PM, 14, 33, 127, 131, 300, 317
Vanichenker, W, 228, 237
Van Kessel, A, 51, 61
Van Kessel Welmers, BAC, 154, 155, 161
VanKeulen, V, 97, 113
Van Kimmenade, A, 313, 319, 321, 329
Van Leeuwen, BH, 70, 86, 271, 272, 274, 283, 291, 292, 293, 294, 296, 297
Van Lier, RAW, 277, 279, 284
Van Neerven, RJ, 280, 286
Van Oosterhout, AJ, 27, 36, 168, 185, 300, 313, 318
Van Oosterhout, AJM, 70, 87, 154, 162
van Reijsen, FC, 52, 63
VanSlyke, J, 217, 222
Vargaftig, BB, 16, 17, 34, 127, 130, 132, 154, 161
Varney, V, 102, 104, 116
Varney, VA, 40, 41, 43, 48, 49
Veber, DF, 309, 318
Vecchi, A, 143, 149
Vega, F, 144, 150
Veiby, OP, 143, 149
Velu, T, 277, 284
Venaille, TJ, 120, 121, 122, 123, 125, 126
Venecie, PY, 97, 99, 100, 101, 113
Venge, P, 3, 30, 31, 51, 55, 58, 67, 102, 116, 127, 130, 131, 242, 257, 299, 317
Vercelli, D, 142, 148
Vercellotti,GM, 97, 113
Verdine, GL, 294, 297
Verhee, A, 60, 68, 71, 88, 169, 170, 171, 174, 175, 186, 190, 194, 197, 200, 202, 206, 219, 220, 246, 259, 311, 314, 315, 319, 320
Verheyen, KCP, 70, 87
Verma, NK, 129, 134
Verrier, B, 248, 249, 261
Vetrie, D, 250, 263
Vietta, ES, 70, 86
Viganali, DAA, 145, 151
Virchow, JC, 53, 55, 57, 64, 65, 66, 130, 134, 291, 296, 299, 317
Vita, N, 144, 150
Volovitz, B, 57, 66, 102, 117
Von Allmen, C, 102, 116
Von der Weid, T, 294, 297
Von Hoesslin, H, 21, 36
Von Mecklenburg, C, 4, 31
Vorechovsky, I, 250, 263

**W**

Wade, E, 294, 297
Wagstrom, CR, 199, 203

Wahli, W, 294, 297
Wakao, H, 191, 201, 228, 232, 233, 234, 237, 238, 249, 250, 254, 262, 263
Walker, C, 53, 55, 57, 64, 65, 66, 99, 104, 115, 117, 127, 128, 130, 132, 134, 291, 296, 299, 317
Walker, S, 60, 67
Wallace, PM, 81, 91
Walls, AF, 58, 66, 127, 131
Walsh, DT, 155, 156, 158, 163
Walsh, GM, 39, 48, 52, 63, 70, 87, 98, 110, 115, 128, 134, 154, 161, 300, 317
Walti, S, 56, 65
Waltmann, P, 52, 62, 70, 87, 154, 155, 161
Wang, HM, 227, 236
Wang, J, 58, 67, 156, 164, 215, 222
Wang, JM, 155, 163, 300, 318
Wang, JY, 248, 261
Wang, P, 324, 329
Wang, S, 217, 222
Wang, SZ, 16, 34
Wang, W, 155, 163
Wang, XJ, 249, 262
Wang, Y, 242, 257, 279, 286
Ward, LD, 218, 223
Wardlaw, AJ, 9, 17, 32, 39, 48, 51, 52, 53, 54, 61, 62, 63, 64, 69, 70, 83, 85, 87, 102, 104, 116, 127, 128, 131, 132, 134, 154, 155, 161, 162, 244, 259, 300, 317
Warne, PH, 230, 234, 237
Warner, JA, 299, 317
Warnock, ML, 130, 134
Warren, DG, 154, 160
Warren, DJ, 70, 86, 167, 184, 268, 282
Warringa, RA, 103, 117
Warringa, RAJ, 52, 62, 154, 161
Wasmoen, TL, 2, 29
Wasserman, SI, 83, 92, 98, 110, 115, 127, 131
Wassom, DL, 5, 8, 31, 99, 115
Wasson, DL, 299, 316
Watanabe, S, 144, 150, 196, 203, 206, 219, 227, 230, 231, 234, 236, 237, 238
Watanabe, T, 248, 251, 261
Watanabe, Y, 227, 236, 247, 260
Watefield, MD, 230, 234, 237
Wathelet, M, 279, 286
Watnick, AS, 27, 36, 154, 158, 162, 163, 244, 259, 300, 313, 314, 318, 325, 329
Watson, C, 140, 147
Watson, CJ, 300, 317
Watson, RM, 76, 81, 82, 84, 90, 91
Wattie, J, 81, 83, 91
Weatherbee, JA, 144, 145, 150, 170, 186
Webb, DS, 249, 262
Webb, GC, 70, 86
Weber, IT, 170, 186
Wegmann, TG, 120, 121, 125, 126
Wegner, CD, 10, 17, 32, 33, 103, 117
Wei, S, 249, 262
Weiler, D, 102, 117
Weinberg, AD, 128, 133
Weinberg, RA, 248, 261
Weiner, HL, 141, 147
Weismann, IL, 73, 89
Weiss, A, 278, 285, 290, 296
Weiss, M, 249, 262
Weiss, SJ, 4, 31, 98, 115
Welham, MJ, 248, 262
Weller, PF, 13, 33, 98, 99, 110, 115
Wells, JA, 171, 187, 306, 310, 318
Wells, T, 144, 145, 150
Wells, TN, 194, 197, 198, 202, 203, 241, 256, 311, 315, 319

Wells, TNC, 156, 158, 164, 169, 170, 171, 172, 174, 175, 176, 177, 178, 180, 181, 182, 186, 187, 195, 202, 301, 303, 310, 314, 315, 318, 319, 320
Wen, Y, 45, 49
Werner, P, 57, 66
Wesp, M, 21, 35
Westbrook, CA, 70, 86, 142, 148
Westland, JKT, 52, 63
Wever, R, 98, 115
Wheatley, CL, 3, 19, 30, 98, 115
White, SR, 14, 15, 33
Whitehorn, EA, 206, 220, 315, 320
Whitsett, JA, 228, 237
Whittle, BL, 129, 134
Widdicombe, JH, 8, 32
Widdowson, KI, 309, 318
Widmer, JB, 208, 221
Widmer, MB, 218, 223, 314, 320
Wiekowski, M, 199, 203
Wiener Kronish, JP, 130, 134
Wierenga, EA, 52, 63, 277, 284
Wignall, JM, 208, 221
Wijdenes, J, 144, 145, 149, 207, 221, 277, 279, 284
Willard, D, 177, 178, 180, 181, 182, 187, 195, 202
Willems, F, 277, 284
Williams, DE, 278, 285
Williams, FM, 155, 163
Williams, FS, 14, 15, 33
Williams, TJ, 54, 59, 64, 70, 84, 88, 155, 156, 157, 158, 163, 164
Williams, WV, 176, 187
Williamson, DJ, 168, 185
Willman, CL, 142, 148
Wills Karp, M, 127, 130, 132
Wills-Karp, M, 15, 33
Willson, TA, 144, 150
Wilson, IA, 190, 200
Wilson, JW, 53, 58, 64, 66, 127, 131
Wilson, S, 98, 114
Wilson, SJ, 55, 58, 61, 66, 127, 131
Winborne, E, 168, 170, 171, 173, 174, 183, 185
Winbourne, E, 246, 247, 260
Wingfield, PT, 168, 169, 185, 186
Winkelmann, RK, 97, 112
Winqvist, I, 3, 30
Wintroub, BU, 107, 118
Witt, A, 27, 36, 154, 162
Witte, OH, 251, 264
Witte, ON, 230, 237, 248, 250, 251, 261, 263
Witthuhn, BA, 230, 238, 251, 252, 264
Wlodawer, A, 241, 256
Wolf, C, 97, 112
Wolf, SF, 139, 146
Wolff, K, 97, 112
Wong, DA, 76, 90, 99, 115
Wong, I, 75, 84, 85, 90
Wood, LJ, 76, 80, 81, 82, 84, 90, 91
Woodcock, J, 60, 68, 88
Woodcock, JM, 175, 187, 190, 191, 196, 197, 201, 254, 265, 315, 320
Wooden, S, 217, 223
Woodland, N, 142, 148
Woolley, MJ, 81, 91
Wrana, JL, 217, 222
Wrighton, NC, 190, 199, 200, 203, 206, 220, 315, 320
Wu, G, 139, 146
Wu, L, 156, 164
Wuthrich, B, 102, 104, 116, 117
Wyllie, AH, 58, 67
Wynn, TA, 140, 147

## X

Xiao, H, 154, 162
Xuan, JC, 170, 186

## Y

Yabuhara, A, 120, 121, 122, 123, 125, 126
Yahara, I, 189, 200, 227, 236
Yamachi, K, 154, 162
Yamada, A, 249, 252, 253, 263
Yamada, K, 278, 285
Yamada, M, 170, 186
Yamada, T, 60, 68, 162
Yamagata, T, 242, 258, 273, 274, 283, 293, 296
Yamage, M, 144, 145, 150
Yamaguchi, M, 99, 115
Yamaguchi, N, 167, 171, 185, 189, 193, 200, 201, 208, 221, 242, 243, 246, 247, 248, 256, 258, 260, 261
Yamaguchi, S, 154, 162
Yamaguchi, Y, 70, 87, 128, 133, 154, 161, 244, 258, 289, 295, 300, 318
Yamamoto, H, 142, 148
Yamamoto, K, 103, 117
Yamamoto, M, 228, 237
Yamamoto-Yamaguchi, Y, 208, 221
Yamamura, KI, 243, 244, 245, 250, 258, 259, 264
Yamanishi, K, 196, 203, 251, 264
Yamasaki, K, 248, 261, 314, 320
Yamashiro, K, 246, 260
Yamauchi, A, 144, 145, 150
Yamauchi, S, 243, 244, 258
Yanocopoulos, G, 207, 218, 221
Yanocopoulos, GD, 207, 220
Yanofsky, SD, 206, 220, 315, 320
Yaoita, Y, 52, 62, 154, 161, 168, 185, 241, 256
Yarsuel, Z, 71, 88
Yasakawa, K, 196, 203
Yasruel, Z, 60, 68, 218, 223
Yasue, A, 102, 116
Yasue, T, 102, 116, 250, 251, 264
Yasukawa, K, 207, 218, 221, 248, 251, 261, 264, 314, 320
Yawata, H, 314, 320
Yazaki, Y, 242, 258, 273, 274, 283, 293, 296
Yazdanbakhsh, M, 299, 317
Ye, ZS, 251, 264
Yeo, EL, 73, 89
Yergeau, DA, 245, 259
Yi, T, 231, 238
Ying, S, 40, 41, 43, 48, 49, 54, 55, 56, 57, 58, 59, 64, 65, 66, 67, 69, 83, 85, 92, 102, 104, 116, 119, 125, 128, 132, 133, 154, 162, 244, 259, 280, 286
Yokoa, T, 230, 231, 234, 237
Yokota, T, 75, 90, 189, 191, 196, 200, 203, 206, 219, 225, 226, 227, 228, 229, 231, 232, 234, 235, 236, 237, 238, 242, 251, 252, 257, 264, 269, 271, 272, 274, 280, 281, 283, 293, 296
Yokouchi, M, 250, 263
Yokoyama, C, 249, 262
Yokoyama, S, 235, 238
Yonehara, S, 189, 200, 227, 236, 242, 248, 250, 251, 261, 264
Yoshida, H, 103, 117
Yoshida, K, 249, 262
Yoshida, N, 145, 151
Yoshida, R, 156, 164
Yoshida, S, 228, 237
Yoshida, T, 154, 158, 163, 244, 245, 259
Yoshida, Y, 167, 171, 185
Yoshie, O, 156, 164
Yoshimoto, T, 140, 147
Yoshimura, A, 232, 238, 250, 263
Yoshimura, K, 154, 158, 163, 244, 245, 259
Yost, BL, 17, 34

Young, A, 120, 125
Young, IG, 27, 37, 51, 52, 61, 62, 63, 68, 70, 84, 86, 87, 88, 128, 129, 130, 133, 134, 142, 148, 154, 158, 161, 163, 165, 167, 184, 185, 242, 245, 257, 259, 271, 272, 274, 279, 283, 286, 289, 290, 291, 292, 293, 294, 295, 296, 297, 300, 318
Young, JDE, 3, 30
Young, P, 168, 170, 171, 173, 174, 183, 185, 246, 247, 260
Young, PR, 246, 260
Yu-Lee, L, 254, 264

**Z**

Zacharakis, B, 191, 193, 201
Zambas, DN, 271, 272, 273, 274, 281, 283
Zamvil, SS, 141, 147
Zanders, ED, 85, 92
Zavodny, P, 199, 203
Zeibecoglou, K, 60, 68
Zek-Kapp, G, 98, 114
Zhang, DH, 174, 271, 283, 293, 296
Zhang, JG, 144, 150
Zhang, Y, 140, 147
Zhao, B, 168, 170, 171, 173, 174, 183, 185, 246, 247, 260
Zheng, WP, 242, 257
Zheutlin, LM, 2, 17, 18, 29, 34, 35, 98, 110, 114
Zhou, L, 144, 145, 150
Zieg, G, 58, 67
Zimmerman, LB, 217, 222
Zlotnik, A, 155, 163
Zon, LI, 206, 219
Zubiaga, A, 290, 291, 296
Zurawski, G, 142, 143, 144, 148, 149, 150
Zurawski, SM, 142, 144, 147, 148, 150
Zurcher, J, 27, 36, 154, 162
Zurcher, JA, 70, 82, 87, 154, 158, 162, 163, 244, 259, 300, 313, 314, 318, 325, 329
Zvala, D, 19, 35
Zweiman, B, 102, 116

# SUBJECT INDEX


## A

Acetylcholine, 14
Acute severe asthma, 52
Adhesion molecules
  CD2, 278
  CD44, 278
  E-selection, 108
  ICAM-1, 108
  LFA-1, 278
  L-selectin, 17, 73
  VCAM-1, 108, 143
  VLA-4, 16, 108, 143, 278
Airway hyperreactivity, 52, 322
Airway narrowing, 52
Alanine scanning, 175
Alanine substitution, 193, 254
Allergen
  challenge, 82
  provocation, 40
Allosteric modification, 174
α-Chain binding, 175, 311
Alternative splicing, 207
Angiolymphoid hyperplasia, 96
*Angiostrongylus cantonensis*, 245
Antagonists, 197, 301
Anti-asthmatic agents, 309
Antibody
  B7-1, 141
  B7-2, 141
  $\beta_c$ chain, 252
  CD3, 292
  CD4, 41
  CD8, 41
  CD25, 41
  CD28, 277
  c-fos, 273
  ECP, 41
  eotaxin, 158
  GM-CSF, 53
  IL-5, 53, 313
  IL-5R-α, 252
  JAK-1, 252
  JAK-2, 252
  JunB, 273
  MBP, 41
  Sch 55700, 325
  TRFK-5, 16, 158, 313
Antigenic dose, 139
AP-1, 273

Apoptosis, 234
Ascaris antigen, 322
*Ascaris suum*, 10, 81
Asthma
  corticosteroid-resistant, 58
  IL-5 receptor expression, 60
  nonatopic, 57
  occupational, 57
Asymetric mutagenesis, 177
ATL-16T cell line, 268, 273
Atopic dermatitis, 99
Atropine, 14
Autoantibody, 243
Axonemes, 8

**B**

Baculovirus, 168
Basophils, 17
$\beta_c$-deficient mouse, 228
$\beta_c$ subunit, 247
β-glucuronidase, 19
β-lactoglobulin, 120
BIAcore, 325
Binding, 193
Bone marrow, 74, 82
B-1 progenitors, 243
Bradykinin-2, 13
Bromo-deoxyuridine, 81
Bronchial hyperreactivity, 11
Bronchoalveolar lavage, 9, 322
Bruton tyrosine kinase, 250
Bullous pemphigoid, 104

**C**

Calcium ionophore, 268
Calmodulin, 18
Calorimetry, 171
Capsaicin, 13
Cathepsin G, 13
Cell-based assays, 302
Charcot-Leyden crystals, 21
Chemokine, 155
Chemotaxis, 145
Chloramphenicol acetyltransferase, 291
Chromosome 5q31, 142
Ciliostasis, 5
*c-myc* proto-oncogene, 248
Colony assays, 72
Conformational change, 174
Conserved lymphokine element 0 (CLE0), 272, 293
Cord blood, 120
Coreceptors
  CD28, 141
  CTLA4, 141
Corticosteroids, 41, 57, 269, 293, 328
Costimulatory molecules
  B7-2 (CD86), 141
  B7-1(CD80), 141
Creola bodies, 21
CTN/NF-1, 293
Cutaneous tissues, 96
Cyclosporin A, 59, 144, 269, 277, 281, 290
Cynomolgus monkeys, 322
Cytokine-deficient, 130

**D**

DC28, 278
Deletion analysis, 270
Dibutyryl cAMP, 291
Downstream repressor elements, 276
*Drosophila*, 168, 217
D10.G4.1 T-cell line, 268, 273, 290

**E**

Early response genes, 232
ECP, 100, 105
Eczematoid dermatitis, 96, 103

EDN, 100, 105, 108
Elastase, 103
EL4-23 cell line, 268
Eosinophil
  activation, 20
  cationic protein, 3
  degranulation, 20
  derived neurotoxin, 3
  $EG2^+$, 53
  infiltration, 20
  major basic protein, 2
  peroxidase, 4
  survival, 53
Eosinophilic vasculitis, 107
Eotaxin, 54, 154
Eotaxin knockout mice, 158
Eotaxin receptor, 156
Ets, 292

F

Fibronectin type III, 190
FK506, 281
FMLP, 99
Forskolin, 290

G

GATA, 242, 274, 292, 293
GL113, 322
Glucocorticoids, 279
Glycosylation, 168
GM-CSF-deficient mice, 229
Gordon phenomenon, 3
Granulocyte colony-stimulating factor, 143
Growth hormone, 190
GST fusion proteins, 253

H

Heparin, 13, 16
Histamine, 14, 40
House dust mite, 120
Humanized antibody, 321
Human palindromic element, 275
Hypergammaglobulinemia, 243
Hyperreactivity, 9, 82

I

ICAM, 303
IgA production, 243
IgE antibody, 9, 119
IgE-mediated, 103
IL-2 receptors, 278
IL-3 knockout mouse, 229
IL-5 deficiency, 128
IL-5 mutant protein, 315
IL-5R$\alpha$ isoforms, 60, 210
IL-5R-deficient mice, 244
Immunotherapy, 44
In situ hybridization, 56
Isothiazolone derivatives, 191, 246, 308

J

JAK kinases, 197, 230, 249
Janus kinase 1, 144
Jurkat cells,268

K

Kallikrein, 13
Kinins, 40

L

Langerhans' cells, 46
Lectin ConA, 290
Leucine zipper, 206
Leukemia cell line, 268
Ligand, 192

$LTC_4$, 110
Luciferase, 272
Lung pathology, 130
Lung macrophages, 20

**M**

Mast cells, 17, 46
MBP, 100, 105, 108
*Mesocestoides corti*, 271
Metalloproteinase, 107
Methacholine, 11, 53, 82
Methylscopolamine receptor, 16
Minigene constructs, 210
*Moraxella cararrhalis*, 243
Mucous secreting cells, 20
Muscarinic receptors, 15
Muscle fasciculation, 8
Mutagenesis, 174
Mutated IL-5Rα, 253

**N**

Nasal biopsies, 45
Nasal late responses, 40
Nasal lavage, 40, 45
Nasal secretions, 40
Negative regulatory element, 275
Neutrophil, 19, 103
NFAT, 273, 292
NF-κB, 294

**O**

octamer element, 274
oncostatin M, 232
optical biosensor, 170
ovalbumin, 120, 128

**P**

PAF, 110
Peptide antagonists, 314
Phorbol myristate acetate, 21
Phosphoramidon, 13
Pilocarpine, 16
PI-3 kinase, 230
Platelet factor 4, 13
Platelets, 19
Pollen, 45
Poly-L-arginine, 13
Poly-L-lysine, 13
Posttranscriptional regulation, 279
Progenitor cells, 71, 81
Proline-rich region, 253
Promoter fragments, 268
Prostaglandin $D_2$, 40
Protease cleavage, 191
Protein kinase A, 278
Proto-oncogenes, 248

**R**

Raf kinase cascade, 234
Random screening, 302
Rapamycin, 281
Ras pathway, 248
Rational design, 311
Receptor activation, 196
Receptor-based design, 312
Receptor binding assays, 303
Receptor variants, 208
Reporter construct, 269
Repressor elements, 275
Respiratory epithelium, 4, 23
Retinoic acid, 75
Rhinitis, perennial, 46
Robotic screens, 304

**S**

Sch 55700, 321
*Schistosoma mansoni*, 140
Signal transduction, 229

Sneeze count, 40
Soluble receptor, 314
Src-family tyrosine kinases, 250
*Staphylococcus aureus*, 243
STAT proteins, 144, 230, 249
Stem cell factor, 143
Stem cells, 73
Stoichiometry, 171, 206, 248
Superoxide anion, 19
Surface markers
  CD25, 52
  CD34, 72
  HLA-DR, 52
  VLA-1, 52

**T**

T-cell hybrid, NIMP-TH1, 268
T-cell line, PER-117, 268
T-helper cell, 137
Theophylline, 18
Tracheal rings, 14
Transgenic mice, 271
TRFK-5, 321
Tunicamycin, 168
Tyrosine kinase, 230

**U**

Ussing chambers, 8

**V**

Vaccinia virus, 129
Vagus nerve, 15
Vascular permeability, 8
VCAM, 303

**X**

XID mice, 250